Clinical Radiology
The Essentials

Clinical Radiology
The Essentials

Richard H. Daffner, M.D.

Professor of Radiological Sciences
Medical College of Pennsylvania

Department of Diagnostic Radiology
Allegheny General Hospital

Clinical Professor of Radiology
University of Pittsburgh
School of Medicine
Pittsburgh, Pennsylvania

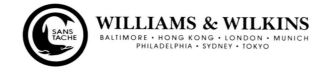

WILLIAMS & WILKINS
BALTIMORE · HONG KONG · LONDON · MUNICH
PHILADELPHIA · SYDNEY · TOKYO

Editor: Timothy H. Grayson
Project Manager: Raymond E. Reter
Copy Editor: E. Ann Donaldson
Designer: Wilma Rosenberger
Illustration Planner: Lorraine Wrzosek
Cover Designer: Wilma Rosenberger

Accurate indications, adverse reactions, and dosage schedules for drugs are provided in this book, but it is possible that they may change. The reader is urged to review the package information data of the manufacturers of the medications mentioned.

Printed in the United States of America

Library of Congress Cataloging-in-Publication Data

Daffner, Richard H., 1941-
    Clinical radiology : the essentials / Richard H. Daffner.
       p.   cm.
    Includes bibliographical references and index.
    ISBN 0-683-02330-6
    1. Diagnostic imaging. 2. Diagnosis, Radioscopic. I. Title.
    [DNLM: 1. Diagnostic Imaging—methods. WN 200 D124ca]
  RC78.7.D53D34 1992
  616.07'54—dc20
  DNLM/DLC
  for Library of Congress   92-12314
                                          CIP

94 95 96
5 6 7 8 9 10

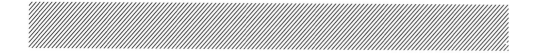

To Alva, Marc, and Scott

Preface

No area of medicine has undergone more dramatic changes as has Diagnostic Radiology in the past two decades. Prior to 1970, the specialty relied primarily on plain film diagnosis supplemented by various contrast examinations for clinical problem solving. The revolution in diagnostic imaging began in the early 1970s with the development of cross-sectional and longitudinal imaging using ultrasound. Almost concomitantly, computerized tomography (CT) was developed. Soon, rapid improvements in technology afforded us the ability to directly image areas of the body that previously were accessible only to the surgeon's knife. In the early 1980s, magnetic resonance (MR) imaging was perfected. Improvements in MR technology have resulted in quality images that eclipse even those made by CT. Magnetic resonance is now the primary investigative tool for the central nervous system and for imaging the internal anatomy of joints.

Although the majority of studies are produced by ionizing radiation (x-rays and nuclear imaging), the use of such nonionizing forms of energy such as ultrasound and magnetic resonance has resulted in our referring to our specialty as *Diagnostic Imaging* rather than *Diagnostic Radiology*. The specialty is in a constantly evolving state. Improvements in computer technology have resulted in three-dimensional imaging and digital imaging. With this last area, digital processing of data will carry the specialty into the next century. The days of film/screen imaging are numbered. Furthermore, picture archiving and computer storage (PACS) is now a reality and will become more generally available in the next few years.

This book is intended for the medical student beginning clinical rotations. It is a sweeping revision of the *Introduction to Clinical Radiology: A Correlative Approach to Diagnostic Imaging* written by the author in 1978. The revision has accounted for the radical changes in how we approach clinical imaging that have occurred in the last 12 years.

In writing this book, I have chosen an orientation based on clinical problem solving. Many of the radiology texts for medical students list the radiographic signs of various conditions as isolated facts without attempting to correlate them with the pathophysiology that produces them. Diagnostic imaging is true detective work. The image represents the patient at that particular point in time. By one's knowledge of anatomy and by observing the changes that the disease has produced, it is possible for one to identify the pathologic process(es) that produced those changes. It is thus my goal to show that by recognition of a radiographic pattern, it is possible to define the pathophysiologic process producing that pattern.

The first chapter provides an overview of diagnostic imaging, listing the "menu" of types of studies available to help solve clinical problems.

The physical basis for each type of study is briefly stated. The second chapter discusses radiographic contrast agents. The third is devoted to a subspecialty area of Diagnostic Imaging known as interventional or invasive radiology. The remainder of the book consists of individual chapters describing imaging of the lungs, heart, breast, abdomen, gastrointestinal tract, urinary tract, obstetrics and gynecology, the musculoskeletal system, and the brain and spinal cord.

Each of the clinical chapters is divided into three sections: technical considerations, anatomic considerations, and pathologic considerations. The *technical considerations* portion of each chapter includes the type of examination performed for that area, the use of special views, and a description of how that particular examination may be of help in clinical problem solving. The *technical considerations* include such things as proper identification of the film with regard to the patient, laterality, an analysis of proper density, exposure parameters and the presence of motion.

The *anatomic considerations* portion reviews pertinent anatomy of the region being studied. No attempt is made to be encyclopedic; rather, the approach is very brief but covers all of the essentials. It is important for you, the reader, to recognize that the images that you are viewing are two-dimensional representations of three-dimensional structures. You must remember the adage that if you know the gross appearance of a structure, you can easily predict its radiographic or other imaging appearance.

The *pathologic considerations* include those pathophysiologic alterations of normal anatomic structures that produce the abnormalities seen on the images. Logic tells us that there are a limited number of ways for a disease to affect an organ. Similarly, there are limitations in the way an organ responds to that disease process. For example, in the gastrointestinal tract, a mucosal tumor appears the same whether it is located in the esophagus, stomach, small intestine, or colon. The same holds true for other lesions of this system. Furthermore, an extrapolation may be made to other tubular structures in the body—airways, urinary tract, and blood vessels. Once the reader recognizes the pattern of a lesion, he/she will recognize it anywhere in the body, even if it is in an unusual location.

Throughout the text, the reader is reminded that he/she has a large variety of imaging studies that may be performed on his/her patient. The choice of study should be based on the analysis of the history, physical findings, economics, and good judgment. Please remember that many of these studies are expensive.

The reader will find that the text emphasizes certain types of imaging examinations and makes little or no mention of others. The goal of the author is to provide you, the reader, with state-of-the-art imaging information. Thus, CT and MR are recommended in many instances over a nuclear imaging study. This reflects the fact that CT and MR have superseded many of the nuclear imaging studies performed in the past.

There is a list of suggested additional readings at the end of each chapter. The majority of these are of current textbooks in the various subspecialties of diagnostic radiology. The reader is referred to them for a more in-depth discussion of individual topics. Most of these books should be available in either the medical school library, hospital library, or departmental library.

Finally, it is my hope that the book will be easily read and understood. Learning should be fun. It has been my intent to keep it that way in this book.

Richard H. Daffner, M.D.

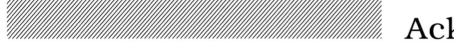 # Acknowledgments

No book of this nature may be produced without the cooperation of a large number of contributors. The author wishes to acknowledge the following individuals for their help in producing this book: Mustafa H. Adatepe, M.D., Irwin Beckman, D.O., Farhad M. Contractor, M.D., Nilima Dash, M.D., Ziad L. Deeb, M.D., Andrew L. Goldberg, M.D., Gilbert H. Isaacs, M.D., Maroon B. Khoury, M.D., Paul M. Kiproff, M.D., Anthony R. Lupetin, M.D., Kook Sang Oh, M.D., William E. Rothfus, M.D., and Rolf L. Schapiro, M.D., Chairman of the Department of Diagnostic Radiology at Allegheny General Hospital, who provided case material and consultation on the manuscripts in their areas of expertise.

I appreciate the contributions of Patricia Prince, R.T., R.D.M.S., and Kelli Swango, R.T., R.D.M.S., for the obstetrics/gynecology ultrasound cases.

I would like to thank Peter Stracci, M.D., of the Department of Cardiology, for case material and consultation, and Alex Bellotti, Mary Jane Bent, and Bill Brattina of the Department of Creative Services for the photography. In addition, I would like to thank Kevin Kennedy, also of the Creative Services Department, for the artwork.

I would also like to thank Maggie Cauley for her unflagging perseverance in the preparation of the manuscript.

Finally, I especially thank my wife, Alva, for her encouragement and support during the long months of preparation of this work.

Contents

Chapter 1

Overview and Principles of Diagnostic Imaging

HISTORICAL PERSPECTIVES

Wilhelm Conrad Roentgen, a Dutch physicist, discovered a form of radiation that now bears his name, the roentgen ray, in 1895. He called this new form of unknown radiation, which was invisible, could penetrate objects, and caused fluorescence, "X-strahlung" (x-rays) because initially he did not understand its nature. Roentgen was doing experiments with cathode ray tubes, and studying their behavior in a completely darkened room. He noticed that when the tube was operating, there was a faint glow on the table of his laboratory. He discovered the glow was caused by a fluorescent plate that he had inadvertently left on the bench. When he reached for the plate, he was shocked to see the image of the bones of his hand cast onto the plate. His meticulous work investigating his discovery provided the world with an understanding of this new form of radiation. For his monumental work he was awarded the Nobel Prize in physics in 1901.

The first recorded diagnostic use of x-rays was in 1896. In the 1st decade of the discovery of the roentgen ray, the physical effects of x-rays on patients were also observed. It was not long before a new medical specialty, radiology, was born. Traditionally, radiology was divided into two distinct disciplines, diagnostic and therapeutic. The only common area between these disciplines was the use of ionizing radiation. As each field continued to develop and grow in complexity, it became apparent that separation of the two specialties was needed. Today, one trains in either diagnostic radiology, or radiation oncology.

The last quarter of a century has brought changes and developments in diagnostic radiology that far surpassed those made the nearly 75 previous years. These newer developments have revolutionized medical diagnosis, making areas of the body previously inaccessible to nonsurgical examination clearly visible. Furthermore, the ability to accurately image all areas of the body made it possible for interventional and biopsy procedures to be performed using newer methods of diagnostic imaging for guidance. Previously, these procedures would have required surgical exploration.

The realm of diagnostic radiology encompasses a variety of modalities of imaging that may be used individually or, more commonly, in combination to provide the clinician with enough information to aid in making a diagnosis. Diagnostic imaging includes plain film radiography, contrast-enhanced radiography, computerized tomography, magnetic resonance imaging, and diagnostic ultrasound. The first three of these imaging forms utilize x-rays. Nuclear radiology involves the detection of emissions from radioactive isotopes in various parts of the body; magnetic resonance and ultrasound do not have any associated ionizing radiation. A brief introduction to each type of examination is necessary at this point for the reader to understand how these modalities are used in clinical problem solving.

RADIOGRAPHY
Definition

X-rays, or roentgen rays, are a form of electromagnetic radiation or energy of extremely short wavelength. The spectrum of electromagnetic radiation is illustrated in Figure 1.1. X-rays in the diagnostic range are in the spectrum of short wavelengths. The shorter the wavelength of an electromagnetic radiation form, the greater its energy and, as a rule, the greater the ability to penetrate various materials.

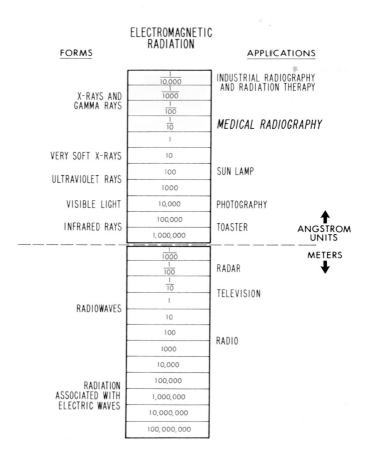

Figure 1.1. Spectrum of electromagnetic radiation. The numbers represent the wavelength of the particular radiation. The shorter the wavelength, the greater the energy associated with that radiation.

X-rays are described in terms of particles or packets of energy called quanta or photons. Photons travel at the speed of light. The amount of energy carried by each photon depends on the wavelength of the radiation. This is measured in electron volts. An electron volt is the amount of energy an electron gains as it is accelerated through a potential of 1 volt.

An atom is ionized when it has lost an electron. Any photon that has about 15 or more electron volts of energy is capable of producing ionization in atoms and molecules (*ionizing radiation*). X-rays, gamma rays, and certain types of ultraviolet radiation are all typical ionizing radiation forms.

Production of X-Rays

X-rays used in diagnostic radiology require a vacuum and the presence of a high potential difference between a cathode and an anode. In the basic x-ray tube, electrons are boiled off the cathode (filament) by heating it to a very high temperature. To move these electrons toward the anode at an energy sufficient to produce x-rays, a high potential, up to 125,000 volts (125 kV), is used. When the accelerated electrons strike the tungsten anode, x-rays are produced.

Production of Images

Image production by x-rays results from attenuation of those x-rays by the material through which they pass. Attenuation is the process by which x-rays are removed from a beam through absorption and scatter. In general, the greater the density of the material, i.e., the number of grams per cubic centimeter, the greater its ability to absorb or scatter x-rays (Fig. 1.2). Absorption is also influenced by the atomic number of the structure. The denser the structure, the greater the attenuation, which results in less blackening of the film (fewer x-rays strike the film). Less-dense structures attenuate the beam to a lesser degree and result in more blackening of the film (more x-rays strike the film) (Fig. 1.3).

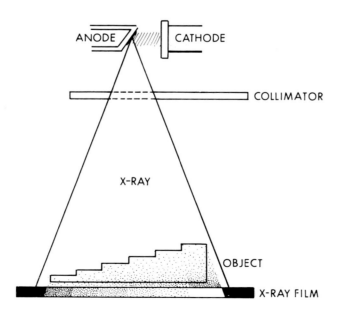

Figure 1.2.   Relationship between density and absorption of x-rays. The denser a particular material is, the greater its ability to absorb x-rays. The net result of greater absorption is less darkening of the film.

Figure 1.3.   Differential absorption of x-rays depends on the composition of various tissues. Denser tissue absorbs more x-rays; less dense tissue transmits more x-rays. The resultant radiographic image is essentially a "shadowgram."

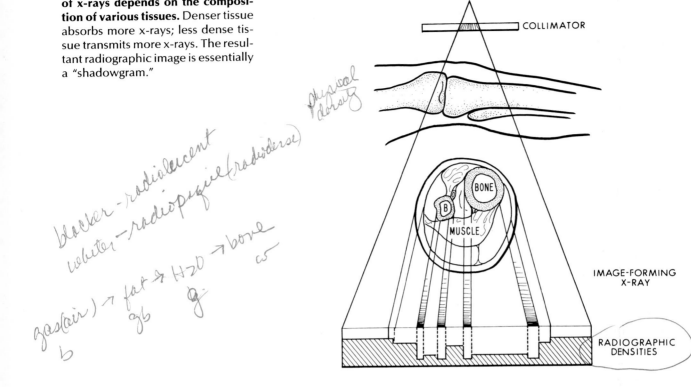

It is important to differentiate between two types of "density" that you will hear mentioned when discussing radiographs with radiologists or other colleagues—physical density and radiographic density. Physical density is the type of density just described. *Radiographic density* is a term that refers to the degree of blackness of a film. *Radiographic contrast* is the difference in radiographic densities on a film. The radiographic density of a substance is related to its physical density. The effect on film or other recording media occurs "paradoxically"; structures of high physical density produce less radiodensity and vice versa. Structures that produce more blackening on film are referred to as being *radiolucent*; those that produce less blackening are called *radiopaque* or *radiodense*. There are four types of radiographic densities; these are, in increasing order of physical density, gas (air), fat, water, and bone (metal). Radiographically these appear as black, gray-black, gray, and white, respectively.

Recording Media

The type of recording medium with which you are most familiar is x-ray film. X-ray film consists of a plastic sheet coated with a thin emulsion that contains silver bromide and a small amount of silver iodide. This emulsion is sensitive to light and radiation. A protective coating covers the emulsion. When the film is exposed to light or to ionizing radiation and then developed, chemical changes take place within the emulsion, resulting in the deposition of metallic silver, which is black. The amount of blackening on the film depends entirely on the amount of radiation reaching the film and, therefore, on the amount attenuated or removed from the beam by the subject.

Other recording media include the fluoroscopic screen/image intensification system, photoelectric detector crystals, xenon detector systems, and computer-linked detectors that measure actual attenuation. These last detectors are linked to magnetic tape or disks in the computer.

A fluoroscopic screen is a screen coated with a substance (phosphor) that gives off visible light (or "fluoresces") when it is irradiated. The brightness of the light is proportional to the intensity of the x-ray beam striking the plate and depends on the amount of radiation removed from the beam by the object irradiated. In its most common use today, the fluorescent screen is combined with an electronic device that converts the visible light into an electron stream that amplifies the image (makes it brighter) by converting the electron pattern back into visible light. This system allows the radiologist to see the image clearly without necessitating dark adaptation of the eyes, as is necessary in "conventional" (non-image-enhanced) fluoroscopy. This technology has been adapted for military use for nighttime security and warfare.

The detection of photons emitted by radioisotopes is accomplished with sodium iodide crystals. These crystals respond, when irradiated, by emitting light whose brightness is related to the energy of the photons striking them. Photodetectors convert the light into an electronic signal, which is then amplified and converted into a variety of display images.

Computed tomography (CT) scanners and digital radiography units utilize electronic sensors that actually measure the attenuation coefficient of tissue through which the x-ray beam has passed and converts this mathematical value into a digitalized shade of gray. The data are fed into a computer that plots the location of each of those measurements to produce the computer image. This is recorded on magnetic tape or disks and is displayed on a TV monitor or made into a hard copy (film) by the multiformat camera.

Image Quality

There are physical and geometric factors that affect the radiographic image. These include thickness of the part being irradiated, motion, scatter, magnification, and distortion.

The thickness of the part will determine how much of the beam is removed or attenuated. This was explained earlier. Thus, an obese patient requires more x-rays for adequate penetration than does a thin patient; bone requires more x-rays for penetration than does the surrounding muscle.

Motion of a part being radiographed results in a blurred nondiagnostic image. Motion may be overcome by shortening the exposure time. One way of decreasing the time of exposure is to enhance the effectiveness of the recording medium. This may be done by using intensifying screens. An intensifying screen is a device coated with a fluorescent material that gives off visible light when struck by x-rays. This light exposes the film. Cassettes (film holders) containing screens are used for about 99% of diagnostic x-ray work. This has the advantage of reducing the exposure time during which motion could occur. Improvements in screen technology have allowed us to obtain detailed examinations without increasing radiation dosage. This has been particularly advantageous for mammography.

Scatter is produced by deflection of some of the primary radiation beam; this can produce fog on the film and is undesirable. To eliminate as much scatter as possible, a grid that has alternating angled slats of very thin radiolucent material combined with thin lead strips is used (Fig. 1.4). This results in the removal of much of the scatter. To prevent the lead strips from casting their own shadows as they absorb radiation, the whole grid is moved very quickly during the exposure, eliminating these lines. This system is known as the Bucky-Potter system, after the two men who invented it.

The radiographic image is a two-dimensional representation of a three-dimensional structure. Consequently, some structures will be farther from the film than others. Geometrically, x-rays behave similar to light. Hence, magnification of objects will occur when they are some distance from the film. The farther an object is from the film, the greater the magnification; the closer the object is to the film, the less the magnification (Fig. 1.5). This has considerable importance in evaluating structures such as the heart on chest radiographs. On the standard chest radiograph, the x-ray beam enters through the back of the patient and exits from the front (posterior to anterior [PA]). Since the heart is located anteriorly, there will be relatively little magnification. However, on an anterior to posterior (AP) radiograph of the chest, the beam enters from the patient's front and exits through the back. Hence, there is somewhat greater magnification of the heart because of its distance from the film. The best rule to follow to reduce the undesirable effect of magnification is to have the part of greatest interest closest to the film. This will give the truest image of the region of interest.

Distortion occurs when the object being radiographed is not perfectly perpendicular to the beam. The radiographic image of an object depends

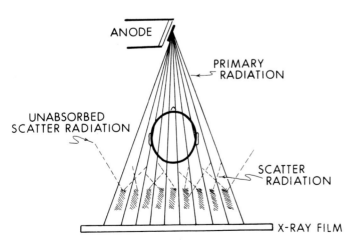

Figure 1.4.   Grid function. A grid absorbs scattered radiation. Angling of the lead strips permits only the primary x-ray beam to pass through.

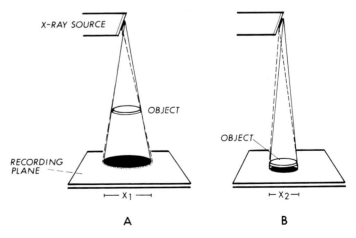

Figure 1.5.   Magnification and image sharpness. A, the object is farther from the film, resulting in a larger image. However its margin is not as distinct as in **B. B,** the object is closer to the film, resulting in a smaller and sharper image than in **A.**

on the sum of the shadow produced by that object when x-rayed. Changes in the relationship of that object to the x-ray beam may distort its radiographic image (Fig. 1.6). For diagnostic clarity, therefore, it is best to have the part of major interest as close and as perpendicular to the film as possible.

Plain film radiography is the bread and butter of the diagnostic radiologist. The term "plain film" means that no contrast material is used to en-

RADIATION SOURCE

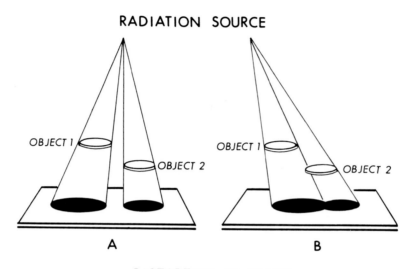

DISTORTION OF IMAGE

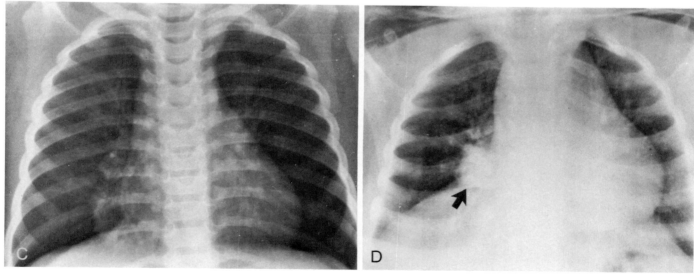

Figure 1.6.   Distortion. The shape of an object on a radiograph depends on the angle at which the radiographic beams strikes it. **A,** two objects of similar size cast distinct images when the x-ray beam is nearly perpendicular. The difference in size is the result of magnification. **B,** angling the x-ray beam while the objects remain in the same relationship to one another results in an overlapping image that is not a true representation of the actual objects. **C,** a PA radiograph of the chest in a patient with right middle lobe pneumonia. **D,** lordotic view of the same patient made with the patient bending backward toward the film. Note the change in the appearance of heart, ribs, and the infiltrate, which now appears as a mass adjacent to the heart border on the right (*arrow*).

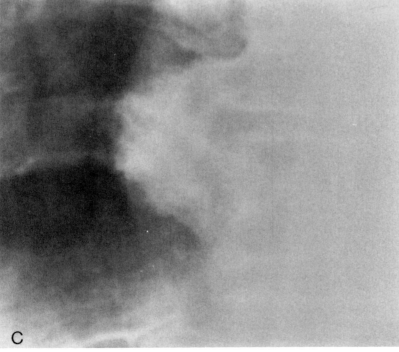

Figure 1.7.   The value of chest fluoroscopy. A, a PA chest radiograph shows a "mass" through the cardiac shadow to the right of midline (*arrow*). **B,** a lateral view shows the mass to be posterior (*arrow*). **C,** fluoroscopic spot film shows the density in question to be bone spurs bridging the thoracic vertebral bodies. There was no tumor.

hance various body structures. In performing plain film examinations, the natural contrast between the basic four radiographic densities—air, soft tissue (water), fat, and bone—is relied on to define abnormalities. Examples of plain film studies with which you are familiar include chest radiographs, plain films of the abdomen, and skeletal films.

Plain film radiography has its special modifications: fluoroscopy and tomography. Fluoroscopy is a useful modality for visualizing the diaphragm, heart motion, valve calcification within the heart, and localization of chest masses (Fig. 1.7).

Conventional tomography is a mode of imaging in which the x-ray tube and the film move in concert to produce a blurred image. The objects in the focal plane, or fulcrum, however, remain in sharp focus (Fig. 1.8). Tomography blurs out unwanted structures while keeping the object of interest in clearer focus. It is most useful in evaluating the lungs (Fig. 1.9), kidneys, and bony structures. Tomography will improve contrast, but it will not create contrast where there is none to begin with.

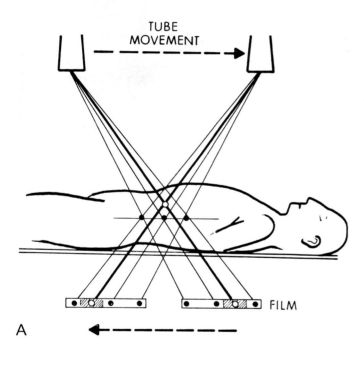

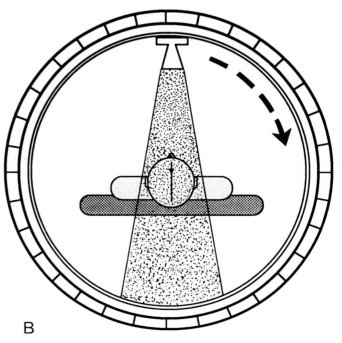

Figure 1.8. Principles of tomography. A, conventional tomography. The x-ray tube and the film move in opposite directions. The focal point (open circle) remains in sharp focus, whereas the other images are blurred. **B,** computerized tomography. In the modern CT scanner, the x-ray tube rotates within the gantry. Instead of film, detectors measure the amount of radiation removed from the x-ray beam.

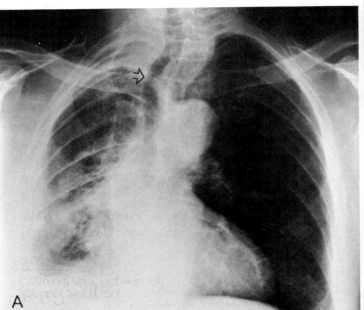

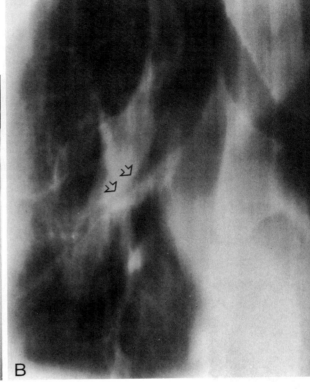

Figure 1.9.   Utilization of conventional tomography. A, frontal chest film shows a mass in the hilar region. There is peripheral pneumonia. Volume loss on the right side is evidenced by deviation of the trachea (*arrow*). **B,** tomogram through the hilum demonstrates a mass encroaching upon the bronchus intermedius (*arrows*). This neoplasm produced obstructive atelectasis in the right lung.

CONTRAST EXAMINATIONS

Plain film radiography is adequate for situations where natural radiographic contrast exists between body structures such as the heart and lungs or the bones and adjacent soft tissues. To examine structures that do not have inherent contrast differences from the surrounding tissues, it is necessary to use one of a variety of contrast agents. The vast majority of contrast studies are of the gastrointestinal tract, urinary tract, and blood vessels.

The most common contrast material used for gastrointestinal examinations is a preparation of barium sulfate mixed with other agents to produce a uniform suspension. These products are available as premixed powders or liquids. They may be administered alone or in combination with air, water, or an effervescent mixture that produces carbon dioxide. These gas-enhanced studies are referred to as "air contrast" studies (Fig. 1.10). Administration of these preparations is either by mouth (antegrade) or by rectum (retrograde).

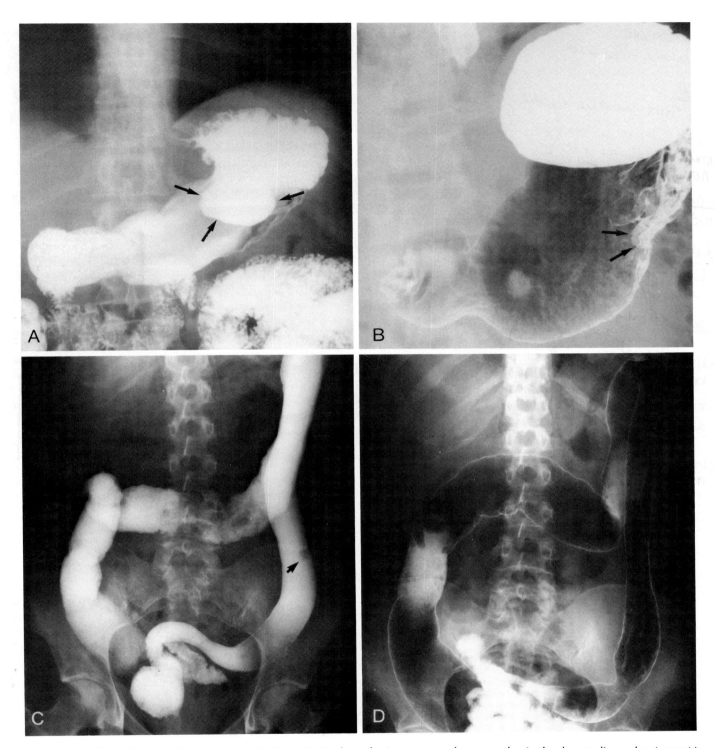

Figure 1.10.   Gastrointestinal contrast examinations. A, single-contrast examination of the stomach demonstrates a large gastric ulcer (*arrows*). **B,** double-contrast examination shows a tumor along the greater curvature (*arrows*). **C,** single-contrast barium enema shows a polyp in the descending colon (*arrow*) in a patient with ulcerative colitis. Note the loss of haustral markings. **D,** an air-contrast barium enema in the same patient.

GI Barium sulfate
if leakage - H20 soluble

Gallbladder -
oral → blood → liver → bile → gallblad.

Urography (intravenous urogram)
- ionic H2O soluble salts IV
nonionic agents

Angiography (IV, IA)
H2O soluble agents → vessel

Lymphatic - lymphangiography
iodinated form of poppy seed oil
into L. vessels.

Sinogram - (fistulogram)
H2O soluble agents (chemical pneumonia)

*Oil soluble where there is
bronchopleural fistula

Sialography
oil contrast (iodinated
poppy seed oil

myelography (cord or nerve root compression
nonionic, iodinated, H2O-soluble

In addition to barium preparations, water-soluble agents are available for studying the gastrointestinal tract whenever there is a possibility of leakage of the contrast material beyond the bowel wall. Although barium is a chemically inert substance, it produces a severe desmoplastic reaction in tissues. Water-soluble agents, on the other hand, do not produce this type of reaction and are absorbed from the rupture site to be excreted through the kidneys. The water-soluble agents, however, are not without hazard, since they can cause a severe chemical pneumonia if aspirated. Water-soluble agents also cost more and hence are not used on a routine basis.

Gallbladder studies are performed by oral-administration drugs that are removed from the bloodstream, conjugated by the liver, excreted in the bile, and transported to the gallbladder, where concentration takes place. This results in visualization of this structure.

Urography is the radiographic study of the urinary tract. The contrast agents used for this study are primarily the ionic water-soluble salts of diatrizoic or iothalamic acids or the nonionic agents (iopamidol, iohexol). The common term for this study is the intravenous urogram (IVU). An older and less appropriate term is intravenous pyelogram (IVP). The physiology of these agents will be discussed in the next chapter.

Angiography is the study of the vascular system. Water-soluble agents similar to those used for urography are injected either intraarterially or intravenously, and a rapid sequence exposure is made to follow the course of the contrast material through the blood vessels (Fig. 1.11).

The lymphatic system may be studied by injecting an iodinated form of poppy seed oil into the lymph vessels on the dorsum of the foot or the hand. The resultant study shows the flow of lymph from the limb to the re-

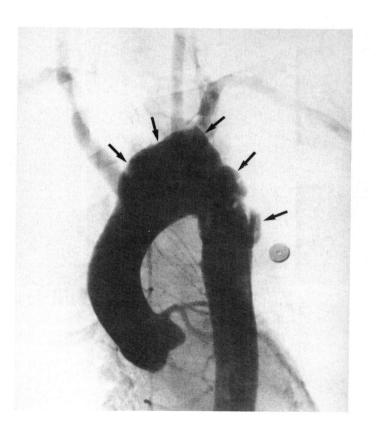

Figure 1.11. Arteriogram in a patient with posttraumatic rupture of the aorta. This is a subtraction film in which black and white are reversed to improve contrast. Note the irregularity and ballooning of the aortic arch at the site of injury (*arrows*).

gional lymph nodes and then to the deep lymphatic system. These studies are infrequently used today to stage patients with malignancies. They have been largely superseded by computerized tomography.

A sinogram (fistulogram) involves the injection of contrast material through an abnormal sinus tract into the body. Water-soluble agents are commonly used for these studies. In evaluating an empyema cavity in the chest where there is a danger that a bronchopleural fistula may be present, an oil-soluble material such as Dionosil is used because water-soluble contrast material entering the bronchial tree could produce a severe and often fatal chemical pneumonia.

Sialography is the study of the salivary glands to evaluate patients with suspected salivary tumors or ductal obstructions. As with lymphangiography, an oily contrast material (iodinated poppy seed oil) is injected into the duct, which has been cannulated.

Diseases encroaching on the spinal canal may be studied by myelography. The main indication is evidence of cord or nerve root compression. The most common lesion is a herniated nucleus pulposus from a lumbar disc. Myelography is performed by inserting a needle between the spinous processes of a lumbar vertebra and entering the subarachnoid space. It may also be performed by puncture of the cisterna magna when there is a complete block within the vertebral canal and it is necessary to inject contrast medium above the lesion. Cerebrospinal fluid may be removed for study at this time. Nonionic, iodinated, water-soluble compounds are injected under fluoroscopic monitoring in varying amounts, and the patient is positioned for the study. Figure 1.12 shows a myelogram

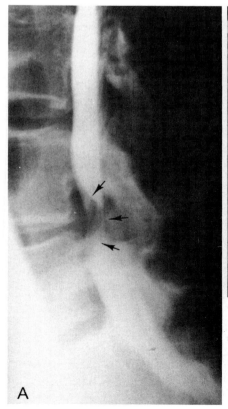

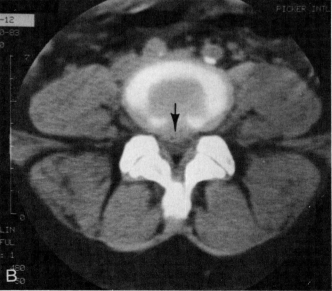

Figure 1.12. Herniated intervertebral disc. A, a myelogram shows compression of the subarachnoid space by the herniated disc material (*arrows*). **B,** CT scan in the same patient shows the herniated disc (*arrow*).

taken in a patient with a herniated lumbar disc. Note the compression of the thecal sac by the herniated material. Myelography is often combined with computerized tomography. The development of magnetic resonance imaging, however, has decreased the number of myelograms performed today, as compared with a decade ago.

COMPUTERIZED TOMOGRAPHY

Under ordinary circumstances, the fleshy organs of the body such as the heart, kidneys, liver, spleen, and pancreas are considered to be of uniform radiographic density, like water, which produces a gray appearance on conventional radiographs. However, these tissues vary somewhat in their chemical properties and it is possible, using computer-enhancing techniques, to measure these differences, magnify them, and display them in varying shades of gray or in color; this is the basis of computerized tomography.

In CT (Fig. 1.13), an x-ray beam and a detector system moves through an arc of 360°, irradiating the subject with a highly collimated (restricted) beam. This allows the detector system to measure the intensity of radiation passing through the subject. The data from these measurements are analyzed by a computer system where various shades of gray (CT numbers) are assigned to different structures based on their absorption or attenuation coefficients. The computer reconstructs a picture based on geometric plots of where these measurements were taken. Although this system of diagnosis was developed in the early 1970s, the reader may be interested to know that the mathematical formula for the reconstruction of images based on measurements of their points in space was actually developed in 1917 by the mathematician, Radon.

The information obtained with CT systems is displayed on a television screen (CRT) and recorded on magnetic tape on disc. Once the information has been recorded, it is possible to alter the visual intensities of the

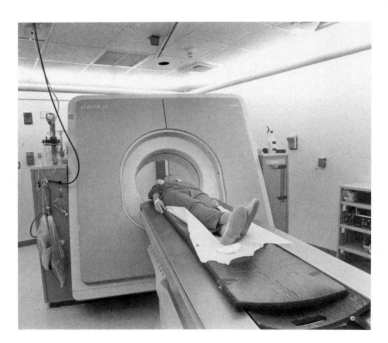

Figure 1.13.   Typical CT scanner. In this case, the gantry is tilted for improved visualization of the patient's brain.

various densities on the reading console (Fig. 1.14). The data from the television screen may be recorded further on x-ray film using a device known as a multiformat camera.

To enhance the appearance of certain viscera or vascular neoplasms, contrast material is injected intravenously. The contrast agent used is identical to that used in urography or arteriography.

Cranial scanning is performed for the evaluation of patients with a variety of neurologic findings. This study is particularly useful in defining and localizing brain tumors (primary or metastatic) and in evaluating patients with neurologic emergencies such as intracerebral hemorrhage or subdural hematoma. Figure 1.15 shows the head scan of a patient with a meningioma. Notice how well the tumor is defined against the normal brain tissue. Figure 1.16 shows a patient with a subdural hematoma. Note the compression of normal brain tissue by the hematoma.

Scanning the rest of the body is particularly useful in evaluating visceral neoplasms (Fig. 1.17). Other uses include studies of patients with abdominal trauma, investigation of patients with suspected pancreatic disease, mediastinal studies for defining the extent of tumors, evaluation of patients with Hodgkin's disease/lymphoma for staging purposes, diagnosis of intraabdominal abscess (Fig. 1.18), and scanning the musculoskeletal system for a variety of bone and soft tissue disorders (Fig. 1.12**B**).

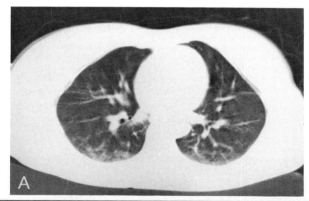

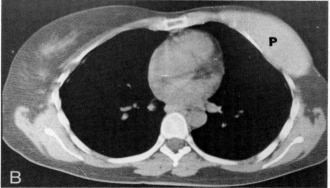

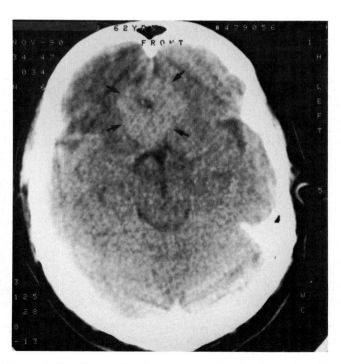

Figure 1.14. The effects of changes in window settings. A, image of a patient's thorax made at a window setting to enhance the lungs. **B,** the same section at soft tissue windows. Note the difference when compared with **A.** There is a breast prosthesis *(P)* on the left.

Figure 1.15. Brain CT shows a mass in the frontal region (*arrows*).

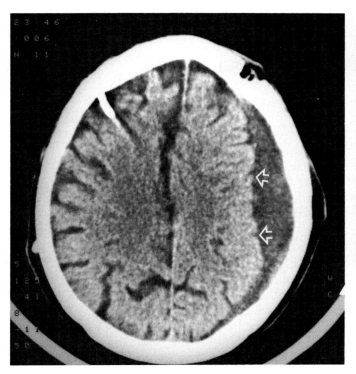

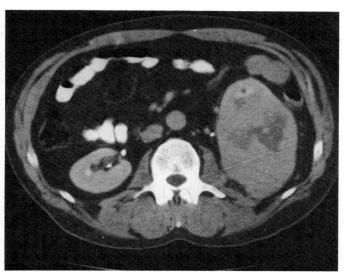

Figure 1.17. Abdominal CT showing a renal carcinoma on the left. Note the difference in kidney size and loss of the normal parenchymal appearance when compared with the right.

Figure 1.16. Subdural hematoma on the left. Note the compression of the left side of the brain by the low-density hematoma (*arrows*). There is loss of the sulci on the left as the result of compression. Compare with the right.

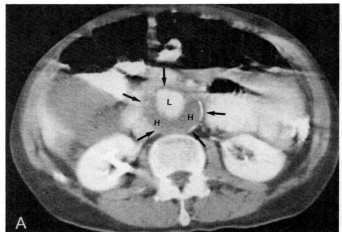

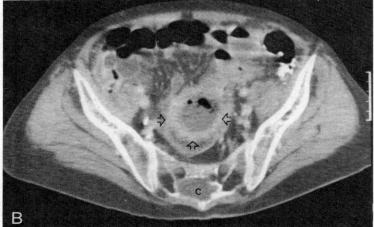

Figure 1.18. Abdominal aortic aneurysm and perirectal abscess in the same patient. A, a CT scan through the abdomen shows a large abdominal aortic aneurysm (*arrows*). Note the central enlarged lumen *(L)* and the more peripheral hematoma *(H)* and the calcification of the wall on the left side. **B,** further down, there is a gas-containing mass (*arrows*) in the perirectal region. Incidental note is also made of a large subarchnoid cyst in the sacrum *(C).*

NUCLEAR IMAGING

Nuclear medicine traditionally has two divisions, nuclear imaging (radiology) and laboratory analysis. The diagnostic radiologist is concerned with the imaging aspect. The use of isotopes for laboratory purposes and for evaluation of physiologic functions will not be discussed. However, the reader should be aware that the laboratory aspect of nuclear medicine is an area equally as important as the imaging aspect.

The principles of nuclear imaging depend on the selective uptake of certain compounds by different organs of the body. These compounds may be labeled with a radioactive substance of sufficient energy level to allow detection outside the body. The ideal isotope is one that may be administered in low doses, is nontoxic, has a short half-life, is readily incorporated into "physiologic" compounds, and is relatively inexpensive. At the present time, technetium-99m fulfills most of these requirements.

The *half-life* of an element is the time necessary for its degradation to one-half of its original activity. There are actually three types of half-lives: physical, biologic, and effective. The physical half-life is that time period in which the element would "decay" on its own. This occurs naturally whether the element is sitting on the laboratory shelf or has been administered to a patient. Biologic half-life concerns the normal physiologic removal of the substance to which the isotope has been attached. For example, the sodium pertechnetate commonly injected for nuclear scanning is excreted in the urine and into the gastrointestinal tract. Although the physical half-life of technetium-99m is approximately 6 hours, the biologic half-life is less. The effective half-life is a mathematical derivation based on a formula combining biologic and physical half-lives. It measures the actual time the isotope remains effective within the body.

Nuclear imaging is performed either on a static or on a dynamic basis. Static studies include the thyroid, liver, and renal scans. Dynamic studies include rapid sequence flow to the skeleton and perfusion-diffusion studies of the lung. Table 1.1 lists common types of scans (Figs. 1.19 to 1.23). Equipment for detecting the uptake of isotopes and for recording their images includes the gamma camera and the tomographic scanner.

There are basically five mechanisms of isotope concentration within the body:

1. Blood pool or compartmental localization (e.g., cardiac scan);
2. Physiologic incorporation (e.g., thyroid scan, bone scan);

Table 1.1.   Isotope Scans and Common Indications

Type of Scan	Figure No.[a]	Common Indications
Lung	1.19	Pulmonary embolism
Liver	1.20	Metastases, masses
Bone	1.21	Metastases
Thyroid	1.22	"Goiter" nodules
Heart	1.23	Myocardial function and perfusion

[a]Scan illustrated in these figures.

Figure 1.22. Thyroid scan showing a nodule as a photopenic area in the right lobe of the thyroid.

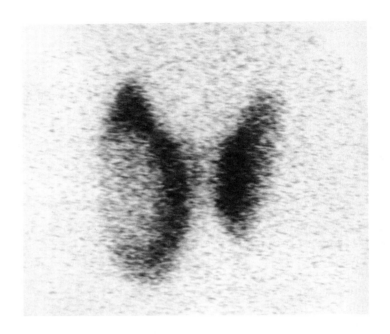

Figure 1.23. Cardiac scan with thallium. A, Resting scan over the apex of the heart is normal. **B,** During exercise, there are photopenic areas within the heart muscle, indicating lack of perfusion.

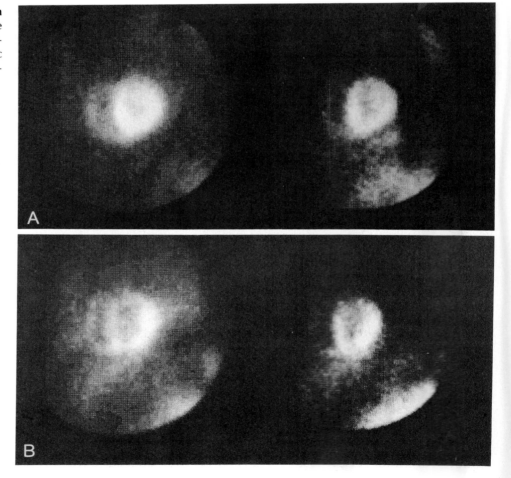

3. Capillary blockage (e.g., lung scan);
4. Phagocytosis (e.g., liver scan);
5. Cell sequestration (e.g., spleen scan).

Conventional nuclear scans utilize isotopes that produce gamma or x-radiation. Positron emission tomography (PET) scanning uses cyclotron-produced isotopes of extremely short half-life that emit positrons. Positron emission tomography scanning is used to evaluate physiologic function of organs such as the brain on a dynamic basis. Areas of increased brain activity will show selective uptake of the injected isotope.

MAGNETIC RESONANCE IMAGING

Magnetic resonance (MR) imaging is a noninvasive technique that does not use ionizing radiation. In the parameters used for medical imaging it is without significant health hazard. Magnetic resonance imaging is based on the principles described by Bloch and Purcell in an experimental procedure they designed to evaluate the chemical characteristics of matter on a molecular level. For their work, Bloch and Purcell were awarded the Nobel prize for physics in 1962. Damadian began investigating the possibilities of using MR for imaging in 1971. The development of computer imaging algorithms for CT accelerated the development of MR for medical diagnosis.

Magnetic resonance uses radiofrequency radiation in the presence of a high magnetic field to produce high-quality images of the body in any plane. The nucleus of any atom with an odd number of nucleons (protons and neutrons) behaves like a weak magnet in that they align themselves with a strong magnetic field. If a specific radiofrequency signal is employed to perturb the nucleus under study, its relationship to the external magnetic field is altered and it will generate a radio signal of its own having the same frequency as the signal that initially disrupted it (Fig. 1.24). This signal can then be amplified and recorded and this forms the basis for MR. Although many nuclei may be used for MR, the most common is hydrogen because of its abundance in tissue and its sensitivity to the phenomenon of magnetic resonance.

Magnetic resonance has the ability to display structures in a transverse or axial fashion, similar to CT. However, MR has the additional advantage of being able to produce images in virtually any plane. The common display parameters used are sagittal and coronal planes. Furthermore, MR has the advantage of being able to highlight the pathologic changes in different tissues through contrast manipulation. This is accomplished by altering the pattern of radiofrequency pulses in a study. The MR image reflects the strength or intensity of the MR radiofrequency signal received from the sample. Signal intensity depends on several factors such as hydrogen density and two magnetic relaxation times (T1 and T2). The greater the hydrogen density, the more intense (bright) the MR signal will be. Tissues that contain very little hydrogen such as cortical bone, flowing blood, and air-filled lung, generate little or no MR signal and appear black on the images produced. Tissues high in hydrogen, such as fat, have high-signal intensity and appear white.

A detailed explanation of T1 and T2 is beyond the scope of this text. However, in simple terms, these two measurements reflect quantitative al-

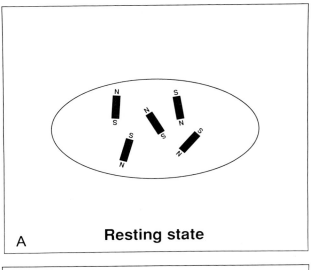

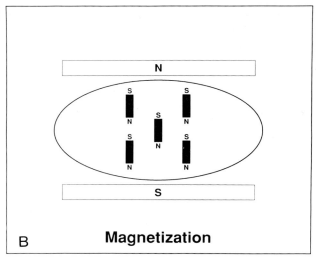

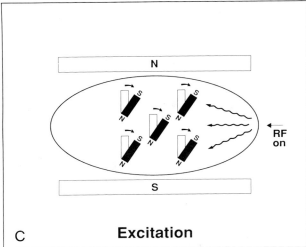

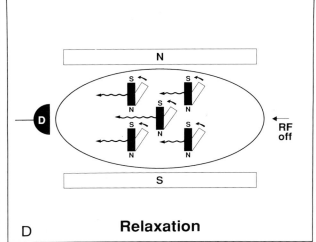

Figure 1.24.   Principles of MRI. A, in the resting state, the molecules in the body behave like small bar magnets and are arranged in a random fashion. **B,** following the magnetization, the molecules align themselves along the plane of magnetization. **C,** excitation. A pulsed radiofrequency *(RF)* beam deflects the molecules as they absorb the energy from that beam. **D,** relaxation. When the radiofrequency beam is switched off, the molecules return to their preexcitation position giving off the energy they absorbed. This may be measured with a detector *(D).*

terations in MR signal strength due to interactions of the nuclei being studied and their surrounding chemical and physical milieu. T1 is the rate at which nuclei align themselves with the external magnetic field after radiofrequency stimulation. T2 is the rate at which the radiofrequency signal emitted by the nuclei decreases after radiofrequency perturbation.

Figure 1.25 shows a typical MR unit. Magnetic resonance is presently used primarily for studying intracranial (Fig. 1.26) and intraspinal (Fig. 1.27) pathology, and for evaluating abnormalities of the musculoskeletal system (Figs. 1.28 and 1.29) and the heart. Less commonly, it is used to evaluate abdominal visceral problems.

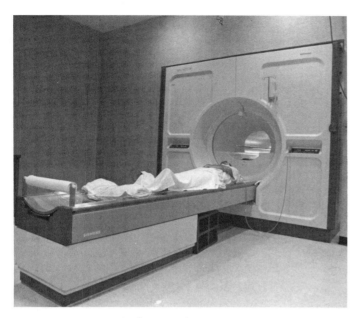

Figure 1.25. A typical MRI unit.

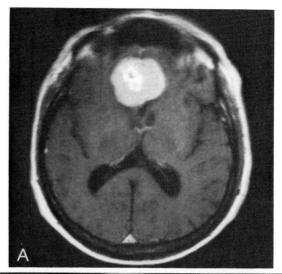

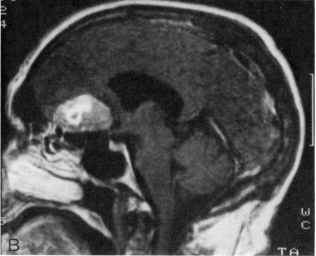

Figure 1.26. An MRI of meningioma. (This is the same patient as in Fig. 1.15). **A,** axial image shows the tumor to much better advantage. Note the internal structure of the tumor compared to Fig. 1.15. **B,** direct sagittal section. Computed tomography is not capable of scanning in this plane.

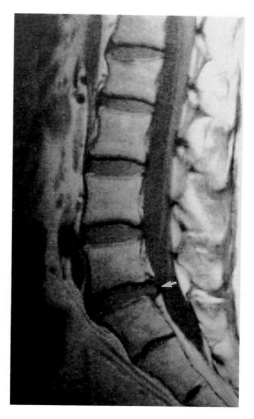

Figure 1.27. Herniated intervertebral disc at L-5. A T1-weighted MRI image shows posterior herniation of disc material (*arrow*).

Figure 1.28. Metastatic disease of the spine. Sagittal MRI examination shows areas of low signal (dark) as well as compression in two vertebrae. Other scans showed the tumor to encroach upon the subarachnoid space.

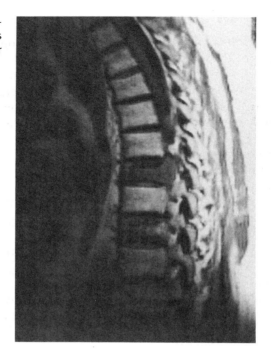

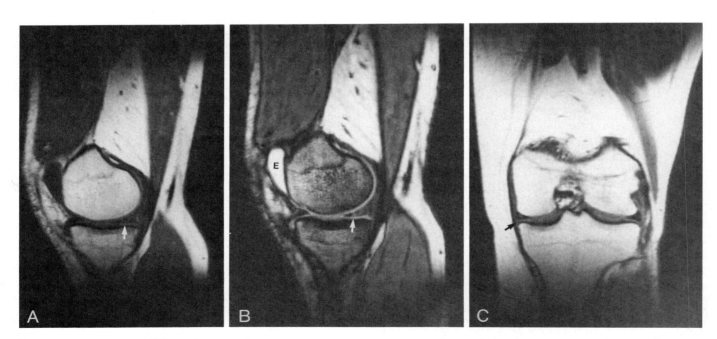

Figure 1.29. A torn medial meniscus. A, the MR image at T1-weighting shows fragmentation of the posterior horn of the medial meniscus *(arrow).* **B,** the same patient at gradient echo parameters shows the torn meniscus to better advantage *(arrow).* Note the suprapatellar joint effusion *(E).* **C,** a coronal view shows a mensicocapsular separation medially *(arrow).*

DIAGNOSTIC ULTRASOUND

Diagnostic ultrasound is a noninvasive imaging technique utilizing sonic energy in the frequency range of 1 to 10 MHz (1,000,000 to 10,000,000 cps). This is well above the normal human ear response of 20–20,000 Hz. Ultrasound is a nonionizing form of energy. Echoes or reflections of the ultrasound beam from interfaces between tissues with different acoustic properties yield information on the size, shape, and internal structure of organs and masses. However, ultrasound is greatly reflected by air-soft tissue and bone-soft tissue interfaces, limiting its use in the chest and musculoskeletal system.

Both pulsed and continuous wave ultrasound are used. Pulsed ultrasound is used principally for static cross-sectional images in the abdomen or pelvis. The transducer transmits ultrasound waves for approximately 1 μsec and then acts as a receiver for the returning echoes for approximately 1 msec. More commonly, real-time ultrasound techniques are used to perform dynamic imaging (moving picture) of moving objects such as the fetus in utero or the pulsating aorta. This technique also permits rapid and efficient screening of a body region. The continuous wave or Doppler method is used primarily to record the dynamics in periodically changing regions such as the fetal heart or blood vessels. Figure 1.30 shows the components of an ultrasound machine.

Three display modes are commonly used (Fig. 1.31). In amplitude mode (A-mode), information is displayed on a CRT as vertical spikes. The height or amplitude of a spike is related to the size of the echo; the distance from the initial or transducer spike is related to the depth of the reflecting

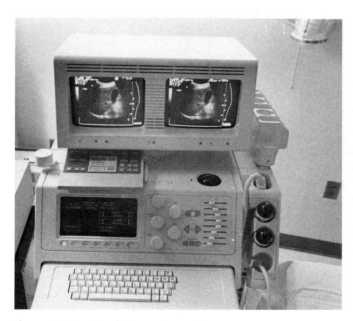

Figure 1.30. An ultrasound machine.

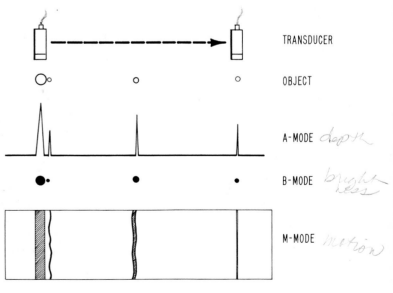

Figure 1.31. Ultrasound display modes. Three modes are demonstrated when the transducer passes over objects of varying size. See text for details.

interface from the transducer. Amplitude mode is now used very infrequently for echoencephalography to detect any shift of midline brain structures.

In brightness mode (B-mode), information is displayed as dots, the brightness of which corresponds to the strength of the corresponding echo. The location of the dot is proportional to the distance of the reflecting interfaces from the transducer. Since this constitutes only a single line on the CRT (corresponding to the line of sight of the transducer), one can build up a cross-sectional image or B-scan by a composite of many such lines obtained during a scan. The images can then be displayed over a wide range of gray scale or shading (Figs. 1.32 and 1.33). In particular, the difference in acoustic properties of various tissues is seen as a difference in the gray scale display of these tissues. Brightness mode and real-time ultrasound techniques are used extensively to evaluate the abdominal viscera, the fetus, and the heart.

Motion mode (M-mode) is used in echocardiography to study the dynamic changes of the cardiac structures. Essentially the base line is moved at a constant rate on the CRT screen. The cardiac structures form patterns in the M-mode relating to their motion.

An important advantage of ultrasound is the absence of ionizing radiation and the relatively lower cost of the equipment. However, a great deal of technical skill is required to perform a study.

Because ultrasound is unable to cross a tissue-gas or tissue-bone boundary, it is not useful for evaluating the lung or the skeleton. Furthermore, bony and gas-containing structures can obscure other tissues lying deeper to them.

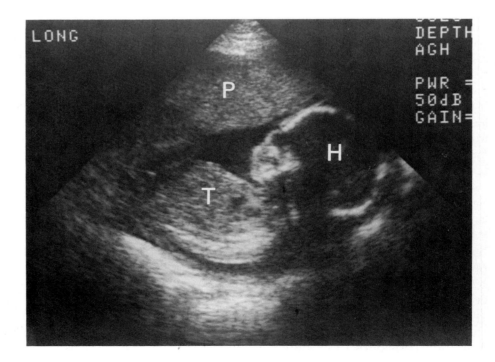

Figure 1.32.   Uterine ultrasound at 22 weeks of gestation. Note the placenta *(P)*, fetal head *(H)*, and torso *(T)*. Ultrasound has become a primary diagnostic tool in obstetrics.

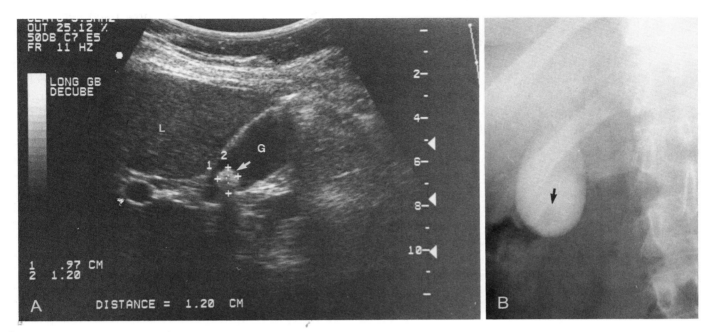

Figure 1.33.   Image of gallstones. A, ultrasound examination in the longitudinal plane shows a gallstone measuring 0.97 × 1.20 cm (*arrow*) in the dependent portion of the gallbladder *(G).* The liver *(L)* lies immediately above the gallbladder. **B,** oral cholecystogram in the same patient shows the lucent gallstone (*arrow*).

THE "RADIOLOGIC RESTAURANT"

The preceding discussion outlined a large variety of studies available to you, the clinician, to solve different clinical problems. You have a large "menu" of studies that can be performed to evaluate your patient. The first choice you must make is the exact approach you wish to take toward this evaluation. Three approaches are currently in use: the "shotgun," the algorithmic, and the directed.

The *shotgun approach* is one that is all too often employed. It takes little thought to order a battery of diagnostic laboratory and imaging studies for each patient in the hope that one or more of those tests will provide important diagnostic information on your patient. This approach is often modified toward the specific complaint to give some economy of selected tests.

The *algorithmic approach* follows a more orderly selection of studies based on symptoms and the results of each study (Fig. 1.34). While thought is required by the clinician, and it is possible to be selective in the studies, it is also possible that unnecessary studies will be performed, just because they are in the protocol. For example, a patient with an acute back strain usually needs no radiographs and may be treated conservatively with rest, heat, and antiinflammatory agents. Unfortunately, these patients often receive a complete radiographic evaluation of their lumbar spines.

The *directed approach* is a carefully thought-out process in which the clinician has performed a careful history and physical examination and then considers the diagnostic possibilities in that patient. He/she chooses diagnostic studies based on *probability of diagnostic yield, safety,* that is, choice of invasive or noninvasive study, *radiation dose, cost,* and also *medicolegal aspects.* I personally prefer this approach and stress it daily to my consulting clinicians. Table 1.2 lists common imaging procedures, their cost, and their radiation dose.

Figure 1.34.   Algorithm for evaluation of low back pain. The clinical, laboratory, and/or imaging findings will determine the next step. Imaging studies are highlighted.

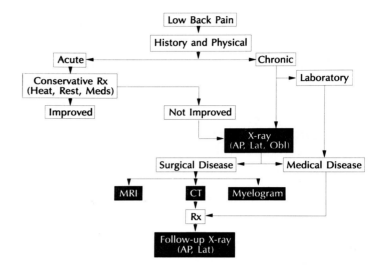

Table 1.2.   Common Imaging Examinations, Their Cost and Radiation Dosage

Examination	Cost[a]	Dose (mR)
Chest (Pa, Lateral)	$130	108
Abdomen (Supine, Upright)	130	1460
Femur	140	60
Pelvis	140	545
Wrist	110	4
Cervical (5 View)	150	194
Lumbar (5 View)	200	884
Mammogram	200	300
Upper Gastrointestinal	300	1700[b]
Barium Enema	300	4700[b]
Intravenous Urogram	330	595/image
Abdominal Aortoiliac Angiogram	1500	151/image
Cranial CT	700	4400
Chest CT	800	1500
Abdominal CT	830	3500
Lumbar CT	850	3000
Abdominal Ultrasound	500	0
Pelvic (Obstetric) Ultrasound	550	0
Cranial MR	1200	0
Lumbar MR	1200	0
Pelvic MR	1200	0
Bone Scan (Isotope)	300	1000 bone, 260 whole body
Lung Scan (Isotope)	300	900 lung, 61 whole body

[a]1992 figures (includes technical and professional charges).
[b]Includes fluoroscopy time.

THE RADIOLOGIST AS A CONSULTANT

The complexity of today's diagnostic imaging studies make it imperative that the radiologist be more than an interpreter of x-rays. As the practice of radiology has become more organ-system oriented in larger hospitals, radiologists have gravitated to subspecialty areas through extra training following residency. Thus, large radiology groups have members who are specialists in neuroimaging, angiography and invasive procedures, body imaging, musculoskeletal imaging, pulmonary imaging, trauma, gastrointestinal imaging, uroradiology, pediatric radiology, and nuclear imaging. As such, these radiologists work closely with specific groups of clinicians to solve their special diagnostic problems. These clinicians consult with their radiologic colleagues on a daily basis either for interpretation of studies or to determine the best method of working up a particular diagnostic problem. The radiologic subspecialists are often on call to perform studies after normal working hours. They make themselves available to consult on request with the clinician. They often participate in multidisciplinary conferences such as the Surgery-Radiology-Pathology conference, and lecture the clinicians on topics of mutual interest.

You should learn to make use of this most valuable resource, the radiologist. Keep in mind, however, that he/she can best help you when informed of clinical or laboratory data on a patient. This means that requests for diagnostic studies should contain pertinent clinical information. The radiologist may thus be able to tailor an examination to the exact needs of the patient as well as you, the clinician. This will result in time saved in both the studies obtained as well as the hospital stay. A secondary benefit will be cost containment—a topic of current importance. Many studies provide similar information. There is little benefit in ordering expensive studies that will duplicate the diagnostic information. Remember, your prime consideration is for the welfare of your patient. Consultation with the radiologist is as important for helping that patient as consulting with any other specialist.

Suggested Additional Reading

Curry TS III, Dowdy JE, Murry RC. Christensen's physics of diagnostic radiology. 4th ed. Baltimore: Williams & Wilkins, 1990.

Eisenberg RL. Radiology. An illustrated history. St. Louis: Mosby Year Book, 1991.

Gottschalk A, Hoffer PB, Potchen EJ, eds. Diagnostic nuclear medicine. 2nd ed. Baltimore: Williams & Wilkins, 1988.

Grainger RG, Allison DJ, eds. Diagnostic radiology. An Anglo-American textbook. New York: Churchill Livingstone, 1992.

Moss A, Gamsu G, Genant HK. Computed tomography of the body with magnetic resonance imaging. 2nd ed. Philadelphia: WB Saunders, 1991.

Runge VM. Magnetic resonance imaging: clinical principles. Philadelphia: JB Lippincott, 1991.

Sandler MP, Patton JA, Shaff MI, Powers TA, Partain CL. Correlative imaging: nuclear medicine, magnetic resonance, computed tomography, ultrasound. Baltimore: Williams & Wilkins, 1989.

Stark DD, Bradley WG Jr, eds. Magnetic resonance imaging. 2nd ed. St. Louis: Mosby Year Book, 1991.

Chapter 2

Radiographic Contrast Agents

We are able to recognize various structures within the body either because of their inherent radiographic density (such as bone distinguished from muscle) or because they contain one of the basic natural materials (e.g., air). However, since most of the internal viscera are of the radiographic density of water or close to it, it is necessary to introduce into these structures a material that will outline walls, define anatomy, and demonstrate any pathologic conditions. The first chapter briefly mentioned these agents and some of the studies for which they are used. This chapter will deal with their physiology and pharmacology, define indications and contraindications for their use, and discuss the treatment of reactions to them.

BARIUM PREPARATIONS

Barium sulfate (USP), in one of its many forms, provides the mainstay for radiographic examinations of the gastrointestinal (GI) tract. Barium is of high atomic weight, which results in considerable absorption of the x-ray beam, thus providing excellent radiographic contrast. In the usual preparation, finely pulverized barium mixed with dispersing agents is suspended in water. When administered orally or rectally, it provides adequate coating of the GI tract.

Although barium itself is chemically inert, when it is extravasated outside the GI tract, a severe desmoplastic reaction may develop. This is most likely to occur when there is a perforation of the GI tract. In the past, barium mixed with fecal material was deemed to be a rapidly lethal mixture when introduced into the peritoneal cavity. However, studies have shown that the combination of barium and feces is no more lethal than the introduction of feces alone into the peritoneum. However, because of the tendency to produce severe granulomas and adhesions, barium should not be used whenever a suspected perforation exists. In these situations a water-soluble contrast material should be used.

Barium preparations are safe as long as the entire GI tract is patent. Oral barium may be used if an obstruction is present *proximal* to the ileocecal valve, since the contents of the small intestine remain fluid up to that point. If the obstruction is *distal* to the ileocecal valve, the patient is best examined with a retrograde study (barium enema) because once the bowel contents enter the cecum, water is rapidly absorbed. If barium is allowed to remain within the colon for a long time behind an obstruction, it may inspissate and compound the patient's problem.

WATER-SOLUBLE CONTRAST MEDIA

Water-soluble contrast agents are used predominantly for urography, angiography, and contrast enhancement of computed tomography (CT) studies. The most common agents used are the sodium or meglumine salts of diatrizoic or iothalmic acid in concentrations of 60 to 90%.

The common chemical structure of all water-soluble contrast media is triiodobenzoic acid. These agents are referred to as *ionic* media because of their property in solution to dissociate into the sodium or meglumine cation and their iodine-containing anion.

These agents are very hypertonic (three times that of serum), resulting in a fluid shift from the intra- or extracellular to the intravascular space or lumen of the GI tract (depending on the route of administration). Although normal individuals may not suffer any severe long-lasting effects from this shift, patients who are dehydrated or in a precarious state of cardiac and fluid balance are at special risk, particularly for renal failure. Secondary effects from the changes in viscosity and tonicity of the blood include platelet aggregation, changes in blood pressure, change in cardiac output, and changes in pulse rate. As the serum osmolality rises, there may be changes in blood coagulation, with a resultant bleeding tendency.

The extent and severity of these changes will depend on the volume of the agent injected, the speed of injection, and the tonicity and viscosity of the agent. Rapid injection, high-volume injection, and high tonicity and viscosity of the agent are associated with more severe reactions. Fortunately, the majority of these agents are used for urography, where a slower injection rate prevents many of these effects. Occasionally a vagal reaction occurs in which there is vasodilation and systemic hypotension. Bradycardia is encountered rather than tachycardia.

Cardiac changes include bradycardia, a fall in systemic blood pressure, flattening of the T waves, and decreased cardiac output. This occurs especially if the contrast agent is injected directly into the heart. In the kidneys, especially in a dehydrated patient, glomerular and tubular damage may result in temporary impairment of renal function and oliguria.

The goal of reducing the normal physiologic and abnormal adverse effects of the ionic contrast agents led to the development of a new class of water-soluble media. These agents are of two varieties. The first are *nonionic* monomers—variants of triiodobenzene—in which the sodium or meglumine cation has been replaced by a side chain that will not dissociate from the iodine-containing portion of the molecule. This results in a pronounced lower osmolality than the ionic agents.

The second class of low-osmolality agents is an ionic dimer formed by linking two triiodobenzoic acid molecules, one of which contains a sodium or meglumine cation. However, doubling the iodine content in the anionic portion reduces the overall osmolality.

These new lower osmolality contrast media are associated with a lower overall incidence of side effects and mortality than the older ionic agents, and are now used in greater frequency than their ionic counterparts. The main reason for their less than universal adoption is the higher cost (approximately 10 times greater) of the low-osmolality agents. Hopefully, this should change in the future.

The low osmolality contrast media are also used for myelography. In the dilutions used, they provide excellent contrast without excessive density. Thus, they may be used for CT myelography. These agents may produce headache in up to 30% of patients and transient psychologic disturbances due to intracranial flow of contrast in less than 5%. This last complication is reduced by keeping the patient's head elevated after the myelogram.

In addition to their use in angiography, urography, myelography, and arthrography, these same agents may be injected into sinus tracts or used in diluted form to examine the GI tract when there is a suspected perforation. They do not cause any of the undesirable side effects that barium is known to produce when outside the GI tract. However, there is one important contraindication for water-soluble contrast media: suspected communication between GI tract and the tracheobronchial tree (tracheoesophageal fistula). As mentioned in Chapter 1, water-soluble materials are extremely irritating to the tracheobronchial mucosa and produce a severe chemical pneumonia that may result in death. A barium or oil-soluble preparation should be used when airway communication is suspected.

Excretion of these agents is by pure glomerular filtration within the kidney. The material is removed intact by the glomeruli. In patients with chronic renal failure, however, the material may be secreted into the bile or small bowel by a process known as "vicarious excretion."

AGENTS USED TO VISUALIZE THE BILIARY TREE

The agents used for cholecystography are iopanoic acid (Telepaque), iocetamic acid (Cholebrine), sodium tyropanoate (Biloqaque), and calcium or sodium ipodate (Oragrafin). These agents are ingested orally, absorbed in the duodenum, conjugated as a glucuronide salt in the liver, and excreted in the bile. The material is then stored and concentrated within the gallbladder. In their native form, these agents are not water-soluble, allowing for their absorption from the GI tract. In the conjugated form, they are water-soluble and are not reabsorbed on passage through the bowel.

AGENTS USED TO ENHANCE MAGNETIC RESONANCE (MR) IMAGING

Despite the wide variety of pulse sequences available for MR imaging difficulties still exist for differentiation between neoplasm and chronic cerebral infarction, tumor and perifocal cerebral edema, or recurrent herniated intervertebral disc and surgical scar. For these reasons, a number of *paramagnetic* contrast agents have been developed for intravenous use during MR imaging. To date, gadolinium-diethylenetriaminepentaacetic acid (Gd-DTPA) is most commonly used. Gadolinium was chosen because of its strong effect on the relaxation time in the scanning sequence. Chelation with DTPA has reduced the inherent toxicity of the free Gd ion. In diagnostic doses, Gd-DTPA increases the signal in vascular structures, similar to the effect of conventional water-soluble contrast media.

OIL-SOLUBLE AGENTS

Oil-soluble agents such as propyliodone (Dionosil) are used for bronchography. The material is inert within the tracheobronchial tree and provides adequate coating and definition of the structures. It may be used for esophagography in suspected esophago-airway fistulas. Ethiodized oil (Ethiodol) is an oily agent used for lymphangiography. It also may be used for sialography (study of the salivary ducts) or hysterosalpingography (study of uterine cavity and fallopian tubes).

ADVERSE REACTIONS TO CONTRAST MATERIAL AND THEIR MANAGEMENT

The incidence of adverse reaction to iodinated contrast material is variable and unpredictable. The Subcommittee on Treatment of Adverse Reactions of the Committee on Contrast Media from the International Society of Radiology reviewed the data from 150,000 case reports. They found that the overall incidence of adverse reactions was 5%. Serious reactions were reported to vary between 1:1000 and 1:2000, with fatalities occurring from 1:13,000 to 1:40,000. Although many adverse reactions occur in patients with no previous allergic history, the study revealed that a patient with a history of allergy has a risk of reaction that is twice that of the general population. If the patient has a history of a previous reaction to contrast media, the chances of another reaction are three times greater than that of the general population. Pretesting with a small injection of the contrast medium was found to have little or no value in identifying patients who would later react. Similarly, pretreatment with antihistamines and steroids in patients with known allergies to contrast material were shown to be ineffective.

Two recent studies from Japan and Australia on 337,647 patients reevaluated the incidence of adverse reactions (including death) from ionic and low osmolar contrast media. The studies revealed that the overall incidence of adverse reactions from ionic contrast material was 12.7% and from nonionic (low osmolar) contrast it was 3.1%. Severe reactions occurred in 0.22% and 0.04% of each group respectively. There was one death in each group, but no causal relationship to the contrast medium was found. The conclusions of the studies were that nonionic (low osmolar) contrast media significantly reduced the incidence of severe and potential life-threatening reactions and their general use to increase the overall safety for contrast media examinations was recommended.

Types of Adverse Reactions to Contrast Media

There are three basic types of adverse reactions to contrast media: mild, intermediate, and severe. Mild or minor reactions (nausea, vomiting, sneezing, flushing, diaphoresis, feeling of warmth, and occasional headache) resolve without therapy. Intermediate reactions are those that require therapy for the patient's symptoms, but are not life-threatening. These include urticaria, angioneurotic edema, and wheezing. Severe reactions include cardiovascular collapse, which may be associated with pulmonary edema, laryngeal edema, and apnea. There may be central nervous system depression. Death may result if proper treatment is not instituted immediately.

Table 2.1 lists signs and symptoms of reactions to contrast agents in order of increasing severity.

Treatment of Adverse Reactions to Contrast Material

Before instituting treatment, the severity of the reaction and the body systems involved should be carefully evaluated. The patient's vital signs should be monitored. Once a determination has been made regarding the organ system involved and the nature and severity of the reaction, proper treatment may be instituted. After successful treatment of a reaction of any kind, the type of reaction, severity, and mode of treatment should be entered in the patient's permanent medical record. In addition, a notation should be made on the patient's x-ray folder that he/she has had an allergic reaction, and the type of reaction should be stated. Furthermore, the patient's referring physician should be notified immediately whenever a reaction occurs.

Mild reactions require careful observation of the patient and reassurance by the radiologist that the symptoms are not serious and will resolve quickly. Most of these symptoms will pass within a few minutes. Anxiety is believed to play a key role in the development of minor reactions.

The intermediate reactions are treated by intravenous administration of 25 to 50 mg of diphenhydramine (Benadryl). This may be augmented by 0.3 to 0.5 ml of a 1:1000 solution of epinephrine subcutaneously. Cimetidine (Tagamet) is a histamine antagonist and may be used as a bolus injection of 300 mg instead of Benadryl or epinephrine. In the majority of the cases, the patient will respond favorably within several minutes; hives

Table 2.1.   Signs and Symptoms of Reactions to Contrast Material

Type	Cardiovascular	Respiratory	Cutaneous	GI	Nervous	Urinary
Mild	Pallor Diaphoresis Tachycardia	Sneezing Coughing Rhinorrhea	Erythema Feeling of warmth	Nausea Vomiting Metallic taste	Anxiety Headache Dizziness	
Intermediate	Bradycardia Palpitations Hypotension	Wheezing Acute asthma attack	Urticaria (hives) Pruritis	Abdominal cramps Diarrhea	Agitation Vertigo Slurred speech	Oliguria
Severe	Acute pulmonary edema Shock Congestive heart failure Cardiac arrest	Laryngospasm Cyanosis Laryngeal edema Apnea	Angioneurotic edema	Paralytic ileus	Disorientation Stupor Coma Convulsions	Acute renal failure

begin to fade, wheezing subsides, and the patient appears less apprehensive. The use of steroids for intermediate types of reaction is controversial. Some authorities believe that a 100 mg bolus of prednisolone is useful in treating the more severe type of intermediate reaction.

Severe reactions require immediate recognition and evaluation of the patient's cardiopulmonary status. Cardiopulmonary resuscitation (CPR) equipment should be readily available in any area where contrast media are used. Furthermore, the radiologist and the technical staff should be well trained in the techniques of CPR. In general, the radiologist is the first physician called to the scene when a reaction occurs. Proper treatment of a severe reaction follows the "ABCD system":

A. Airway open
B. Breathing restored
C. Circulation maintained
D. Drug and definitive therapy

Once the initial CPR has begun, a code/crash team should be summoned. The principles and practice of CPR are a subject with which the reader should be familiar and will not be covered further in this book. The reader should never inject contrast agents unless familiar with CPR and the management of reactions.

A vagal type of reaction has been recognized as a distinct complication of the use of contrast material. This reaction may be recognized by the presence of hypotension and bradycardia rather than tachycardia, the latter occurring in the anaphylactoid reactions. Treatment of patients with vagal reactions is by the use of 0.5 to 1.0 mg of atropine intravenously.

Adjunctive procedures that should be performed before the patient has a reaction and that may aid in the later treatment of a reaction include

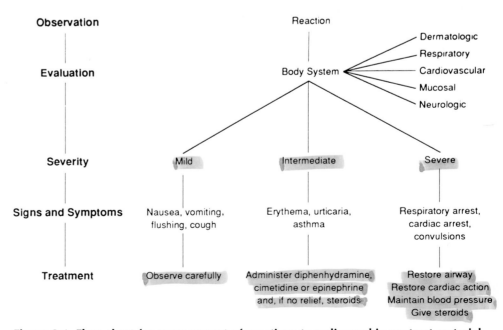

Figure 2.1. Flow chart for management of reactions to radiographic contrast material.

recording the patient's pulse and blood pressure and noting the cardiac rhythm. In addition, the use of a scalp vein-type needle-tubing combination that is taped in place to the forearm will ensure a ready channel of access to the patient's bloodstream in the event of an emergency.

Figure 2.1 is a flow chart of steps to follow in managing a patient who has had a reaction to contrast material.

Summary

The basic types of radiographic contrast materials have been discussed along with their indications and uses. Of prime importance is the recognition that these agents, when injected intraarterially or intravenously, may cause severe life-threatening reactions. The types of reactions, their recognition, and their treatment were briefly discussed. The reader is advised to be thoroughly familiar with the technique of CPR.

Suggested Additional Reading

American College of Radiology. Manual iodinated contrast media. Reston, VA: 1991.

Bush WH, Swanson DP. Acute reactions to intravascular contrast media: types, risk factors, recognition, and specific treatment. AJR 1991;157:1153–1161.

Cohan RH, Dunnick NR, Bashore TM. Treatment of reactions to radiographic contrast material. AJR 1988;151:263–270.

Katayama H, Yamaguchi K, Kozuka T, et al. Adverse reactions to ionic and nonionic contrast media. Radiology 1990;175:621–628.

Katzberg RW. The contrast media manual. Baltimore: Williams & Wilkins, 1992.

McClennan BL. Ionic and nonionic iodinated contrast media: evolution and strategies for use. AJR 1990;155:225–233.

Palmer FG. The RACR survey of intravenous contrast media reactions final report. Australas Radiol 1988;426:32:426–428.

Chapter 3

Interventional Radiology

Interventional or invasive radiology is the subspecialty of diagnostic radiology in which diagnostic examinations are performed by percutaneous puncture. It is also known as interventional or surgical radiology. The origins of this subspecialty date to the work of Seldinger, who, in 1953, first reported the technique that now allows one access to many organ systems percutaneously (Fig. 3.1). Interventional radiology was confined primarily to cardiovascular studies in its first 2 decades. Improvements in imaging such as the development of high-resolution image-intensified fluoroscopy, biplane fluoroscopy, and refinements in catheter and guidewire technology, began in the late 1960s. In the early to mid-1970s, the development of ultrasound and computerized tomography (CT) and subsequent development of digital subtraction angiography (DSA) launched the subspecialty into areas previously known only to surgeons. The development of low osmolar contrast material was an additional benefit.

Invasive radiology is no longer confined to arteriography. This exciting subspecialty is the most labor-intensive in diagnostic radiology and includes biopsy procedures, percutaneous puncture, decompression and drainage procedures, balloon dilations (angioplastic procedures), extraction techniques, vascular chemotherapy, and vascular embolism.

Invasive radiology has also had a dramatic impact on medical practice. Many patients now undergo diagnostic or therapeutic procedures in a radiologic suite rather than having general anesthesia and surgery, which were standard methods of treatment of the same abnormalities in years past. This has had a significant impact on the patient, who may now have a procedure performed with relatively little risk compared to that associated with general anesthetic and surgery. Furthermore, the high-risk patient, who is a poor surgical risk, may be treated for many conditions through interventional radiologic techniques. Finally, many patients now undergo a preliminary therapeutic radiologic procedure prior to surgery, particularly through embolization of certain vascular lesions.

Let us now briefly describe some of the techniques and their indications.

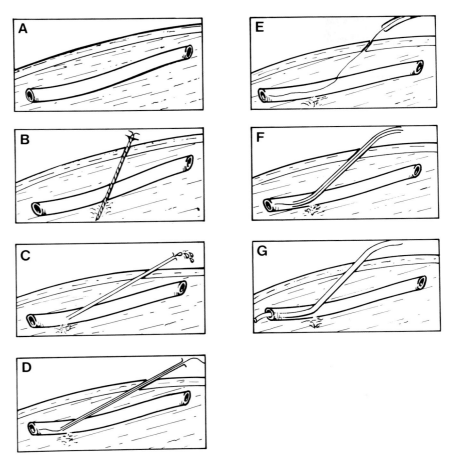

Figure 3.1.   Seldinger technique. This technique is the basis of percutaneous access for most interventional procedures. **A,** the vessel before puncture. **B,** a two-part needle consisting of a central stylet and an outer sheath punctures the vessel through both walls. **C,** the stylet is removed and the sheath is withdrawn until blood is obtained. **D,** a guidewire is fed through the sheath into the vessel. **E,** the sheath is removed and a catheter is threaded over the guidewire. **F,** the guidewire and catheter are advanced in the vessel. **G,** the guidewire is removed, leaving the catheter in the vessel ready for injection or infusion of medication.

ANGIOGRAPHY

Angiography is primarily performed to evaluate the patency and distribution of blood vessels throughout the body. It is used almost exclusively for assessment of the heart and great vessels, the peripheral circulation, and the cranial circulation. Cardiac angiography is performed almost exclusively by cardiologists. The remaining procedures are performed by radiologists. Before the development of CT, ultrasound, or magnetic resonance imaging, angiography was much more frequently performed to diagnose suspected neoplasms in the abdominal viscera and to denote the effects of those neoplasms on the normal vessels. For these reasons, angiography is less frequently performed today. Angiograms are now obtained to evaluate vascular malformations, aneurysms (Fig. 3.2), arteriovenous

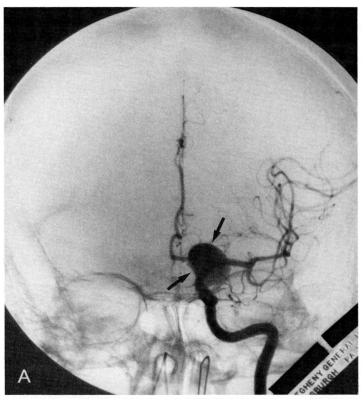

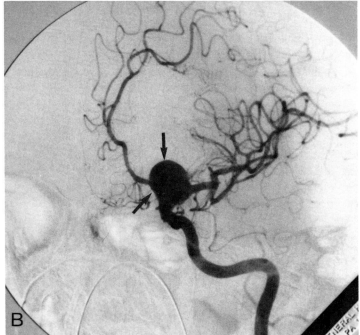

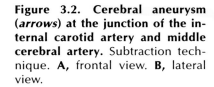

Figure 3.2. Cerebral aneurysm (*arrows*) **at the junction of the internal carotid artery and middle cerebral artery.** Subtraction technique. **A,** frontal view. **B,** lateral view.

fistulas, thromboembolic phenomena (Fig. 3.3), arteriosclerotic vascular disease (Fig. 3.4), and posttraumatic vascular injury (Fig. 3.5). Complications of angiography occur in less than 1% of patients and include pericatheter bleeding, hematoma, pseudoaneurysm formation, arteriovenous fistula, arterial occlusion, and spasm.

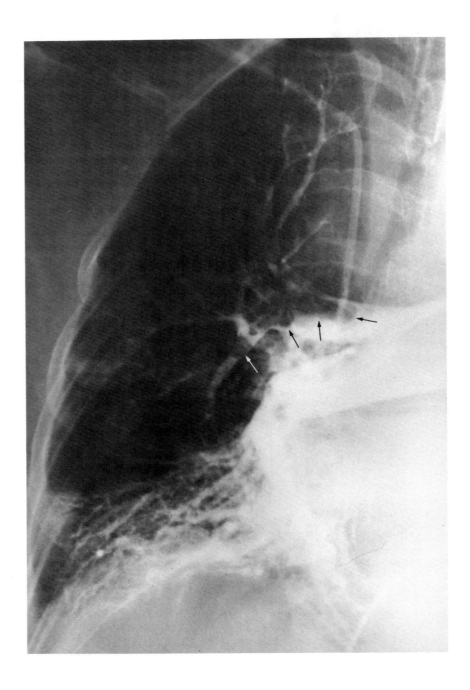

Figure 3.3. Pulmonary thromboembolism. There are multiple lucent filling defects (*arrows*) in the right upper lobe pulmonary artery. Note the paucity of peripheral filling in the upper lobe as compared with the lower lobe.

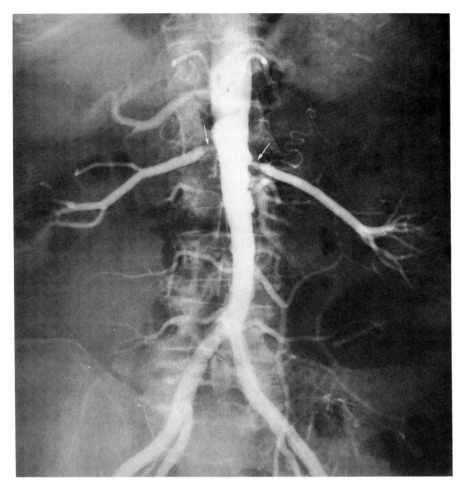

Figure 3.4.   Atherosclerotic disease of the abdominal aorta in renal arteries. Note the irregularity of the abdominal aorta on the left side beneath the renal arteries. Note the stenosis of both renal arteries near their origin (*arrows*).

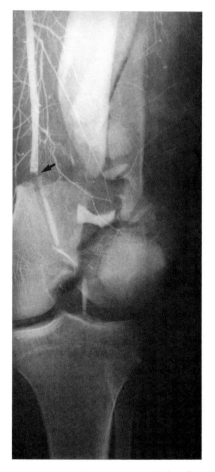

Figure 3.5.   Transection of the distal femoral artery (*arrow*) at the site of a distal femoral fracture. There is partial filling of the remainder of the vessel.

PERCUTANEOUS BIOPSY

Biopsy procedures are performed using a variety of needles (Fig. 3.6) throughout the body. Percutaneous biopsy has prevented countless surgical operations where the sole purpose of that procedure was to obtain tissue. Biopsy should be performed using whatever imaging modality shows the lesion to best advantage. However, most procedures are performed using CT guidance because this gives the best overall depth control (Fig. 3.7). Large skeletal lesions that are very apparent on plain radiographs may undergo biopsy under fluoroscopic control.

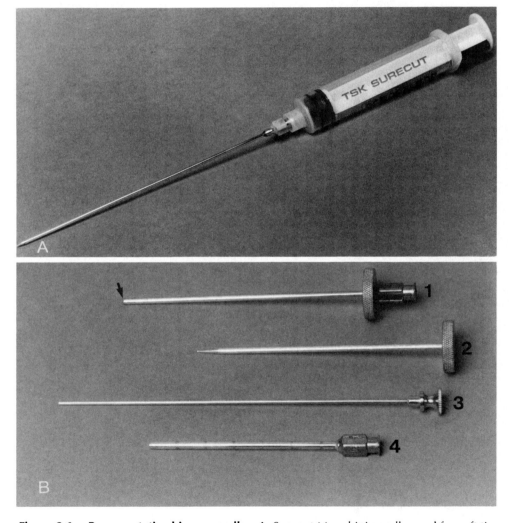

Figure 3.6.   Representative biopsy needles. A, Surecut Menghini needle used for soft tissue lesions. **B,** Ackerman bone biopsy set. 1. Toothed (*arrow*) biopsy needle. 2. Trocar. 3. Clearing rod. 4. Outer, depth-marked sheath.

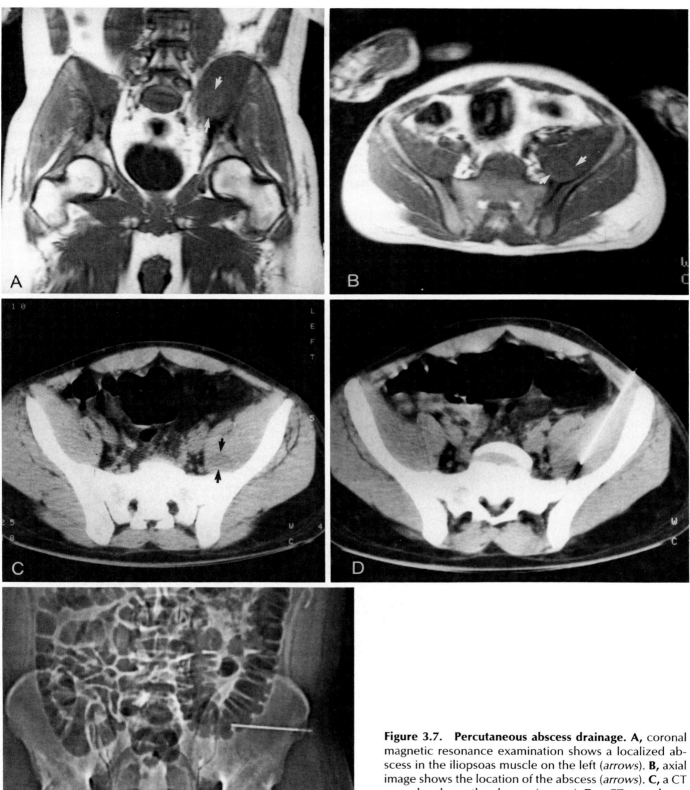

Figure 3.7. Percutaneous abscess drainage. A, coronal magnetic resonance examination shows a localized abscess in the iliopsoas muscle on the left (*arrows*). **B,** axial image shows the location of the abscess (*arrows*). **C,** a CT scan also shows the abscess (*arrows*). **D,** a CT scan shows the placement of the drainage needle in the abscess. **E,** scout view shows the position of the needle. Compare this location with abscess as shown in **A.**

DECOMPRESSION AND DRAINING

Decompression and/or drainage is performed as a variation of the Seldinger technique. A needle is placed into the fluid collection using ultrasound or CT control. A drainage catheter is then introduced into the fluid-filled space (Fig. 3.8). The catheter is either taped or sutured in place and then attached to a vacuum bottle for further drainage. A variation of this technique involves the placement of stents into the ureter through percutaneous nephrostomy or into the biliary tree following percutaneous transhepatic cholangiography (Fig. 3.9).

Improvements in catheter technology and imaging systems have resulted in radiologists now being able to perform extraction procedures for biliary and renal stones as well as foreign bodies. The procedure is a variant of the decompression procedure, with the exception being the use of an extraction instrument through the catheter within the lumen of the occluded duct.

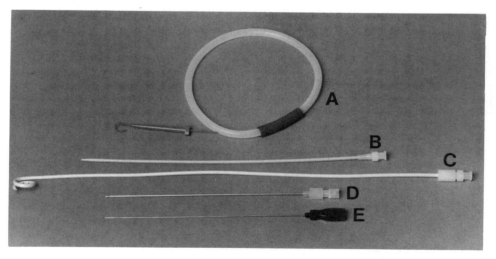

Figure 3.8. Percutaneous neophrostomy set. A, guidewire. **B,** dilator. **C,** pigtail drainage catheter. **D,** needle and stylet. **E,** thin-walled needle.

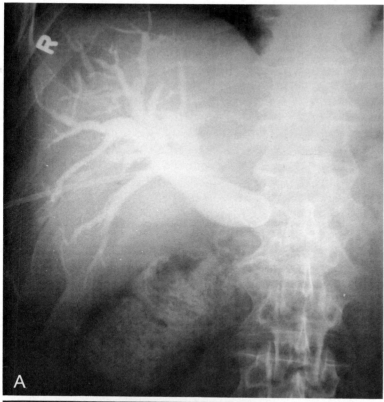

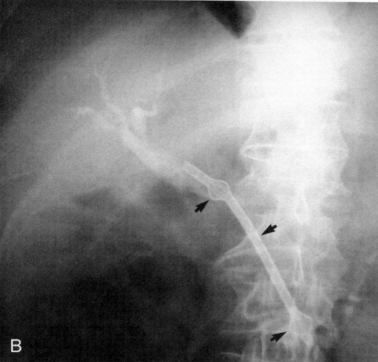

Figure 3.9. Placement of biliary stent in obstruction of the common bile duct. A, injection of contrast through a catheter following percutaneous transhepatic cholangiography shows complete obstruction of the common bile duct near the catheter tip. Note the dilation of the biliary tree. **B,** following placement of a stent (*arrows*), there is decompression of the biliary tree.

IMAGE-GUIDED AND VASCULAR THERAPY

Image-guided therapy is a technique in which radioactive therapeutic agents and drugs are precisely deposited in various anatomic locations using the techniques and skills of the interventional radiologist.

Vascular chemotherapy relies on selective arterial catheterization to deliver a high concentration of chemotherapeutic agents into the feeding vessels of a tumor. This procedure is often used as a prelude to the surgical removal of the tumor. A variation of this procedure involves the introduction of vasoconstrictor agents such as vasopressin into the feeding vessels that are responsible for gastrointestinal tract hemorrhage. Finally, thrombolytic agents may be introduced intravascularly for such conditions as pulmonary embolism, deep venous thrombosis, coronary thrombosis, and peripheral arterial thrombosis.

BALLOON DILATION

Interventional dilation or transluminal angioplasty using special dilating catheters (Fig. 3.10) is used to dilate stenotic blood vessels. This procedure was originally introduced by Dotter and Judkins in 1964. However, it was nearly 2 decades later before refinement in the technique and catheter technology resulted in its widespread use. The procedure is used for a variety of peripheral arterial stenotic lesions (Fig. 3.11) as well as coronary arterial stenosis. The degree of success approaches that achieved by surgery.

Figure 3.10. Catheters used for angioplasty. A, entire catheter. **B,** close-up of tip (inflated).

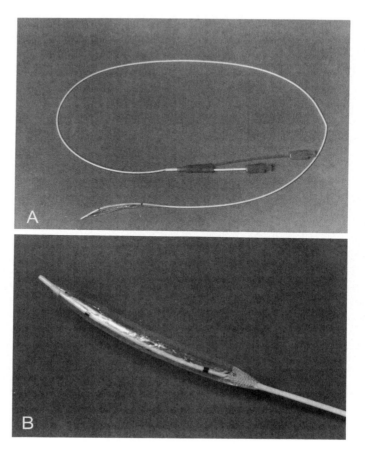

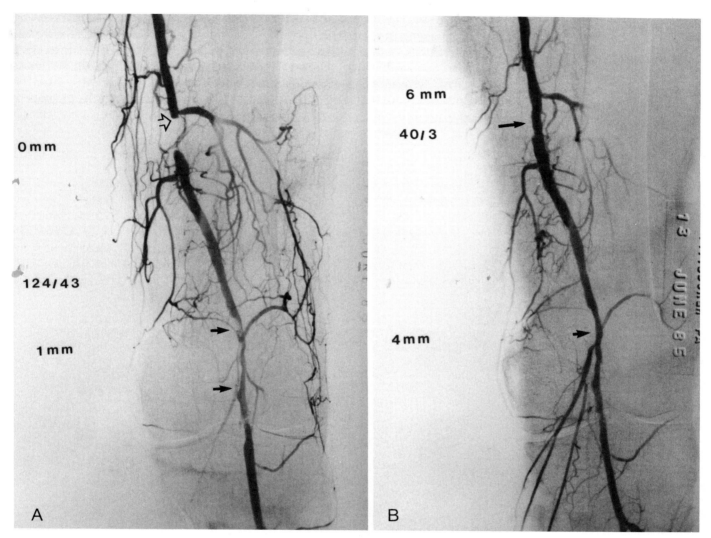

Figure 3.11.   The effect of femoral angioplasty (subtraction technique). A, before angioplasty, there is complete occlusion of a segment of the femoral artery (*open arrow*). The distal vessels fill through collaterals. There is an area of stenosis of the popliteal artery (*solid arrows*). Prior to angioplasty, there is no lumen at the occluded area, and a 1-mm lumen at the distal le-sion. The gradient is 124/43. **B,** following angioplasty, flow is re-established through the occluded area (*long arrow*). There is also improved flow through the distal stenotic area (*short arrow*). The proximal lumen now measures 6 mm and the lower measures 4 mm. The gradient is now 40/3. Note the less prominent appearance of the collateral circulation.

EMBOLIZATION

Embolization procedures involve the deliberate occlusion of arteries, veins, or abnormal vascular spaces by the introduction of various embolic materials through a selectively positioned catheter. The procedure is particularly advantageous to high-risk patients who otherwise might have to undergo surgery for the occlusion of these vessels. A variety of autologous and artificial materials are used. These procedures are used for acute bleeding (Fig. 3.12), embolization of neoplasms, arteriovenous malformations (Fig. 3.13), and for prevention of further pulmonary thromboembolism by using an inferior vena cava filter (Fig. 3.14). Embolization procedures require the utmost of care to ensure that the embolized materials do not end up in vessels other than those desired.

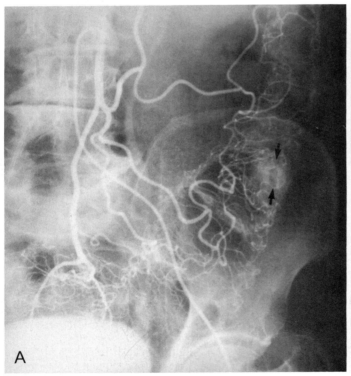
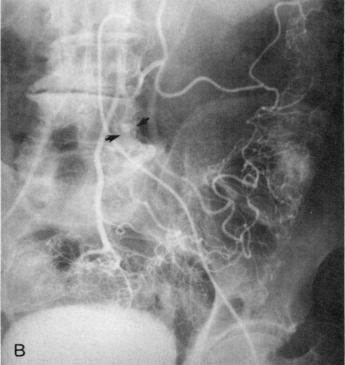
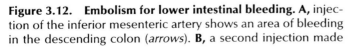

Figure 3.12. Embolism for lower intestinal bleeding. A, injection of the inferior mesenteric artery shows an area of bleeding in the descending colon (*arrows*). **B,** a second injection made following infusion of an occlusive material (*arrows*) shows marked diminished flow to the area of bleeding.

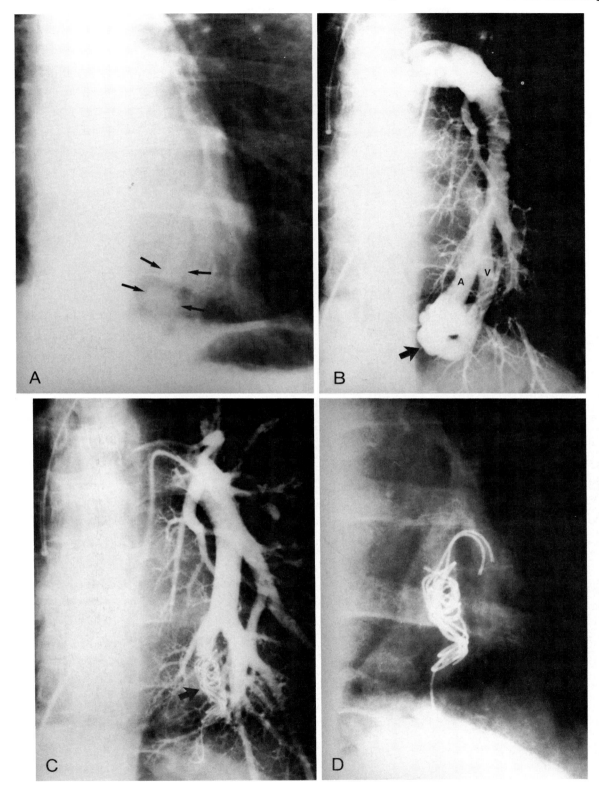

Figure 3.13. Embolism of a pulmonary arteriovenous malformation. A, cone-down view of the left lower lobe shows the mass-like A-V malformation (*arrows*). **B,** pulmonary arteriogram shows the arterial *(A)* and the venous *(V)* branches of the malformation (*arrow*). **C,** arteriogram following embolism of an occluding coil (*arrow*) through a catheter. Note that there is no flow of contrast into the malformation. **D,** radiograph of the left lower lobe following embolization shows the coil in place.

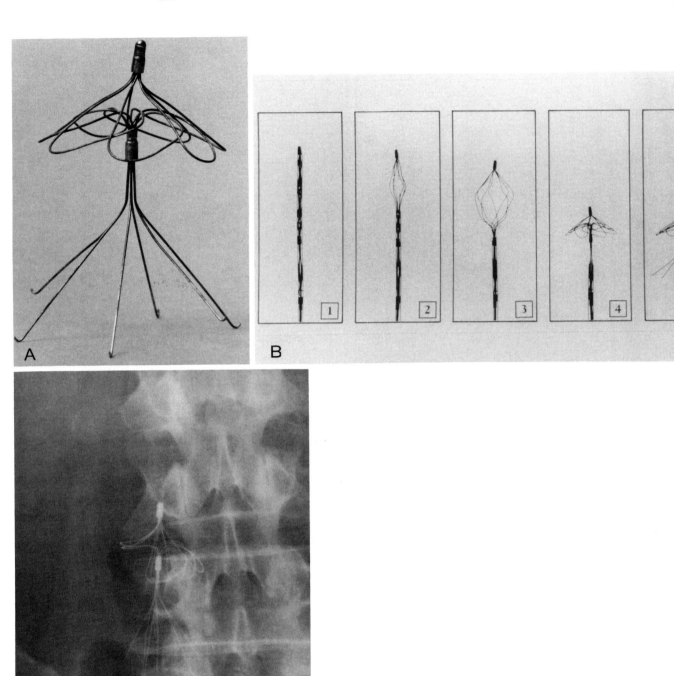

Figure 3.14. Simon-Nitinol inferior vena cava filter. **A,** photograph of the filter. **B,** photographs showing deployment of the filter from its catheter (Courtesy of Cardiomedics, Inc.). **C,** radiograph showing the filter in place.

Summary

Interventional radiology is an exciting new subspecialty in which a variety of diagnostic and therapeutic techniques are used through percutaneous puncture. In many instances, an invasive radiologic procedure may be performed instead of a surgical procedure, thus saving the patient exposure to anesthesia and the risks of surgery.

Suggested Additional Reading

Castañeda-Zuniga WR, Tadavarthy SM. Interventional radiology. 2nd ed. Baltimore: Williams & Wilkins, 1991.

Kadir S. Current practice of interventional radiology. St. Louis: Mosby Year Book, 1991.

Wojtowycz M. Interventional radiology and angiography. St. Louis: Mosby Year Book, 1990.

Simon- Nitinol IVC filter

PA

claercals superimposed over upper
+ slanted c̄ medial
drawing over upper

AP

Chapter 4

Pulmonary Imaging

The chest radiograph is the examination you will be requesting and observing with the greatest frequency. In addition, it is the examination that you will most likely be reviewing alone. Chest radiographs account for more than half of all the examinations performed in any radiology practice. One of the reasons for this is that the chest is the "mirror of health or disease." Besides giving information about the patient's heart and lungs, the chest film provides valuable information about adjacent structures such as the gastrointestinal (GI) tract, the thyroid gland, or the bony structures of the thorax. Furthermore, metastatic disease from the abdominal viscera, head and neck, or skeleton frequently manifests itself in the lungs.

TECHNICAL CONSIDERATIONS

Once you have assured yourself that the radiograph presented is that of the correct patient, the film should be analyzed for density, motion, and rotation. A determination should be made as to whether the entire thorax is displayed. Be sure that the technologist has not cut the costophrenic angles off the film. On a properly exposed radiograph, the thoracic vertebrae should be barely discernible through the image of the heart. The medial ends of the clavicles should be equidistant from the patient's midline, indicating no rotation.

The next step is to decide what type of examination has been performed. The ordinary chest radiograph is made with the patient in the erect position with the anterior portion of the chest against the film cassette. The x-ray tube is positioned 6 feet behind the patient, and the horizontal beam enters from the back (posterior) and exits through the front (anterior): the PA radiograph. If the patient turns completely around and the beam enters from the front, the film is termed an AP film. Figure 4.1**A** is a PA erect film of a young patient; Figure 4.1**B** is an AP erect film of the same patient. Note the differences.

In general, the following are features that commonly identify PA chest radiographs: identification markings, if present, are oriented so that the observer may read them without reversing the film; the clavicles are superimposed over the upper lungs and are slanted with the medial aspect lower than the lateral; and the posterior portions of the cervical and thoracic ver-

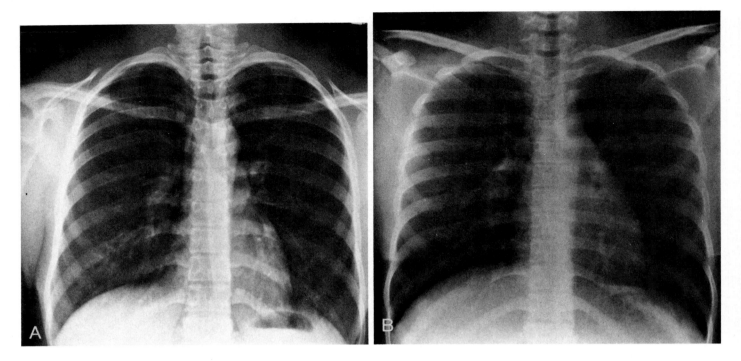

Figure 4.1. **Normal chest radiograph. A,** PA view. **B,** AP view (see text for description).

tebrae (neural arch, articular processes, apophyseal joints, and laminae) are more clearly visible. The following findings suggest an AP radiograph: identification marks and writing are reversed; the heart appears slightly large; the clavicles are usually higher; and there is demonstration of the bodies and Luschka joints of the lower cervical vertebrae.

One of the most important technical considerations in evaluating the chest radiograph is the determination of whether or not the film is in optimal inspiration. Figure 4.2, a film of a healthy man, was deliberately made in forced expiration. Failure to observe that the film was a poor inspiratory *result* could easily lead to a mistaken diagnosis of congestive heart failure. After all, the heart appears large and rather poorly defined, the pulmonary vessels appear slightly prominent, and there is apparent blunting of both lung bases, suggesting fluid. Figure 4.3 is a maximal inspiratory film of the same individual; it is perfectly normal.

There are many reasons why a film may not be obtained in full inspiration. Massive obesity is a mechanical cause; pain in a patient postoperatively results in voluntary restriction; the cardiac patient with congestive heart failure is unable to displace the edema fluid in the "water-logged" lungs; and the patient with chronic restrictive lung disease cannot expand his/her chest to expected maximum because of scarring and loss of compliance in the lung tissues. For all these reasons, the term "*poor inspiratory result*" is used rather than "*poor inspiratory effort.*" In most instances, these patients will have made a good inspiratory *effort,* but the *result* is poor.

A film is considered to be in optimal inspiratory result when we are able to see the diaphragm crossing the 10th rib or interspace posteriorly or

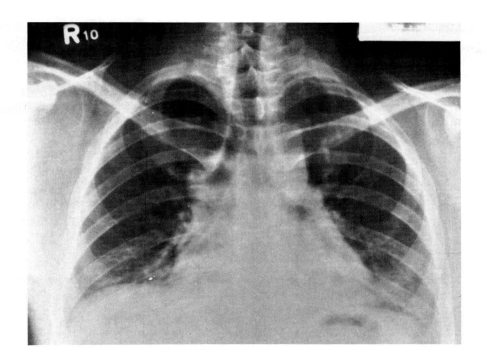

Figure 4.2. Expiratory chest radiograph. This film was made in deliberate expiration. There is elevation of the diaphragm, crowding of the lower lung markings, and apparent heart enlargement. (Compare with Figure 4.3.)

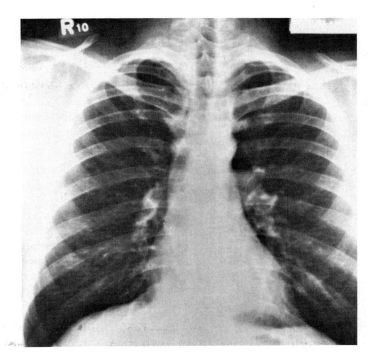

Figure 4.3. Normal inspiratory chest radiograph. (This is the same patient as in Fig. 4.2.) Note the differences in full inspiration.

the 8th rib anteriorly. The reader is cautioned not to fall into the pitfall of diagnosing "nondisease" in a patient with a poor inspiratory film.

Interestingly enough, there are certain circumstance in which it is desirable to have a film deliberately taken in expiration. These include evaluation of the patient with a suspected foreign body in a bronchus, a "ball-valve" type of bronchial obstruction, or a suspected pneumothorax. In the first instance (Fig. 4.4), the PA inspiratory film is normal; the expiratory film demonstrates no change in the volume of the lung on the obstructed side. The normal lung decreases in volume, and the mediastinum swings toward the normal side. In the second instance, the pneumothorax is enhanced by the decrease in lung volume (Fig. 4.5).

Rotation of the patient or angulation may result in distortion of normal anatomic shadows. As mentioned previously, you should be able to detect rotation by observing the position of the medial ends of the clavicles.

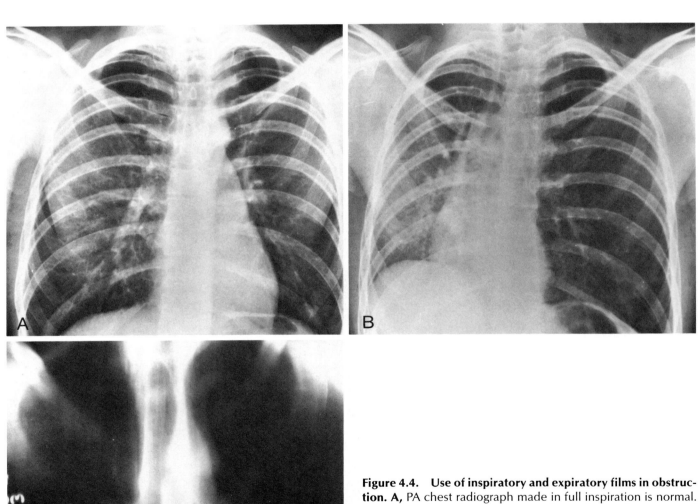

Figure 4.4. Use of inspiratory and expiratory films in obstruction. A, PA chest radiograph made in full inspiration is normal. **B,** radiograph made in expiration shows the mediastinum and heart to shift to the right. There is no volume change on the left. These findings indicate an obstructing lesion in the mainstem bronchus on the left. **C,** tomogram of the tracheobronchial tree shows an obstructing lesion (*arrow*) in the left mainstem bronchus.

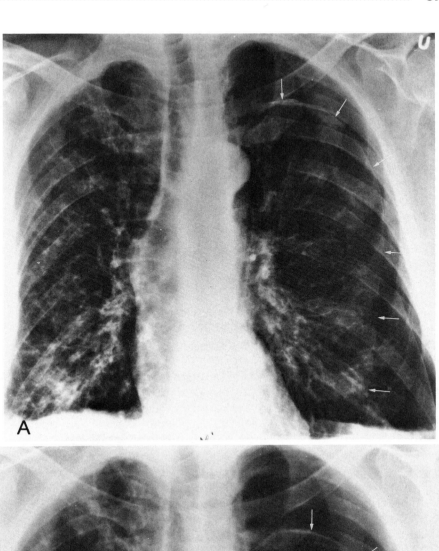

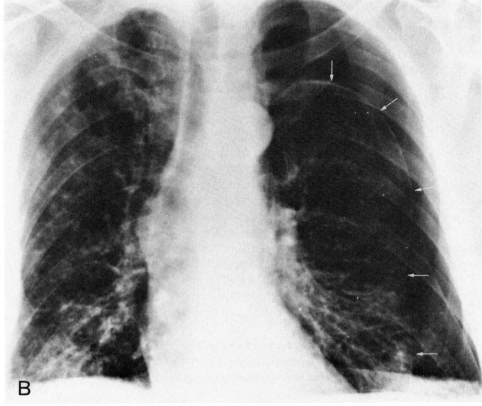

Figure 4.5. Use of inspiratory and expiratory film in pneumothorax. A, inspiratory film shows a pneumothorax on the left (*arrows*). **B,** expiratory film shows enlargment of the pneumothorax (*arrows*).

Lordotic views have been advocated as a means of examining lesions in the lung apices. The examination is made by having the patient lean backward toward the film while a horizontal beam is used to make the exposure. We do not use this view frequently because anterior lesions are often not demonstrated by this technique. An alternative to a lordotic view, a coned-down view of the apex of the lung, is more useful for suspected upper lobe lesions.

Another technical consideration is the analysis of radiographs made by portable technique. Studies of this kind are performed on severely debilitated or gravely ill patients who are unable to come to the x-ray department. In reviewing these films, it is important to recognize the circumstances under which they were made. There may be slight motion on the film (the patient cannot hold his breath), the patient may be rotated, or the patient may sag down against the pillow, with the result that a lordotic view of the chest is obtained. This is easy enough to detect because the heart assumes an egg-shaped configuration, the ribs appear tapered, and the clavicles are seen above the ribs.

Many portable films are obtained with the patient supine. This can result in a redistribution of blood to the upper lobes of the lung. Since this is an early sign of congestive heart failure, the reader again is cautioned to observe whether this film was performed with the patient in the upright position or in the supine position. The presence or absence of an air-fluid level in the gastric air bubble may aid in determining upright versus supine positioning. Our technologists routinely use a vial of (radiopaque) potassium iodide solution to indicate the degree of erectness. An upright film will have a sharp fluid meniscus; a recumbent film will not.

Occasionally it may be useful to use a film with the patient lying on one side (decubitus position). This study is primarily used in patients suspected of having pleural effusions to determine if the effusion will layer out. The technique may also be used to "clear" a portion of the lung base that is obscured by fluid. Unfortunately, loculated effusions often do not shift with changes in patient position.

A final technical consideration is the use of old films to compare with the current study. Many individuals have abnormal chest x-rays from inactive or old diseases. The most common conditions encountered are old, healed granulomas, scarring, and chronic obstructive pulmonary disease. Without the old radiographs for comparison, the patient may have to undergo extensive (and expensive) evaluation that may include a biopsy. Every effort should be made to obtain old studies. *Every* current study should be compared with a previous one.

Although chest radiography is the mainstay for diagnosing thoracic disease, all the other imaging modalities are also used. Chest fluoroscopy is a valuable, but unfortunately infrequently used technique for confirmation and localization of suspected lung nodules. This procedure is simple to perform, takes little time, is inexpensive, and has relatively low radiation exposure. Fluoroscopy is also useful for evaluating cardiac and diaphragmatic motion.

Tomography of the lungs and mediastinum is used to evaluate lung nodules, hilar masses, and lesions of the airways. It has been replaced for the most part by computerized tomography (CT).

Computerized tomography is an extremely valuable technique for assessing lung nodules and mediastinal masses (Fig. 4.6). It is also useful for evaluating chronic pleural effusions and chronic infiltrates. By far, the most common use will be for suspected primary or metastatic neoplasms. Computed tomography is much more sensitive in detecting the calcification in nodules that would suggest a benign postinflammatory condition.

Magnetic resonance (MR) imaging is now used primarily to evaluate hilar and other mediastinal masses, more peripheral nodules, and vascular lesions (including superior vena cava syndrome). This technique is particularly advantageous over CT because flowing blood has no signal on MR and appears black. Thus, it is possible to differentiate a hilar mass from a dilated pulmonary vessel (Fig. 4.7). The ability of MR to image in sagittal and coronal planes is another distinct advantage over CT, as is the fact that it requires no intravenous contrast to identify vessels.

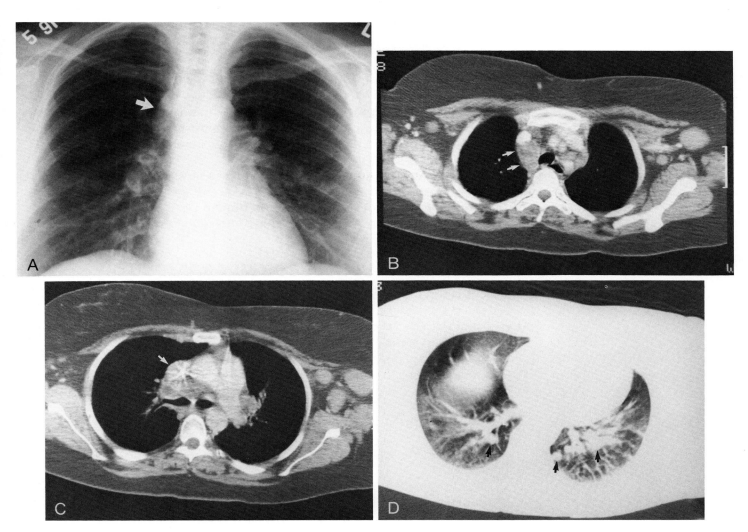

Figure 4.6.   Mediastinal mass. A, PA chest radiograph shows a mass to the right of midline in the upper mediastinum (*arrow*). This is simply a case of "too many bumps." **B,** CT scan through the upper lungs fields show the mass (*arrows*). **C,** another CT section slightly lower shows the mass (*arrow*) adjacent to the superior vena cava. **D,** a section through the lower lung with the window setting for lung parenchyma shows multiple pulmonary nodules (*arrows*).

Figure 4.7.   An MR image differentiation of a hilar vessel from a mass. The mass (*M*) is of higher signal than either of the adjacent vessels. *A*, aorta; *V*, vena cava; *T*, trachea.

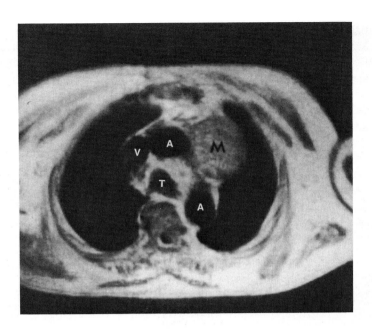

Diagnostic ultrasound is used to diagnose suspected pleural fluid collections, particularly on the right side, where imaging is performed in the transhepatic plane. Ultrasound is not useful for lung lesions because it cannot cross tissue-air borders.

Finally, nuclear imaging is performed to assess pulmonary blood flow and ventilation. It is most commonly used to diagnose suspected pulmonary emboli. The typical ventilation-perfusion (V-Q) scan utilizes xenon-133 by inhalation and technetium-99m labeled macroaggregated albumin particles by intravenous injection.

ANATOMIC CONSIDERATIONS

A logical approach to the interpretation of chest radiographs is predicated on the observer developing an orderly system for scanning films. It matters not whether the review begins from the outside and proceeds inward or vice versa. What is important is that the method is reproduced each and every time that particular type of study is reviewed. Working from the inside outward, observe the following:

1. Trachea and mediastinum
2. Heart and great vessels
3. Lungs
4. Costophrenic angles
5. Pleura
6. Diaphragm
7. Bones and soft tissues

The order of visual scan is illustrated in Figure 4.8, showing a patient who has had a right radical mastectomy and has a congenital anomaly of the left shoulder. Analysis of this film is as follows: "The heart and mediastinal structures are normal. The pulmonary vessels and aorta are normal.

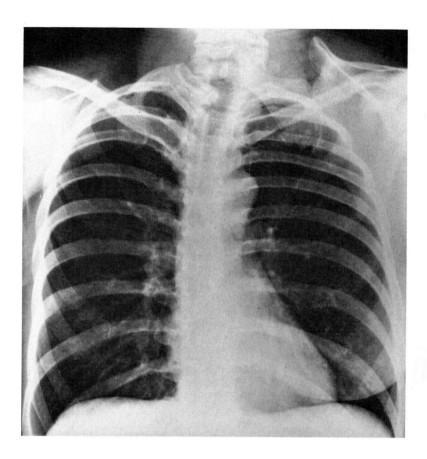

Figure 4.8.   Order of visual scan in a patient with a right radical mastectomy and a left shoulder anomaly. (See text for description.)

The lungs, costophrenic angles, pleura, and diaphragm are normal. The patient has had a right radical mastectomy as indicated by the absence of the right breast shadow and increased lucency (radiability) from the missing pectoralis muscle. A bony anomaly is present in the left shoulder: elevation of the scapula, the presence of an omovertebral bone, and a cleft vertebra at C-6. This particular type of anomaly is called Sprengel deformity."

The lateral chest film should receive the same attention as the PA film and is analyzed in a similar fashion. Consider the lateral chest film in a patient with known esophageal carcinoma (Fig. 4.9): ". . .on the lateral chest film, the trachea is deviated anteriorly by a soft tissue mass that contains an air-fluid level (*arrow*). This is most consistent with the diagnosis of an obstructing esophageal lesion. The cardiac silhouette is normal. The lungs, costophrenic angle, posterior recesses, and diaphragm are normal. There are no significant abnormalities in the spine."

An anatomic review of the structures seen in the chest under normal circumstances will now be covered in the same order as the film analysis.

The trachea is a midline structure whose air shadow stands out in bold contrast to the surrounding soft tissues of the neck and mediastinum. On a well-penetrated film, the carina (bifurcation of the trachea) may be seen at the level of the T4-5 interspace on the frontal film. On the lateral film, the tracheal air column may be seen slowly angling down from the thoracic inlet. The soft tissue line (retrotracheal line) seen on its posterior

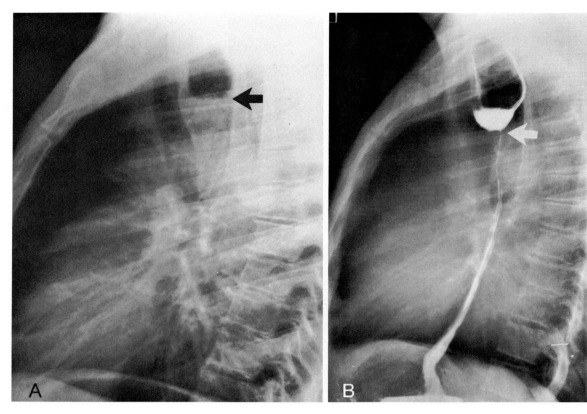

Figure 4.9.   Carcinoma of the esophagus. A, lateral chest radiograph shows an air-fluid level (*arrow*) immediately behind the trachea. There is thickening of the retrotracheal line. Compare with Figure 4.10. **B,** esophagogram shows nearly complete obstruction to the passage of barium (*arrow*).

wall should not be bowed and should not exceed 3 mm in thickness (Fig. 4.10).

The mediastinum, the extrapleural space between the lungs, is the midregion of the thorax. Contained within it are the heart, pericardium, great vessels, trachea, thoracic duct, thymus, fat, numerous small blood vessels, nerves, lymph nodes, and lymphatic vessels. Traditionally, the mediastinum has been divided into four regions—one superior and three inferior components (anterior, middle, and posterior). We may make this division by drawing a horizontal line from the sternal angle (of Louis) back to the T4-5 intervertebral disc (Fig. 4.11). In the living patient, this line cuts through the midportion of the aortic arch. Any structures above this line lie in the superior mediastinum, and any below are in the inferior mediastinum. The anatomic anterior mediastinum is bounded by the sternum anteriorly and by the pericardium posteriorly. The middle mediastinum is located between the anterior and posterior pericardium. The posterior mediastinum is bounded anteriorly by the posterior pericardium and posteriorly by the vertebral column. All three subdivisions of the anatomic inferior mediastinum are bounded inferiorly by the diaphragm.

Although this division may prove satisfactory for the anatomist, radiologists and surgeons prefer to use the *roentgen mediastinum*, a concept proposed by Felson that is far more useful in clinical practice than the ana-

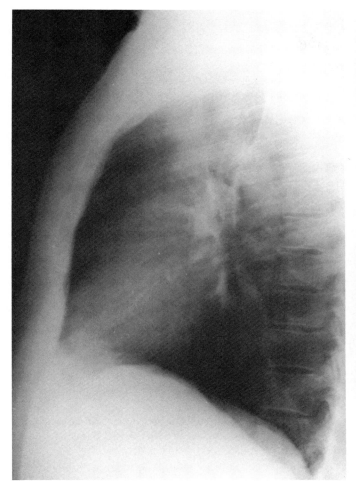

Figure 4.10. Normal Lateral chest radiograph.

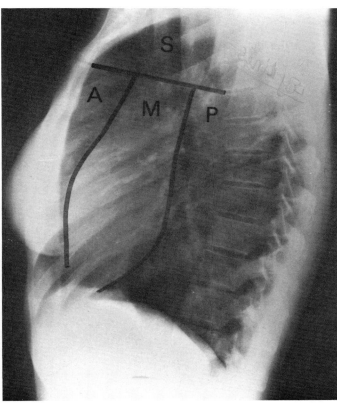

Figure 4.11. Anatomic mediastinum. Anatomically, the mediastinum is divided into anterior (*A*), middle (*M*), posterior (*P*), and superior (*S*), segments.

tomic mediastinum, especially when dealing with neoplasms, since tumors of the mediastinum tend to spread in a craniocaudal manner rather than anteroposteriorly.

To delineate the three parts of the roentgen mediastinum, the following lines may be imagined on a lateral radiograph (Fig. 4.12). Line A-A' begins at the diaphragm just behind the image of the inferior vena cava and extends upward along the back of the heart and in front of the trachea to the neck. The second line, B-B', runs across the body of each thoracic vertebra 1 cm from its anterior margin and extends upward. The area anterior to line A-A' is the anterior mediastinum; the area between lines A-A' and B-B' is the middle mediastinum; and the area posterior to line B-B' is the posterior mediastinum. Pathologic aspects of these compartments will be discussed in the following section.

The anatomy of the heart and great vessels will be described in the next chapter. It is sufficient to say at this point, however, that all lung markings seen on the normal chest radiograph are made by pulmonary ar-

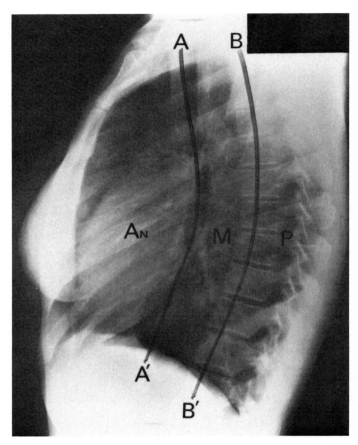

Figure 4.12. **The "roentgen mediastinum."** (See text for description.) *An,* anterior mediastinum; *M,* mediastinum; *P,* posterior mediastinum.

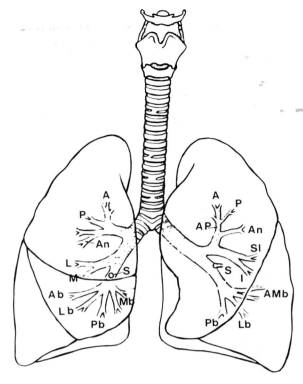

Figure 4.13. **Segmental bronchial anatomy.** Right upper lobe: *A,* apical; *P,* posterior; *An,* anterior. Right middle lobe: *L,* lateral; *M,* medial. Right lower lobe: *S,* superior; *Ab,* anterior basal; *Lb,* lateral basal; *Pb,* posterior basal; *Mb,* medial basal. Left upper lobe: *AP,* apical-posterior; *A,* apical; *P,* posterior; *Sl,* superior lingular; *I,* inferior lingular. Left lower lobe: *S,* superior; *AMb,* anterior-medial basal; *Lb,* lateral basal; *Pb,* posterior basal.

teries and veins and not by bronchi. After all, the blood-filled vessels are of water density; air-filled bronchi, which normally have thin walls, provide no significant contrast to the aerated lungs.

There are three lobes in the right lung and two in the left. Each lobe is divided into anatomic segments supplied by its own bronchus and blood vessels (Fig. 4.13). In the right upper lobe are the apical, anterior, and posterior segments; the middle lobe has medial and lateral segments. The right lower lobe contains a superior segment and, in clockwise fashion, posterior, medial, anterior, and lateral basal segments.

The left upper lobe consists of a fused apical-posterior segment, an anterior segment, and superior and inferior lingular segments. The left lower lobe is similar to the right lower lobe except that the anterior and medial basal segments are fused. A knowledge of the location of these segments is important in localizing disease. The reader is advised of the fact that there is a significant portion of lung contained in the costophrenic recess posteriorly. This recess extends as far down as the level of L-2. Occasionally, tumors occur within the lung in this location. These lesions often will not be seen on chest radiographs but may be detected on an abdominal radiograph (Fig. 4.14) or on CT.

The basic anatomic and functional pulmonary unit is the acinus, the portion of lung distal to the terminal bronchiole where gas exchange takes place. It contains respiratory bronchioles, alveolar ducts, alveolar sacs, and alveoli. Anatomically and radiographically, a consistently recognizable structure results from the grouping of three to five acini together to form the pulmonary lobule. The usual lobule is approximately 1 cm in diameter in the adult. Each of these lobules is surrounded by its own interlobular septa and interstitial structures (Fig. 4.15). Diseases that affect the

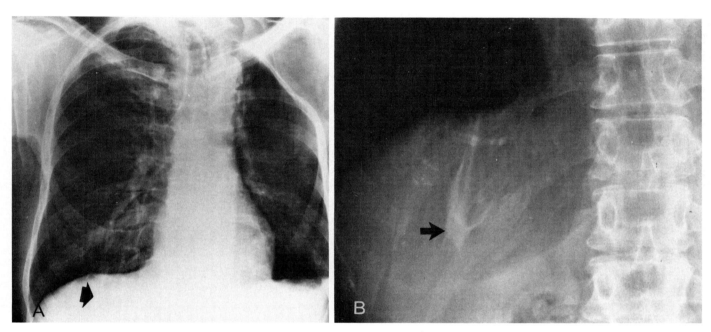

Figure 4.14. Carcinoma of the right lower lobe in an extreme basal segment. A, PA chest radiograph barely shows a lesion beneath the diaphragm on the right (*arrow*). **B,** detailed view from an abdominal radiograph shows an irregular mass (*arrow*) in an extreme basal segment of the right lower lobe.

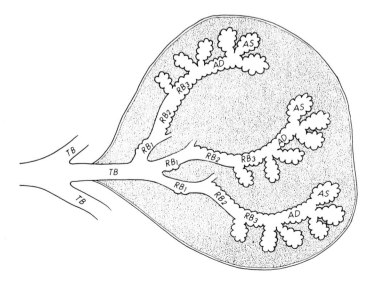

Figure 4.15. The pulmonary lobule. This consists of a terminal bronchiole (*TB*), several levels of respiratory bronchioles (*RB*), alveolar ducts (*AD*), and alveolar sacs (*AS*). Each acinus is surrounded by its own interstitial structures and interlobular septum.

Septal/KERLEY Lines =
edematous or thickened
interlobular septa.

esp. periphery.

air spaces are referred to as having an acinar- or alveolar-type pattern; diseases that affect the interstitial tissues are referred to as having an interstitial pattern.

The interlobular septa are not seen under normal circumstances. However, when they become edematous or thickened by other pathologic processes, they become visible as faint linear lines known as septal (Kerley) lines (Fig. 4.16).

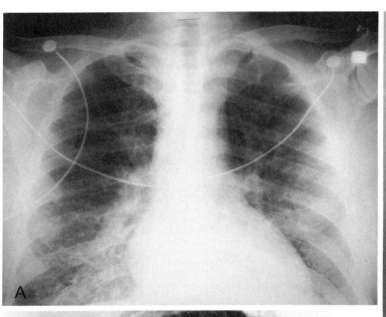

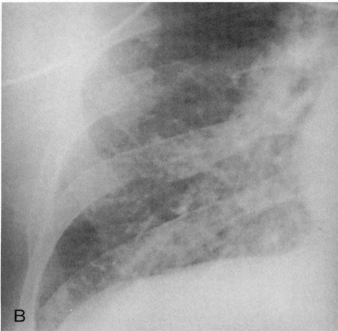

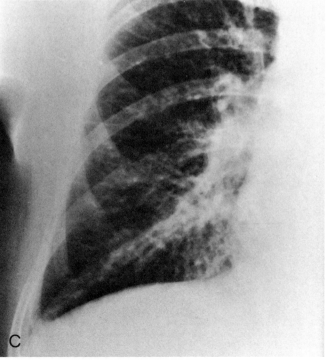

Figure 4.16. Kerley lines in a patient with congestive heart failure. A, AP radiograph shows prominent interstitial markings in both bases with a fine interlacing pattern. **B,** detailed view shows the linear horizontal "Kerley B-lines" in the periphery. **C,** detailed view of another patient shows similar findings.

There are microscopic communications between the distal portions of the bronchiolar tree and surrounding alveoli known as the canals of Lambert. They provide an accessory route for air passage from the bronchioles to the alveoli. Another connection, the pores of Kohn, are small openings in the alveolar wall 10 to 15 microns in diameter. These permit the lung distal to an obstructed bronchus or bronchiole to be ventilated by a process known as collateral air drift.

The pleura consists of two layers, the visceral pleural and the parietal pleura. The visceral pleura encases the lungs. Under normal circumstances the pleura is not visualized with the exception of the normal interlobar fissures (Fig. 4.17). On the right there are two fissures, the oblique (major) and the horizontal (minor). The left lung contains an oblique fissure only. The oblique fissure begins at the level of the fourth thoracic vertebra, extending obliquely downward and forward and ending approximately at the level of the sixth rib anteriorly. The horizontal fissure begins roughly at the level of the sixth rib laterally and extends anteriorly and slightly downward to end near the medial portion of the fourth rib. Occasionally, an accessory fissure may be seen bordering a segment of lung that has become partially or completely separated from its adjacent segments. The best known of these is the azygos fissure, which is created by the downward migration of the azygos vein through the apical pleura of the right upper lobe. In doing so, the vein invaginates a portion of pleura and results in a comma-shaped structure seen in the vicinity of the right upper lobe (Fig. 4.18). It is a normal variant.

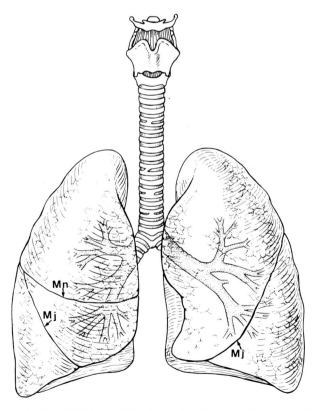

Figure 4.17.   Division of the lungs by fissures. *Mn*, minor fissure; *Mj*, major fissure.

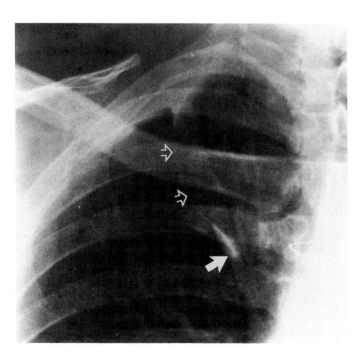

Figure 4.18.   Azygous fissure (*open arrows*) and azygous vein (*solid arrow*). This is a normal variant.

The pleura is frequently involved in inflammatory and traumatic insults to the chest. These may result in areas of thickening along the pleural surface or in the costophrenic or cardiophrenic angles. They may distort these anatomic boundaries.

The diaphragm, which separates the thoracic from the abdominal cavities, is most often seen as a smooth dome-shaped structure on either side. There may be scalloping or irregularities along the diaphragmatic surface, a frequent finding considered to be of little significance. The right hemidiaphragm is slightly higher than the left. Occasionally, gaseous distension of the stomach or colon produces elevation of the left hemidiaphragm above the right. The reason for the lower left hemidiaphragm is the contiguity of the left ventricle with it and not the mass of the liver elevating the right hemidiaphragm.

Soft tissue images commonly visible on the routine chest radiograph are the anterior axillary fold produced by the bulk of the pectoral muscles, soft tissue images along the upper surfaces of the clavicles, images of the sternocleidomastoid muscles in the neck, and breast images. In addition, nipple images are frequently seen over the lower chest radiographs in men.

Bony structures visible on the chest radiograph include the ribs, thoracic vertebrae, lower cervical vertebrae, clavicles, scapulae, and occasionally the heads of the humeri. In addition, the sternum is clearly visible on the lateral chest film. Occasionally, the manubrium projects as a prominence just to the right of the midline. It should not be mistaken for a pulmonary mass. Occasionally, cervical ribs are encountered. An abnormal-appearing rib, in the cervicothoracic region can be considered a cervical rib if the transverse process to which it is articulating points inferiorly. Cervical transverse processes point down; thoracic transverse processes point up (Fig. 4.19).

Figure 4.19. Bilateral cervical ribs (*open arrows*). The cervical transverse processes (*C*) point downward; the thoracic (*T*) point upward.

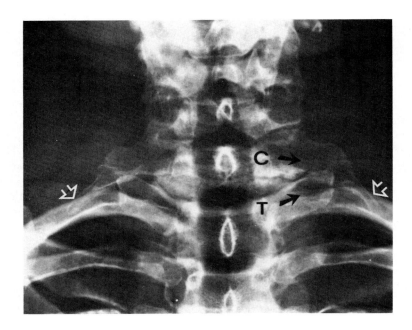

PATHOLOGIC CONSIDERATIONS

This section will discuss six basic pathologic patterns that may alter the normal appearance of the lung. The reader should be aware that any or all of these may be present at one time in the same patient. Furthermore, any of these entities may be combined with abnormalities of the heart and pulmonary vessels. The six abnormalities are as follows:

1. Air space disease—consolidation
2. Atelectasis
3. Pleural fluid
4. Masses
5. Emphysema
6. Interstitial changes

Figure 4.20 illustrates these changes.

Air Space Disease—Consolidation

When the air spaces become filled with fluid (inflammatory exudate, blood, or edema), they lose their normal lucency and become opaque. In pneumonia, the inflammatory infiltrate usually follows normal anatomic

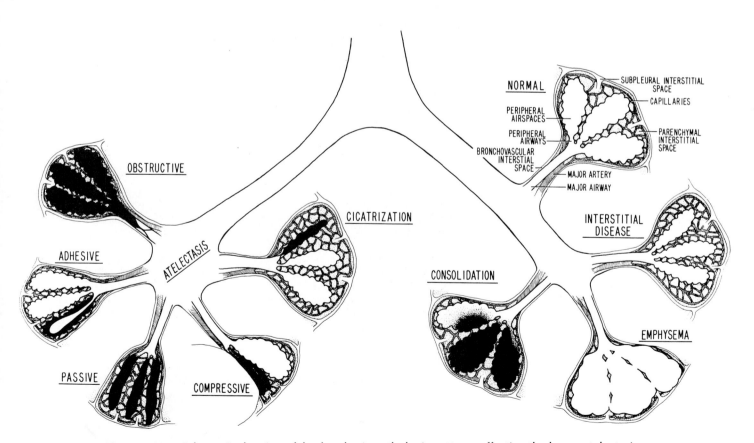

Figure 4.20.   Schematic drawing of the four basic pathologic patterns affecting the lungs, atelectasis (five variations), consolidation, emphysema, and interstitial disease.

planes and has a segmental distribution. By knowing the location of the lung segments and their relationship to the mediastinum and diaphragm, it is possible to accurately localize an area of consolidation by noting the loss of these normal anatomic landmarks.

The basis for visualization of the border of a structure depends on its contiguity with another structure of *different radiographic density.* Hence we see the *silhouette* of the mediastinal structures and the diaphragm because they are of water density and are outlined by the adjacent air density in the lung. Consolidations adjacent to these borders result in the loss of the normal-appearing images or silhouettes. This concept was first described by Fleischner and popularized by Felson as the *silhouette sign.*

Fleischner's famous experiment demonstrating the silhouette sign is illustrated as follows (Fig. 4.21). An empty film box was tilted on end; liquid paraffin was poured into it and allowed to congeal into a triangular density. A second empty film box was taped behind the first box, and both were radiographed (Fig. 4.21**A**). The gray image of the solid paraffin represents a "cardiac border," and the blackness of the air within both boxes represents "aerated lung," creating a model for demonstration of the effects of consoli-

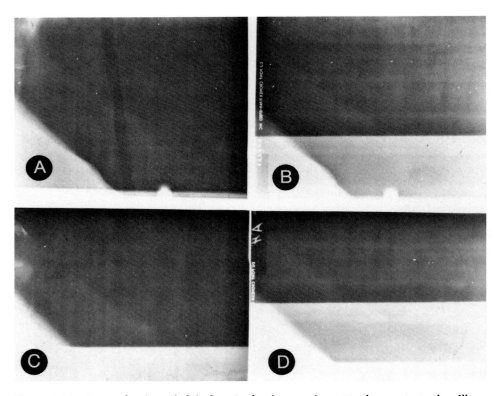

Figure 4.21.   Reproduction of Fleischner's classic experiment to demonstrate the silhouette sign. A, radiograph shows the paraffin in one box with air in the second. **B,** radiograph shows paraffin in one box with mineral oil in the second box. The border of the paraffin is still visible. **C,** radiograph shows mineral oil added to the box with paraffin. The silhouette of the lower portion of the paraffin now disappears. **D,** in radiograph mineral oil is present in both boxes. The only portion of the paraffin obscured is that covered by mineral oil sitting immediately adjacent to it.

dation on the silhouette. The boxes were again radiographed in the upright position after mineral oil (of approximately the same radiographic density as solid paraffin) was poured into the empty box behind the one containing the paraffin (Fig. 4.21**B**). Note the air-fluid level at the border between the mineral oil and the air in the second box. More importantly, the image of the "heart" is still clearly visible because of the air adjacent to its border. Thus, an area of consolidation behind the cardiac silhouette does not cause obliteration of its border.

The mineral oil was then poured out of the back box and into the box containing the paraffin. A radiograph of this (Fig. 4.21**C**) shows obliteration of a portion of the border of the "heart" image because of the contiguity of the two structures of similar radiographic density. This is analogous to pneumonia in the right middle lobe or in the lingula obliterating the cardiac border (Fig. 4.22).

Finally, mineral oil was poured into the second box, with the resultant radiograph shown in Figure 4.21**D**. Note the obliteration of the lower "cardiac" border by the "consolidated" area adjacent to it. However, the upper "cardiac" border is clearly visible along with an air-fluid level behind it because this upper border is still surrounded by air.

In summary, an intrathoracic lesion that is contiguous with the border of the heart, aorta, or diaphragm will result in the loss of that border on the radiograph. This border will not be obliterated unless the lesion is anatomically contiguous with it. These principles apply not only to the PA chest radiograph but also to the lateral view and, in addition, to certain ab-

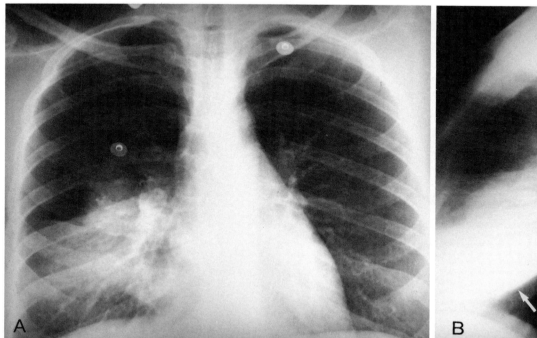
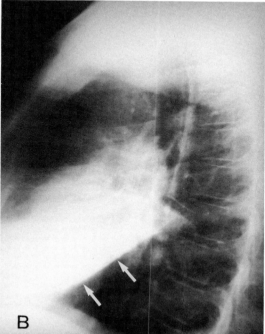

Figure 4.22.   Right middle lobe pneumonia. A, PA radiograph shows the right cardiac silhouette to be obliterated. **B,** lateral radiograph shows the consolidation to involve the middle lobe. Note the sharp definition of the major fissure (*arrows*) on the right side.

dominal radiographs that show loss of the posas margin with retroperitoneal inflammation or hemorrhage.

The following lesions are illustrated: right middle lobe consolidation (Fig. 4.22), right upper lobe consolidation (Fig. 4.23), lingular consolidation (Fig. 4.24), and left lower lobe consolidation (Fig. 4.25).

On the lateral film, we can identify each hemidiaphragm because of a normal-appearing silhouette sign. The anterior portion of the cardiac border lies in contiguity with the left hemidiaphragm. Therefore, the anterior one-third of the left diaphragmatic image is obliterated by the cardiac border. This is the most reliable way to identify the hemidiaphragms (Fig. 4.26). A summary of localization using the silhouette sign is in Table 4.1. Although the localizing signs are extremely useful, the reader is cautioned that they are not always infallible. For example, an area of consolidation in the lateral segment of the right middle lobe will not always obliterate the right cardiac border. It is therefore important to use two views at all times when evaluating patients with lung disease.

The *cervicothoracic sign,* a variant of the silhouette sign, is useful in determining whether a mass that is seen above the level of the clavicles is wholly intrathoracic or mediastinal. If this lesion is seen in its entirety, it must lie *posteriorly* because it is surrounded by air and therefore must be

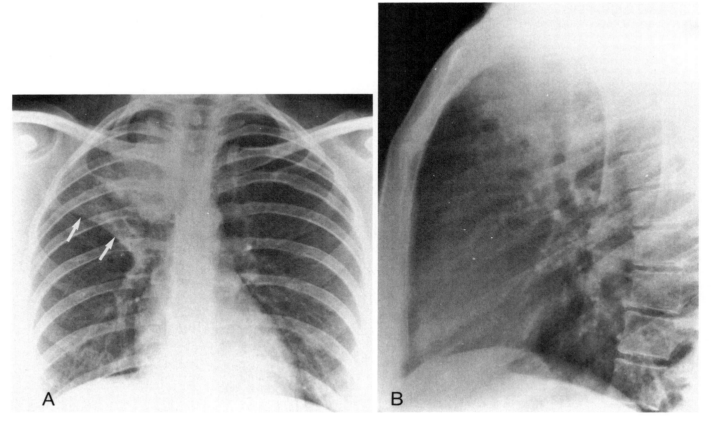

Figure 4.23. Right upper lobe consolidation and atelectasis. A, frontal radiograph shows obliteration of the superior mediastinal silhouette on the right. Volume loss is present as evidenced by elevation of the minor fissure, which is well demarcated (*arrows*). **B,** lateral radiograph shows the upper lobe consolidation.

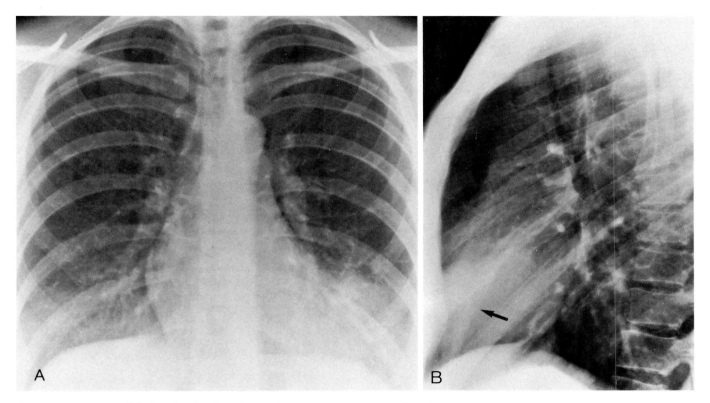

Figure 4.24. Consolidation in the lingula. A, frontal radiograph shows the silhouette of the apex of the heart to be obscured by the overlying consolidation. **B,** lateral radiograph shows the consolidation anteriorly (*arrow*).

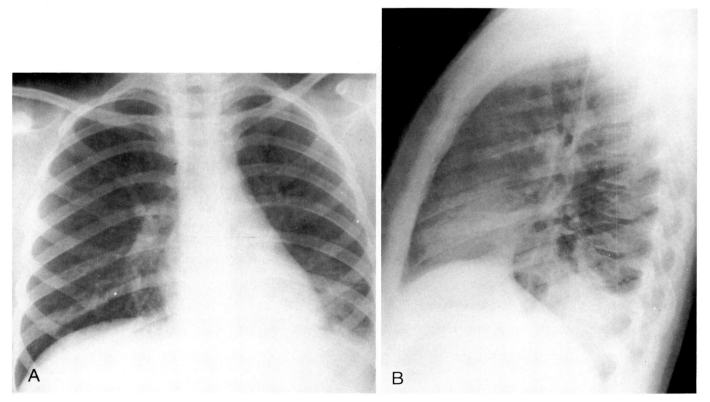

Figure 4.25. Left lower lobe pneumonia. A, frontal radiograph shows the silhouette of the diaphragm on the left to be obliterated. **B,** lateral radiograph shows the posterior consolidation.

Figure 4.26. Normal lateral radiograph showing the diaphragm. (See text for description.)

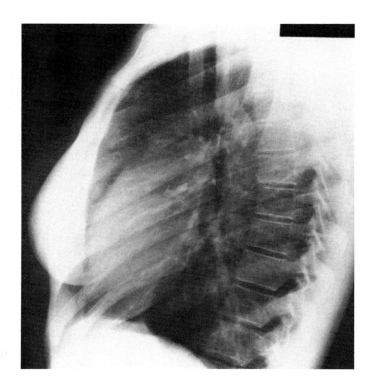

Table 4.1. Localization Using the Silhouette Sign

Structure	Obliteration/ Overlap of Border	General Location	Anatomic Location
Heart	Obliteration	Anterior	Middle lobe Lingula Anterior mediastinum Anterior segment of an upper lobe Lower end of oblique fissure Anterior portion of pleural cavity
	Overlap	Posterior	Lower lobe Posterior mediastinum Posterior portion of pleural cavity
Ascending aorta (right border)	Obliteration	Anterior	Anterior segment, right upper lobe Right middle lobe Right anterior mediastinum Anterior portion, right pleural cavity
	Overlap	Posterior	Superior segment, right lower lobe Posterior segment, right upper lobe Posterior mediastinum Posterior pleural cavity
Aortic knob (left border)	Obliteration	Posterior	Apical-posterior segment, left upper lobe Posterior mediastinum Posterior pleural cavity
	Overlap	Anterior	Anterior segment, left upper lobe Far posterior portion mediastinum or pleural cavity
Descending aorta	Obliteration	Posterior	Superior and posterior basal segments, left lower lobe

entirely within the thorax. If it is located *anteriorly*, its border will be obliterated by the images of the neck structures. Therefore, it is cervicothoracic, lying partially in the anterior part of the mediastinum and partially in the neck. Figure 4.27 illustrates this in a patient with a prominent brachiocephalic artery, the most common cause of this finding.

Another useful sign to indicate consolidation within the lung is the *air bronchogram*. As previously mentioned, normal bronchi are not visible on the chest radiograph. This is because of their thin walls, the fact that they contain air, and the fact that they are surrounded by air within the lung parenchyma. However, parenchymal consolidation that results in a water density in the alveolar spaces in the lung may cause the demonstration of adjacent bronchi, since the air within their lumens will stand out in stark contrast to the dense lung (Fig. 4.28). The formation of the air bronchogram sign is illustrated in Figure 4.29. Plastic tubing sealed at each end was placed in an empty plastic container and radiographed (Fig. 4.29**A**). The walls are barely discernible, since the tubing contains air and there is air surrounding it. Water was then added to the container to cover the tubing (Fig. 4.29**B**). The wall is barely visible. However, the air within the tubing defines its lumen (air bronchogram). Water was then poured into the tubing with the resultant radiographic appearance shown in Figure 4.29**C**.

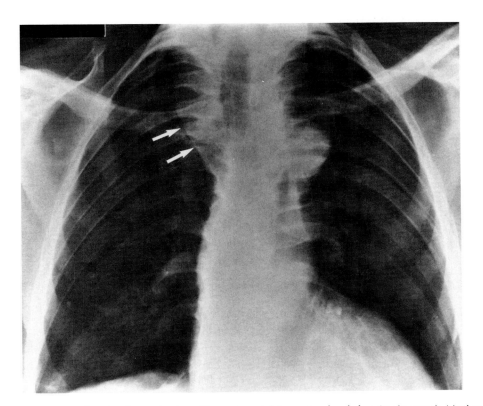

Figure 4.27. Cervicothoracic sign. There is a right paratracheal density (*arrows*). Notice that the image of this density disappears as it crosses the clavicle. This indicates that the structure in question is anteriorly placed and has entered the neck. This is, in fact, the right brachiocephalic artery, which is tortuous in this elderly patient. If this structure were posteriorly located, it would be seen in its entirety above as well as below the clavicle.

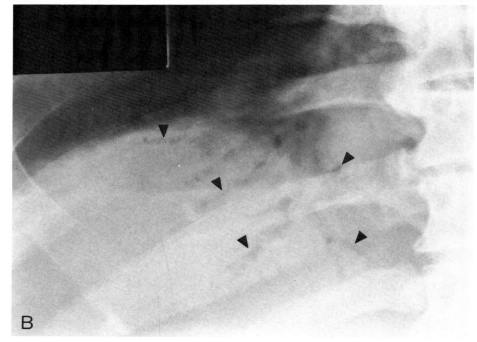

Figure 4.28. Air bronchograms. A, air bronchograms in the right lung (*arrowheads*) in an infant with hyaline membrane disease. **B,** detailed view of the right lower lobe in a patient with pneumonia shows multiple air bronchograms (*arrowheads*).

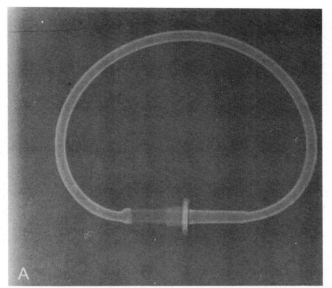

Figure 4.29.   Air bonchogram formation. A, radiograph of a plastic tube shows its walls. **B,** when the tube is submerged in water, the lumen and walls are still visible. This is what would be seen in an air bronchogram. **C,** when water fills the tubing, the lumen is obscured.

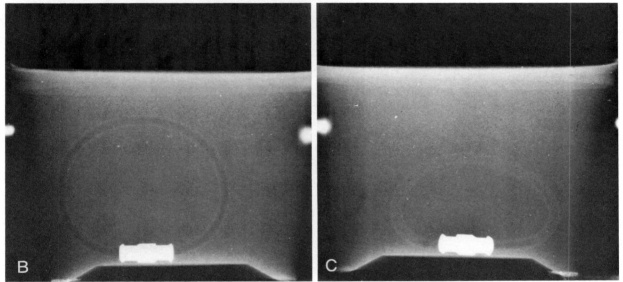

In this illustration there is no difference between the contrast medium inside the tube and the outside (no air bronchogram).

The air bronchogram is a valuable sign that, when present, is virtually diagnostic of air-space (acinar) disease. A pleural or mediastinal lesion may be excluded because there are no bronchi traversing these lesions. Similarly, a mass in the lung would engulf, occlude, or displace bronchi, and therefore the air bronchogram would not occur. If an air bronchogram is seen within a round pulmonary density, the lesion is most likely an inflammatory process, an infarct, a contusion, or, more rarely, an alveolar cell carcinoma or lymphoma. All of these are acinar lesions. Rare exceptions to this rule are bronchiectasis and chronic bronchitis, in which thickening of the bronchial walls may result in tubular air profiles (Fig. 4.30).

Figure 4.30. Thickened bronchial walls produce a tubular pattern in a patient with bronchiectasis.

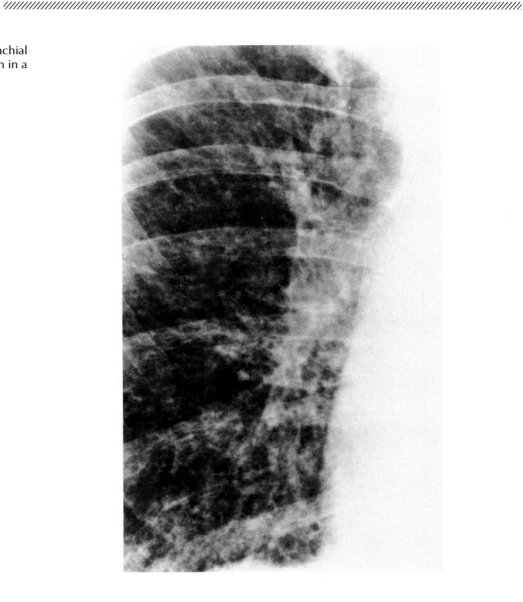

Atelectasis

Atelectasis is a condition of volume loss of some portion of the lung. It may be massive, with complete collapse of an entire lung or, more commonly, less extensive and involve a lobe, segment, or subsegment. Atelectasis results from a number of causes, which are illustrated in Figure 4.20.

Obstructive atelectasis, the most common type, results when a bronchus is obstructed by a neoplasm, foreign body, mucous plug, or inflammatory debris (Fig. 4.31). Quite often, there is associated pneumonia distal to the site of obstruction.

Compressive atelectasis is a purely physical phenomenon in which lung is compressed by a tumor, emphysematous bulla, pleural effusion, or enlarged heart (Fig. 4.32).

Cicatrization atelectasis is produced by organizing scar tissue (Fig. 4.33). This occurs most often in healing tuberculosis and other granu-

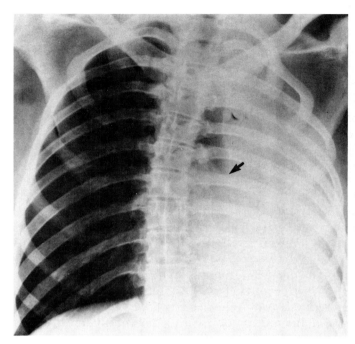

Figure 4.31. Obstructive atelectasis on the left. There is complete collapse of the left lung due to a central obstructing lesion in the left mainstem bronchus (*arrow*). The heart and mediastinum have shifted to the left.

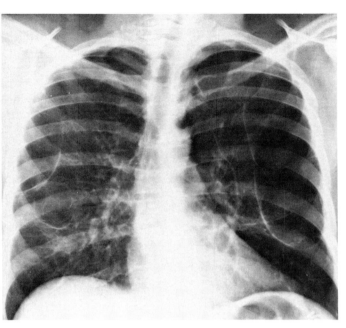

Figure 4.32. Compressive atelectasis with bullous emphysema. The large bullae in each lung compress the remaining lung markings.

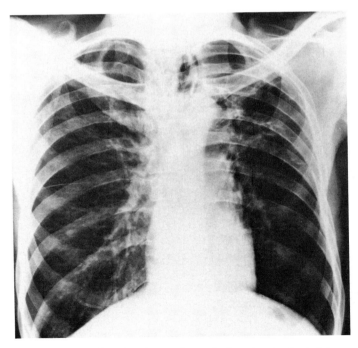

Figure 4.33. Cicatrization atelectasis. Scarring in the left lung has produced atelectatic changes in the left upper lobe. Note the hyperinflation of the lower lobe.

lomatous diseases, as well as in entities such as pulmonary infarct and pulmonary trauma.

Adhesive atelectasis is a unique type of volume loss that occurs in the presence of patent airways. The mechanism involved is believed to be the inactivation of surfactant. A common example of this is hyaline membrane disease.

Passive atelectasis results from the normal compliance of the lung in the presence of either pneumothorax or hydrothorax. The airways remain patent (Fig. 4.34).

The radiographic signs of lobar and segmental collapse are of two types: *direct* and *indirect.* Of the direct signs, displacement or deviation of a fissure is the most reliable, indicating compensatory hyperinflation in an adjacent lobe to take the place of some of the collapsed lung. Other direct signs of collapse are increased opacity, crowding of vessels, and the presence of a silhouette sign. In any patient, one or all of these signs may be present (Fig. 4.35).

Of the indirect signs the most reliable is displacement of the hilar vessels, which shift in the direction of the collapse. Other indirect signs include a shift of the mediastinum, elevation of the hemidiaphragm, compensatory emphysema, herniation of the lung across the midline, and approximation of the ribs. This last sign generally indicates that the collapse has been long-standing. As with the direct signs, any or all of these may occur in a particular patient.

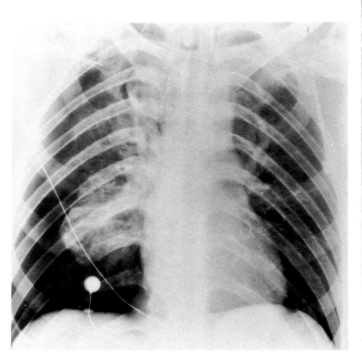

Figure 4.34. **Passive atelectasis.** There is collapse of the right lung in a patient with large pneumothorax on the right.

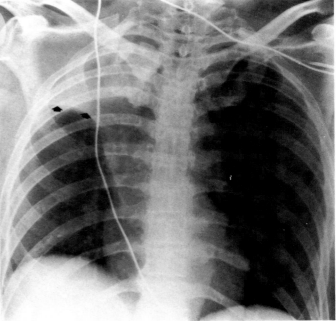

Figure 4.35. **Right upper lobe collapse in a patient with a central lung carcinoma.** There is consolidation in the atelectatic right upper lobe. The minor fissure is elevated (*arrows*). There is a mass in the right hilar region. The mediastinum is shifted to the right.

In general, the upper lobes collapse medially, upward, and anteriorly. On the right side, the most reliable signs are an increase in density with obliteration of the upper mediastinal images on the right and shift of the minor fissure obliquely upward (Fig. 4.35). On the left, the most reliable sign is the presence of increased density near the midline, with preservation of the aortic knob. In both instances the diaphragm is usually elevated. On the lateral view, the major fissure is displaced anteriorly and superiorly (Fig. 4.36).

The right middle lobe and lingula collapse downward and medially, producing haziness adjacent to the cardiac border on the frontal film. A lordotic view orients the atelectatic segment of lung more perpendicular to the direction of the x-ray beam and allows better visualization. On the lateral film, a triangular-shaped density is seen overlying the cardiac silhouette (Fig. 4.37).

The lower lobes collapse posteriorly, medially, and downward. On a frontal radiograph, the classic lower lobe collapse is a triangular-shaped density behind the cardiac shadow. On the lateral film, a fissure shift may

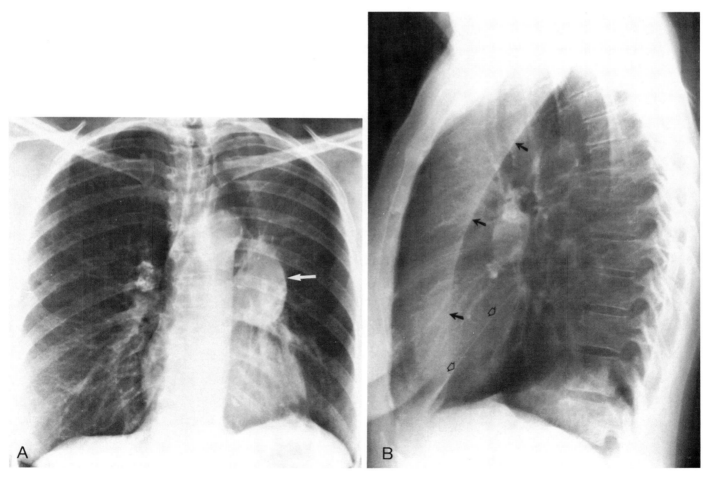

Figure 4.36. Left upper lobe collapse in a patient with a central carcinoma. A, frontal radiograph shows a mass in the left hilar region (*arrow*). Note the shift of the left-sided pulmonary vessels upward. **B,** lateral radiograph shows anterior bowing of the major fissure on the left (*solid arrows*). The normal right-sided major fissure is also shown (*open arrows*).

Figure 4.37. Lingular collapse. A, frontal radiograph shows obliteration of the silhouette of the apex of the heart. **B,** lateral radiograph shows consolidation in the lingula. The major fissure on the left is sharply defined and bowed slightly anteriorly (*arrows*).

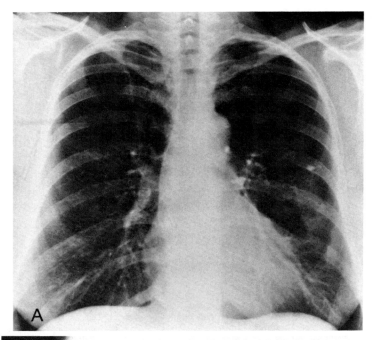

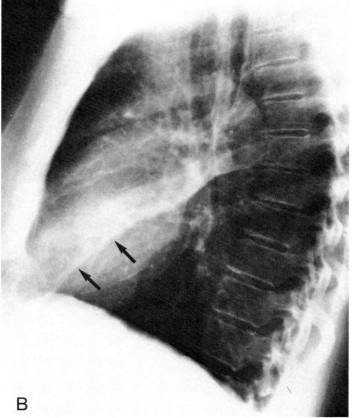

also be appreciated. In total collapse, a wedge-shaped density occurs posteriorly and inferiorly, extending down to the diaphragm (Fig. 4.38). In some instances, lower lobe collapse is difficult to detect on the frontal radiograph. Oblique films are quite useful in making this diagnosis. Because of the orientation of the bronchi, left lower lobe atelectasis is most common.

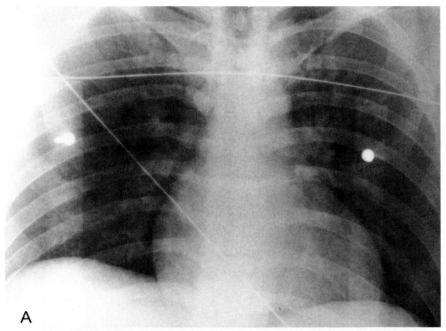

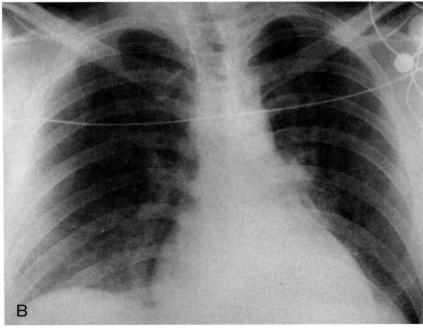

Figure 4.38. Left lower lobe atelectasis. A, admission radiograph shows both lungs expanded and clear. Note the images of both sides of the diaphragm. **B,** 2 days later, the patient has experienced left lower lobe atelectasis. There is increased density behind the heart on the left. The left hemidiaphragm is no longer visible and there is a shift of the hilar vessels downward. Compare with **A.**

Pleural Fluid Accumulation

Pleural effusion is a sign rather than a disease and occurs in a variety of pathologic conditions, including infection, embolism, neoplasm, congestive heart failure, and trauma. Pleural fluid may be either free or loculated within the pleural space. Free pleural fluid occupies the most dependent portion of the pleural cavity and may be demonstrated on the decubitus film (Fig. 4.39**B**). It also can be seen as a meniscus and elevation of the "diaphragm" on an upright film (Fig. 4.39**A**) or as an increase in the overall opacity of one hemithorax on a recumbent film.

Loculation of pleural fluid occurs when fibrous adhesions form. Occasionally, the fluid will collect in a fissure to form a "pseudotumor" or "phantom tumor" (Fig. 4.40). This usually occurs in patients with congestive heart failure and clears with resolution of that condition. A pseudotumor may be recognized by its tapered margins at a fissure.

Other signs of pleural effusion include widening of the pleural space, blunting of the costophrenic angle, and mediastinal shift in massive effusion. It is estimated that up to 300 ml of pleural fluid may be accumulated in the costophrenic sulcus posteriorly before an effusion is apparent on the frontal radiograph.

Patients with unexplained pleural effusion should be carefully studied for neoplasm. In addition to cytologic studies of the fluid itself, it is desirous to clear those portions of the lung that would be obscured by the fluid. To do this, a decubitus or Trendelenberg's position (head down) is used to make the fluid flow away from the lung bases. A more useful, but much more expensive technique, however, is to employ CT, in which the fluid will layer in the horizontal position (Fig. 4.41).

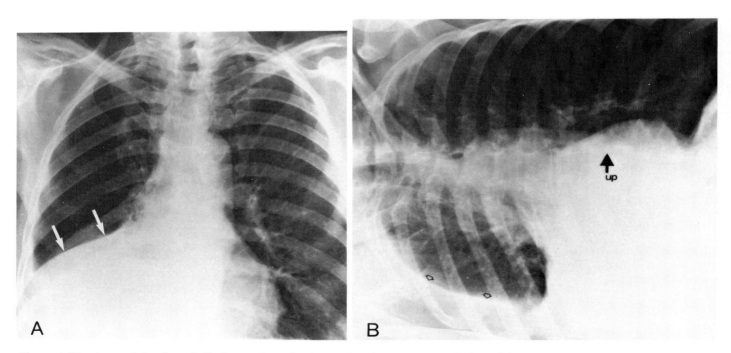

A

B

Figure 4.39. Large right pleural effusion. A, frontal radiograph shows a subpulmonic collection of fluid with a straight border (*arrows*). **B,** a right lateral decubitus film shows most of the fluid layers out (*open arrows*).

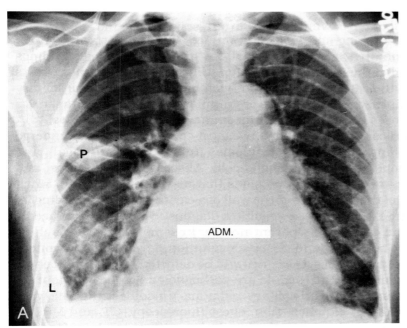

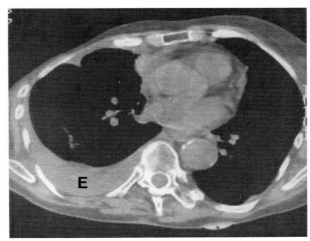

Figure 4.41. Right-sided pleural effusion (*E*) as demonstrated on a CT scan.

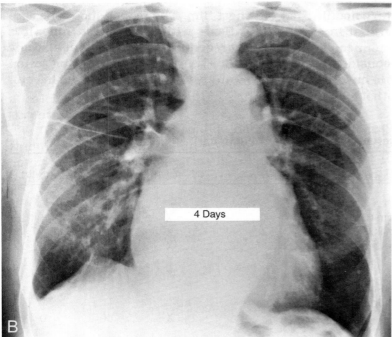

Figure 4.40. Pseudotumor caused by pleural effusion. A, radiograph taken on admission (*ADM*) shows a mass-like collection of fluid along the minor fissure (*P*). There is loculated fluid (*L*) in the right costophrenic angle in this patient with congestive heart failure. **B,** radiograph made 4 days later shows a decrease in the cardiac size. The pleural effusion is also diminished. The pseudotumor is no longer present.

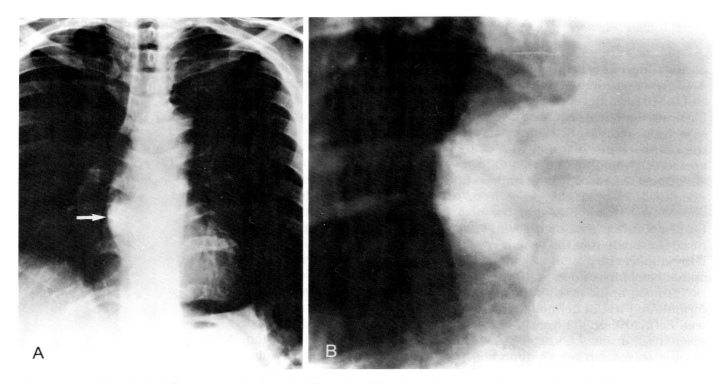

Figure 4.43.   Use of chest fluoroscopy. A, frontal radiograph shows a "mass" behind the heart (*arrow*). **B,** fluorscopic spot film shows the mass to be osteophytes bridging two thoracic vertebrae.

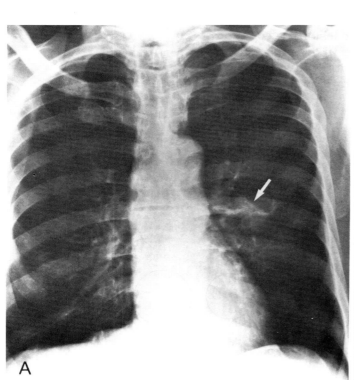

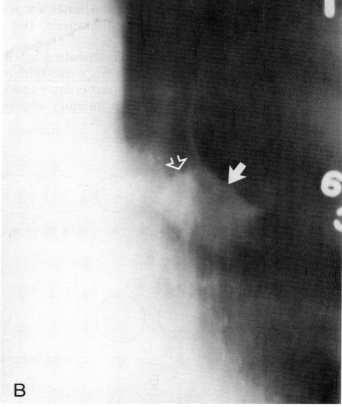

Figure 4.44.   Irregular margin in a lung carcinoma. A, frontal radiograph shows a mass adjacent to the left hilum (*arrow*). **B,** tomogram further defines the mass. There are smooth margins (*solid arrow*) and spiculated margins (*open arrow*), indicating invasion.

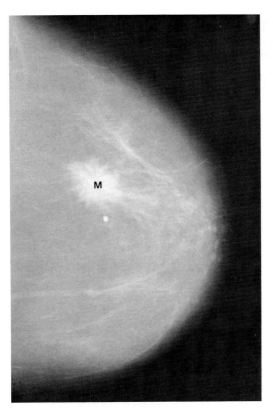

Figure 4.45. Carcinoma of the breast (*M*) showing irregular spiculated margins. Spiculation indicates invasion. Note the similarity to Figure 4.44**B.**

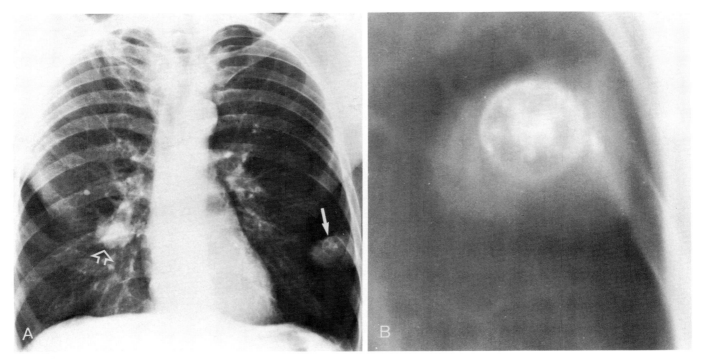

Figure 4.46. Calcification in a lung lesion. A, frontal radiograph shows bilateral lung masses. The mass on the right (*open arrow*) contains no calcification. There is calcification on the left (*solid arrow*). **B,** tomogram of the left-sided mass shows the calcification. This lesion was a granuloma that was later engulfed by a carcinoma.

appear as masses. The demonstration of these vessels supports the diagnosis. Tomography is being replaced, for the most part, by CT.

Computed tomography is most useful in evaluating patients with pulmonary and mediastinal masses (Fig. 4.47). The information gained includes evidence of mediastinal invasion, chest wall invasion, and presence of peripheral nodules. Contrast-enhanced or dynamic CT may be used to differentiate hilar masses from dilated or enlarged pulmonary vessels. The latter will enhance with contrast, while a tumor will not. Computed tomography is also useful for detecting multiple metastases and is also the mainstay for guided percutaneous biopsy (Fig. 4.48).

As previously mentioned, MR imaging of the chest is useful for evaluating suspected mediastinal masses (Fig. 4.7). The flow void easily allows vessels to be distinguished from neoplasm.

Figure 4.47. Lung carcinoma, right upper lobe. A, frontal radiograph shows a mass (*arrow*) just above the right hilum. The mass does not obscure the image of the ascending aorta (*arrowheads*), indicating a location either anterior or posterior to that structure. **B,** CT section shows the mass to be located in the anterior segment of the right upper lobe (*arrow*) adjacent to the pleura.

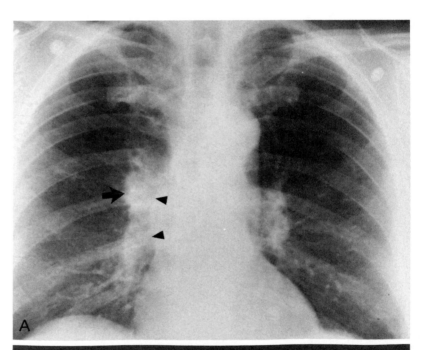

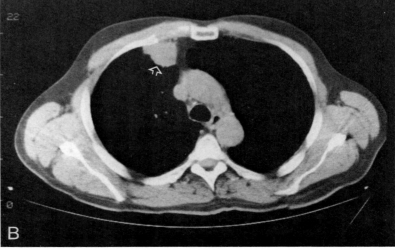

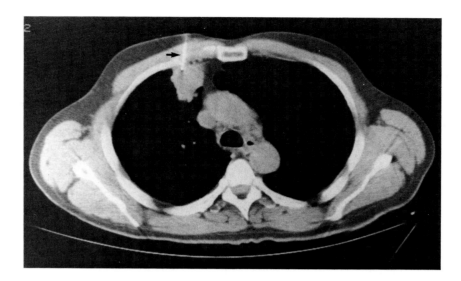

Figure 4.48. Use of CT guidance for biopsy of a lung mass. (This is the same patient as in Fig. 4.47). A needle (*arrow*) has been placed into the mass.

Patients with solitary pulmonary nodules are often submitted to a battery of diagnostic studies, including upper GI, barium enema, intravenous urography, abdominal CT, and metastatic bone surveys. These are performed before histologic confirmation of the lesion in the hope that a primary lesion will be found, thus indicating that the pulmonary lesion is metastatic. The yield from this process is extremely low and results in longer hospitalization and more expense to the patient. The final diagnosis rests on tissue examination. It is now routine to do a biopsy of these lesions percutaneously or transbronchially under fluoroscopic or CT control (Fig. 4.48). If either of these studies fails to provide an adequate answer, thoracotomy with excision of the lesion in toto is the next step.

Mediastinal masses are sometimes difficult to separate from pulmonary parenchymal masses. However, most show extraparenchymal signs such as sharp margins, tapered borders, and convexity toward the lung. The majority of all primary mediastinal masses occur in the anterior compartment, one-third occur in the middle compartment, and the remainder occur in the posterior compartment. Most patients with mediastinal masses are asymptomatic. Table 4.3 lists abnormalities found in each compartment of the "roentgen" mediastinum.

The most common lesions of the anterior mediastinum are lymphomas (Fig. 4.49), thymic lesions (Fig. 4.50), and teratomas. Other anterior lesions that may be seen include foramen of Morgagni hernias (Fig. 4.51) and pericardial cysts (Fig. 4.52).

The majority of masses arising in the middle mediastinum are lymph nodes representing lymphoma, metastatic disease, sarcoidosis (Fig. 4.53), or response to infection.

The most likely cause of a posterior mediastinal mass is a neurogenic tumor (Fig. 4.54). These generally appear as a paraspinous mass and are often associated with changes in the vertebrae or of the posterior ribs. Neurofibromas frequently enlarge the neural foramina. Calcification may occur in neuroblastomas in children.

Bronchogenic carcinoma may appear as a mediastinal mass in *any* compartment. This should always be considered in any adult with a mediastinal mass.

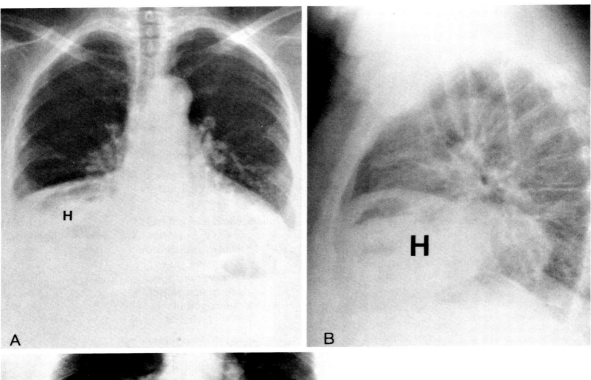

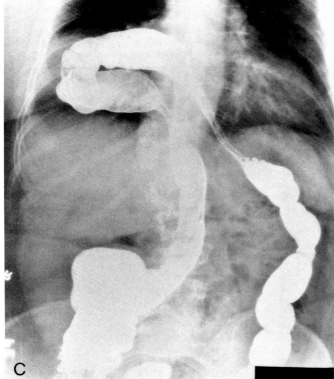

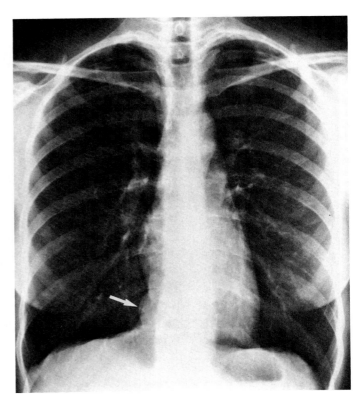

Figure 4.51.   Foramen of Morgagni hernia. A, frontal radiograph shows apparent consolidation in the right lower lobe containing gaseous shadows. This is the hernia sac (*H*). **B,** lateral radiograph shows the gas-containing hernia (*H*). **C,** barium enema shows the herniated colon in the right hemithorax.

Figure 4.52.   Pericardial cyst (*arrow*).

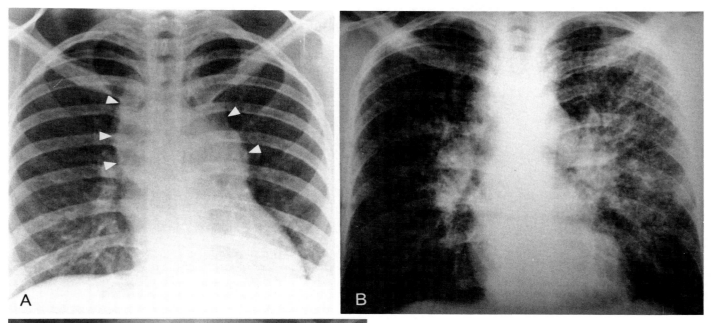

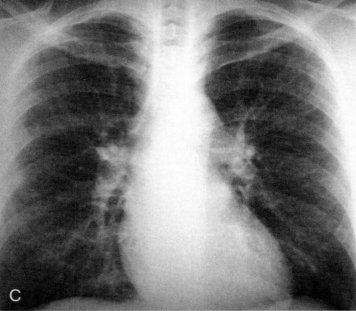

Figure 4.53. Sarcoidosis. A, nodal pattern. There are "too many bumps" (*arrowheads*). **B,** mixed parenchymal and nodal pattern in another patient. Note the enlargement of mediastinal and hilar lymph nodes as well as diffuse interstitial disease, particularly on the left. **C,** the same patient 2 months after treatment. The nodes are smaller and the peripheral lungs are normal.

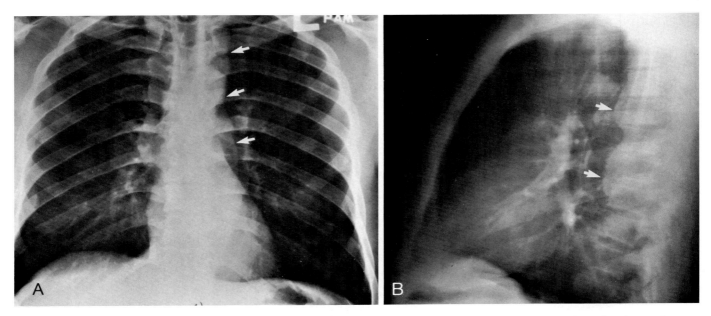

Figure 4.54. Posterior mediastinal widening in a patient with neurofibromatosis. A, frontal radiograph shows lobulation in the left paraspinal region (*arrows*). **B,** lateral radiograph confirms the posterior location of the masses (*arrows*).

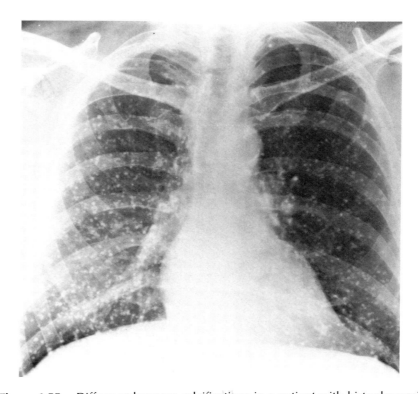

Figure 4.55. Diffuse pulmonary calcifications in a patient with histoplasmosis.

Multiple pulmonary nodules may be granulomas or metastases. If the lesions contain calcium and are widely disseminated (Fig. 4.55), the diagnosis is most likely a granulomatous disease. Multiple large nodules, particularly of varying sizes and with fuzzy borders (Fig. 4.56) usually are metastases. Metastases may also occur in a "lymphangitic" form, resulting in a prominent interstitial pattern (Fig. 4.57).

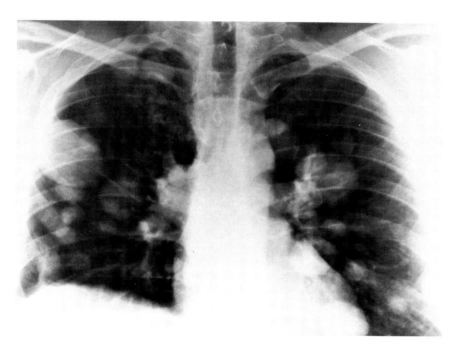

Figure 4.56. Multiple metastases.

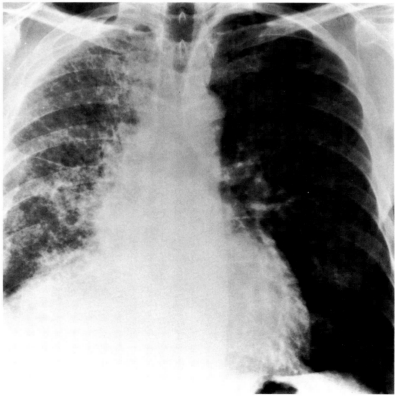

Figure 4.57. Lymphangitic spread of carcinoma. There is enlargement of the right hilum and a prominent interstitial pattern on the right that indicates lymphedema and lymphangitic spread of tumor.

Emphysema

One does not need a chest radiograph to make a diagnosis of emphysema. There are adequate physical findings for that. However, there are certain radiographic findings that corroborate those of the physical examination. A better use of the chest film in the emphysematous patient is to detect localized bullae, peribronchial infiltrates, and pneumothorax or pneumomediastinum.

The radiographic findings of classic emphysema reflect the overinflation, loss of compliance, and parenchymal destruction that denote the pathophysiology of the disease. The most reliable radiographic sign is decreased vascularity. Other signs are hyperlucency; increased retrosternal clear space; increased lung volume; depression, flattening, or reversal of the curvature of the diaphragm; decreased diaphragmatic excursion; presence of prominent central pulmonary arteries with rapid tapering ("marker") vessels; bowing of the sharply defined trachea ("saber trachea"); and vertical cardiac configuration. Bullae may be present to a greater or lesser extent (Fig. 4.58).

Patients with chronic pulmonary disease may not have all the classic findings of emphysema. Some may have prominent interstitial markings, the so-called "dirty lung" seen particularly in smokers. In some younger individuals, the only finding may be hyperlucency, representing early overinflation. Emphysematous changes are often combined with other abnormalities.

Figure 4.58. Bullous emphysema. Note the large bilateral blebs.

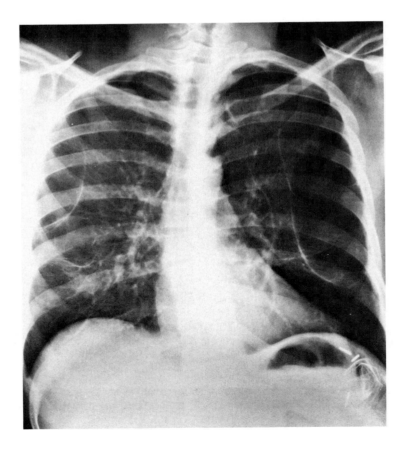

Interstitial and Acinar Disease

Diseases that primarily involve the interlobular connective tissue with or without secondary involvement of the air spaces are called interstitial diseases. They constitute a group of diseases that have recognizable radiographic patterns: linear, nodular, combined lineonodular, and reticular (web-like, "honeycombing"). The etiologies vary and include early congestive heart failure (edema), pneumoconiosis, collagen disease (fibrosis), metastatic neoplastic (lymphangitic) permeation, and primary inflammatory conditions (early viral pneumonia, interstitial pneumonia). Many of these diseases produce some degree of air space or acinar pattern as they progress.

Pure acinar lesions produce a pattern characterized by fluffy margins, coalescence, a segmental or lobar distribution, a butterfly shadow (radiating out from the hila), air bronchograms, and a rapid sequence of onset and clearing. Conditions that produce acinar patterns include acute alveolar edema (pneumonia, congestive heart failure with pulmonary edema, toxic or chemical reaction), bleeding (idiopathic pulmonary hemorrhage), aspiration of any fluid, and alveolar cell carcinoma. A rare condition that produces this pattern is alveolar proteinosis.

It is possible to differentiate many of the more common acinar diseases on the basis of pattern, distribution, and resolution. Pulmonary edema is one of the most common acinar diseases encountered. The causes include congestive heart failure, fluid overload (iatrogenic), narcotic poisoning, central nervous system depression, aspiration, inhalation of noxious gases, uremia, pulmonary thromboembolism, and trauma. Pulmonary edema in the presence of cardiac enlargement is usually of cardiac origin. Edema in the presence of a normal heart is generally due to some other cause. Upper lobe distribution occurs more with neurologic abnormalities. The pattern often changes on a daily basis. In more severe cases, usually of cardiac origin, interstitial edema may also be present.

Pneumonia, on the other hand, may involve any lobe, an entire lung, or be unilateral or bilateral. There are few distinguishing features of the acute bacterial pneumonias. However, those due to an unusual organism tend to produce a more widespread acinar pattern. *Klebsiella* often produces bulging of a fissure away from the consolidated lobe; *Staphylococcus aureus* may produce multiple cavities and pneumatoceles. Pneumonic consolidations, as a rule, clear by slowly fading. The acinar consolidation often remains visible on the chest radiograph after the patient has become clinically better. You should be careful to treat your patient and not the radiograph.

Other acinar processes have the same appearance as pneumonia or pulmonary edema. The pattern and timing of the clearing often may provide clues to their etiology. Consolidation from a lung infarct clears slowly with a gradual reduction in size of the lesion, keeping the same basic shape ("melting ice cube" pattern). Lung contusions from trauma generally clear within 24 to 48 hours. Persistent consolidation (with or without interstitial disease) in these patients may mean the onset of adult respiratory distress syndrome.

Pure acinar disease may frequently be distinguished from pure interstitial disease by pattern recognition. For demonstration purposes, consider the lung to be analogous to a piece of chicken wire, where the wire hexagons represent the interstitial tissues and the spaces represent the air spaces. Under normal circumstances, there is a uniform black background with thin interlacing strands of gray (Fig. 4.59**A**). In acinar disease, the air spaces are filled in. Unless there is total consolidation of a lobe or a lung, an alveolar process will appear as *white dots* (representing the so-called acinar shadows) *on a black background* of aerated lung (Fig. 4.59**B**). If, however, the disease is primarily interstitial, there is thickening of the borders around the acini and the resulting pattern is that of *black dots* (representing aerated acini) *surrounded by a white background* of the thickened interstitial tissue (Fig. 4.59**C**). Combined airway and interstitial disease produce a combined pattern. The following outline lists some of the more common interstitial diseases:

PRIMARY PULMONARY INTERSTITIAL DISEASES

    I. Infectious disorders
        A. Tuberculosis
        B. Histoplasmosis
        C. Coccidioidomycosis
   II. Inhalated disorders
        A. Inorganic dust
           1. Silicosis
           2. Asbestosis

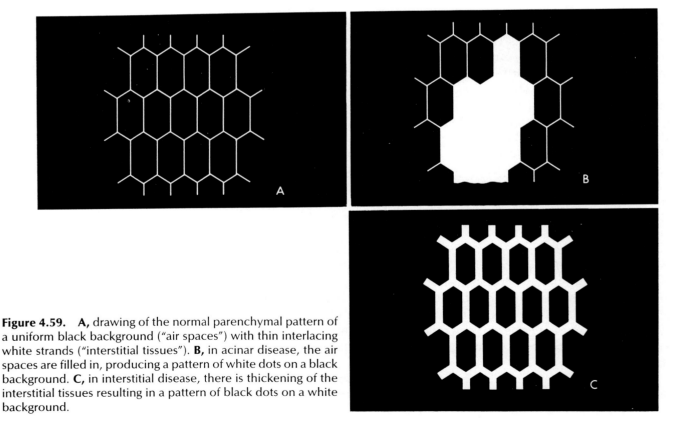

Figure 4.59. **A,** drawing of the normal parenchymal pattern of a uniform black background ("air spaces") with thin interlacing white strands ("interstitial tissues"). **B,** in acinar disease, the air spaces are filled in, producing a pattern of white dots on a black background. **C,** in interstitial disease, there is thickening of the interstitial tissues resulting in a pattern of black dots on a white background.

3. Pneumoconiosis (mixed dust)
4. Siderosis
5. Other inorganic dust diseases
B. Organic dust
   1. Farmer's lung
   2. Mushroom worker's disease
   3. Bagassosis
   4. Other organic dust diseases
III. Miscellaneous
   A. Sarcoidosis
   B. Drug-induced disease
   C. Rheumatoid arthritis
   D. Scleroderma
   E. Hemosiderosis
   F. Chronic thromboembolism
   G. Histiocytosis
   H. Desquamative interstitial pneumonia
   I. Idiopathic interstitial fibrosis (Hamman-Rich's syndrome)

Quite often the presence of ancillary radiologic and clinical findings will be needed to make the correct diagnosis. A good clinical history is also essential, especially if we are entertaining a diagnosis of pneumoconiosis or other industrial exposure. Figures 4.60 through 4.62 show representative examples of pure interstitial disease.

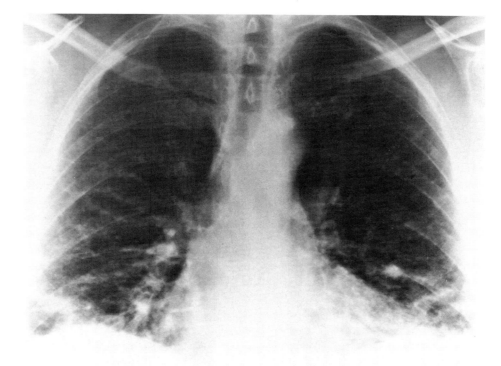

Figure 4.60. Silicosis. There is prominence of the interstitial markings, worse in the lung bases.

Figure 4.61. Diffuse interstitial disease in a chronic smoker. Note the prominent interstitial markings. This is the so-called "dirty lungs" pattern.

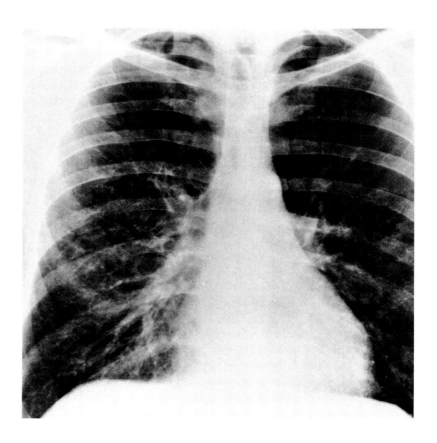

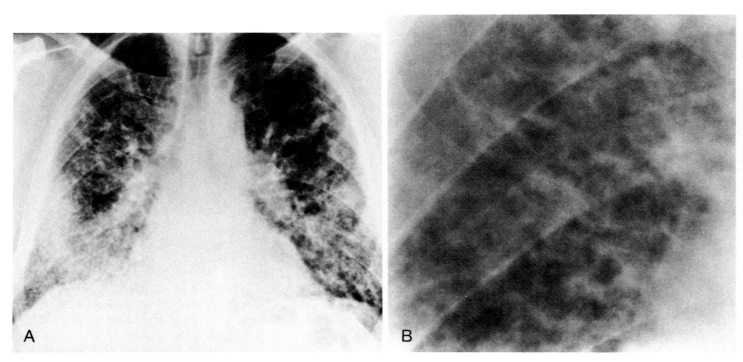

Figure 4.62. Pulmonary fibrosis in "honeycombing." A, frontal radiograph shows extensive interstitial disease with confluent margins (massive pulmonary fibrosis). **B,** detailed view shows the honeycombing pattern.

Pneumothorax

Pneumothorax may result from a variety of causes, including trauma (laceration by fractured rib, stab, or bullet wound) and iatrogenic factors (following thoracentesis, lung biopsy, or placement of subclavian catheter) or may occur spontaneously. The most common radiographic findings are absence of pulmonary vessels extending to the chest wall, a visible pleural line displaced from the chest wall, and increased lucency of one hemithorax. If the patient has a tension-type pneumothorax, air continuously enters the pleural space and builds up pressure, which compresses the mediastinum toward the opposite lung. This may result in severe respiratory distress unless immediately recognized. The most common sign of tension pneumothorax is a shift of the mediastinum away from the abnormal side (Fig. 4.63). This is a true emergency and requires immediate tube decompression. An ancillary sign in tension pneumothorax is depression of the affected hemidiaphragm. A pneumothorax may be enhanced by an expiratory film (Fig. 4.5).

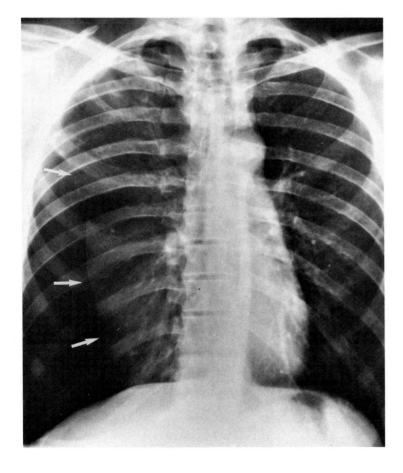

Figure 4.63. Tension pneumothorax. There is displacement of the lung (*arrows*) toward the left.

Pulmonary Embolus

It is estimated that pulmonary embolus is the most common abnormality found in hospitalized patients who die and are examined by autopsy. Fortunately, in most cases, embolism occurs without infarction because of the double blood supply to the lung. Pulmonary emboli are most likely to occur in severely ill patients who are bedridden, in those with venous disease, and in those with chronic congestive heart failure.

Interestingly, there may be few radiographic findings of pulmonary embolus in any particular patient. Clinicians and radiologists should have a high index of suspicion to make this diagnosis since the most common radiographic finding is that of a "normal" chest, which is incompatible with a patient in acute cardiopulmonary distress. Radiographic signs that may be seen, however, include pleural effusion, pulmonary infiltrates, focal atelectasis, elevation of the diaphragm, and hypovascular peripheral lung segments. Infiltration and formation of a "mass" may occur with infarction. With healing, these areas of consolidation shrink in the same pattern as a melting ice cube, retaining its original outline, only becoming smaller.

The radioisotope ventilation-perfusion lung scan is a useful diagnostic procedure in patients strongly suspected of having pulmonary embolus. The lung scan depends on the trapping of radioactive particles in the capillary bed and thus is an index of pulmonary arterial perfusion. Patients with emphysema, pneumonia, pulmonary fibrosis, or pleural effusions may demonstrate abnormal lung scans because of displaced vessels, shunting, and attenuation of the isotope emission, respectively. However, the scan is indeed useful in patients with these conditions if there are areas of decreased perfusion in an otherwise normal area of lung on the radiograph (Fig. 4.64). If a patient who is highly suspected of having a pulmonary embolus can be shown to have perfusion defects in radiographically normal-appearing areas with a normal ventilation scan, the diagnosis is certain. Furthermore, if a patient is shown to have normal perfusion despite the radiographic appearance, you can exclude embolus as a cause for that appearance.

If the isotope scan is equivocal, pulmonary arteriography may be used to confirm the diagnosis of pulmonary emboli. Radiographic findings include filling defects, delayed flow, and a disparity of flow as indicated by the venous phase being present on one side while the arterial phase is still seen on the abnormal side. Pulmonary arteriography does carry considerable hazard, however, and may result in severe arrhythmia or death. It should be reserved for situations where the diagnosis cannot be made by any other means. Figure 4.65 shows a patient with pulmonary embolus diagnosed by arteriography.

Appearance of the Chest After Surgery

Thoracic surgery has made monumental advances in the past 25 years in developing new techniques for cardiopulmonary bypass, lung surgery, coronary revascularization procedures, development of new prosthetic heart valves, heart transplantation, and perfection of new techniques for esophageal bypass surgery. These advances have reduced

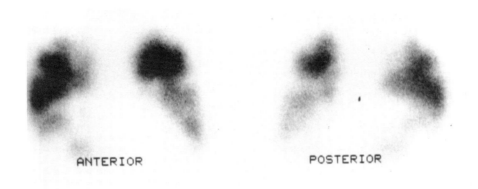

ANTERIOR   POSTERIOR

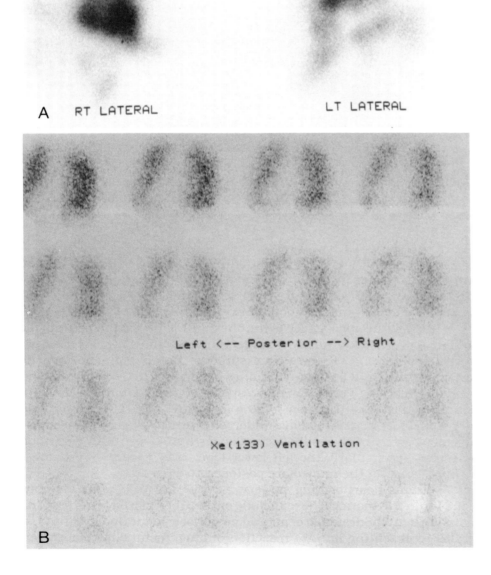

A   RT LATERAL   LT LATERAL

Left <-- Posterior --> Right

Xe(133) Ventilation

B

Figure 4.64. **Pulmonary embolism.** **A,** perfusion scan shows photopenic areas throughout both lungs, representing regions of lack of perfusion. **B,** ventilation scan shows that these areas are normally ventilated.

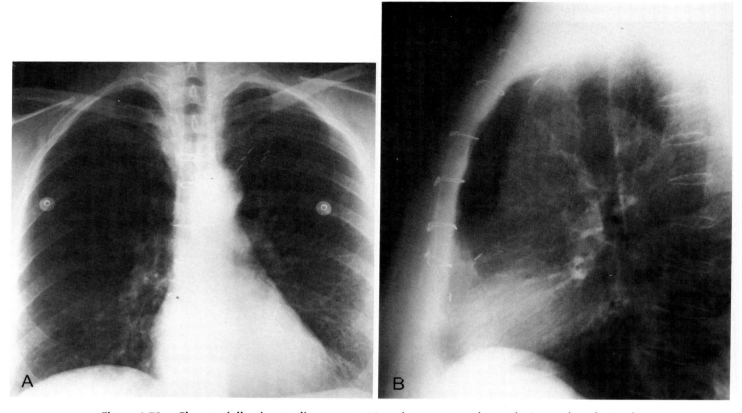

Figure 4.73.   Changes following cardiac surgery. Note the presence of sternal wires and mediastinal vascular clips. **A,** frontal view. **B,** lateral view.

curve to the catheter (Fig. 4.74). Any kinking or odd course of the lead should suggest that the catheter is not in the right position. The pacer box is in the subclavicular area. Epicardial leads are placed along the outside of the heart in the vicinity of the interventricular septum. Generally, these wires go through the diaphragm to the power box, which is in the abdominal wall (Fig. 4.75).

Recently, cardiologists have developed an automatic implantable cardiac defibrillator. This device is implanted either directly on the heart surface or subcutaneously in the anterior chest wall. The leads are attached to the transmitter box that is contained subcutaneously in the abdomen. When ventricular tachycardia or fibrillation occurs, the device automatically discharges a cardioverting shock. Early results suggest success in preventing sudden death from arrhythmias. The device may be recognized on a chest radiograph by the fly swatter-like pad over the heart (Fig. 4.76).

Numerous procedures have been devised for palliation of esophageal disease. There are basically two types, bypass surgery and hiatal hernia repair.

In a bypass procedure, the stomach or a segment of colon may be used to bypass a stenotic segment of esophagus or a neoplasm. The by-

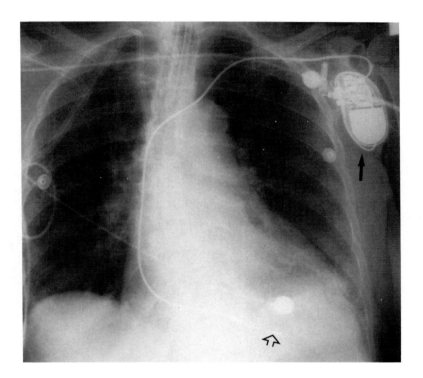

Figure 4.74. Transvenous pacemaker. The pacing box (*solid arrow*) is in the chest wall on the left. The pacing lead enters through the left subclavian vein. The tip of the pacing lead (*open arrow*) is in the right ventricle.

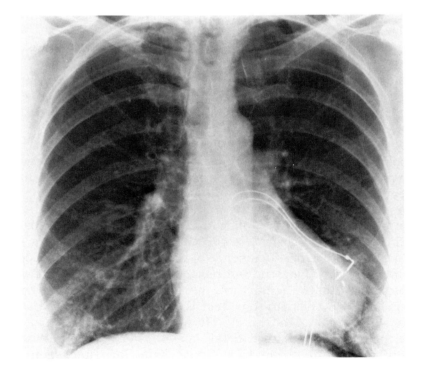

Figure 4.75. Epicardial pacemaker leads on the left side.

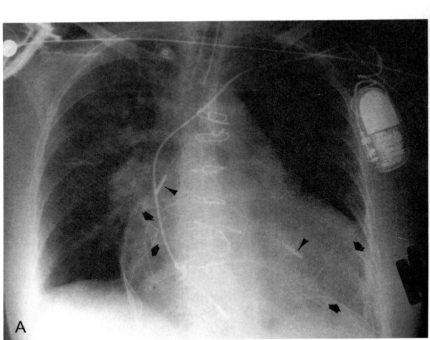

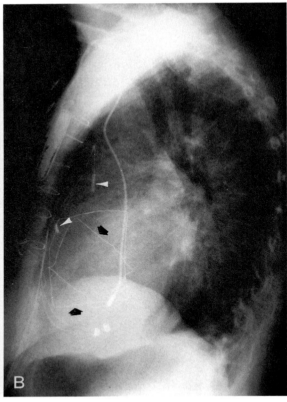

Figure 4.76.   Automated internal cardiac defibrillator. Frontal **(A)** and lateral **(B)** views show the defibrillator pads (*arrows*) over the right atrium and left ventricle. The leads (*arrowheads*) go to the power box in the abdominal wall. Note the pacemaker in place.

passing conduit is often visible on the chest radiograph, as illustrated in Figure 4.77.

Hiatal hernia repair may on occasion show a mass in the immediate postcardiac region. This represents the fundus of the stomach, which has been plicated around the distal esophagus to create a competent esophageal sphincter. Metal clips may be seen in this region.

You should familiarize yourself with the various appearances of the chest postoperatively. Remember, once the patient has recovered and is free of symptoms of the previous disease, we can consider this chest "normal" for that individual.

One additional postoperative appearance with which you should be familiar is that of the patient following radical mastectomy for carcinoma of the breast. Following mastectomy, the affected side appears more lucent. This is because of the absence of the breast shadow and pectoralis major muscle. If we follow the soft tissue lines of the axilla on the normal side, we can see that the axillary fold merges imperceptibly with that of the breast shadow. However, on the affected side, the axillary fold extends up to and crosses over onto the thorax. These findings are illustrated in Figure 4.78. Occasionally, we may see metal clips that were left at the site of nodal resection within the axilla in patients who have undergone radical mastectomy.

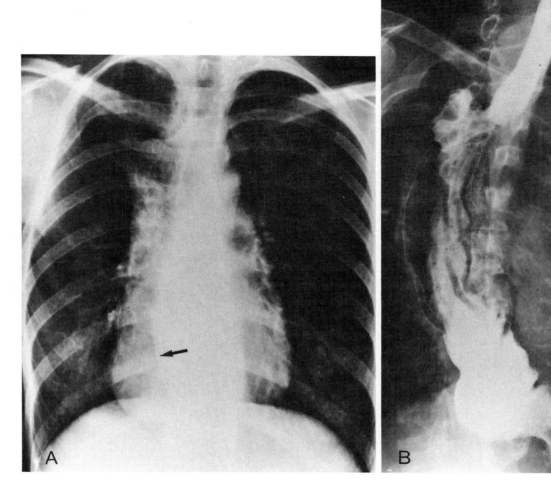

Figure 4.77. Changes following esophagogastrectomy. A, frontal radiograph shows apparent enlargement of the cardiac silhouette. The real cardiac border is seen just to the right of midline (*arrow*). **B,** contrast examination shows the stomach in the right hemithorax.

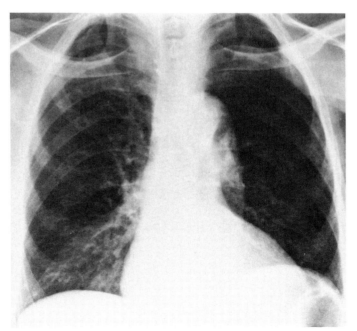

Figure 4.78. Changes following left radical mastectomy. There is hyperlucency in the left hemithorax due to the absence of pectoral tissues. Note the differences in soft tissues between right and left.

Summary

This chapter has described techniques involved in chest radiography. The normal anatomy was described in macroscopic and microscopic terms. The unit of structure and function in the lung is the pulmonary lobule. The mediastinum, its compartments, and its contents were also described in detail.

Pathologic alterations seen in the lung include consolidation, atelectasis, pleural fluid, masses, emphysema, pneumothorax, and pulmonary embolus. Each of these abnormalities produces clearly recognizable patterns. In addition, the concepts of the silhouette sign and air bronchogram were described. The concept of acinar versus interstitial disease was briefly described. Finally, the postoperative appearance of the thorax was discussed.

Suggested Additional Reading

Felson B. Chest roentgenology. Philadelphia: WB Saunders, 1975.

Fraser RG, Paré JAP, Paré PD, Fraser RS, Genereux GP. Diagnosis of diseases of the chest. 3rd ed. Philadelphia: WB Saunders, Vol. 1, 1988; Vol. 2, 1989; Vol. 3, 1990; Vol. 4, 1991.

Freundlich IM, Bragg DG. A radiologic approach to diseases of the chest. Baltimore: Williams & Wilkins, 1991.

Heitzman ER. The lung: radiology—pathologic correlations. St. Louis: CV Mosby, 1973.

Heitzman ER. The mediastinum: radiologic correlations with anatomy and pathology. St. Louis: CV Mosby, 1977.

Mann H, Bragg DC. Chest radiology. St. Louis: Mosby Year Book, 1989.

Reed JC. Chest radiography: plain film patterns and differential diagnoses. 3rd ed. St. Louis: Mosby Year Book, 1991.

Chapter 5

Cardiac Imaging

Cardiovascular radiology is a subspecialty shared by radiologists and cardiologists. Too often the clinician is content to merely have made a diagnosis of "large heart," "congestive heart failure," or "congenital heart disease." It is possible, however, for you as the clinician to recognize certain patterns of disease based on the alterations those diseases produce in the pulmonary vascularity and in specific chambers of the heart. The evaluation of the patient with suspected cardiac disease should be directed along two distinct lines: imaging of anatomic changes and demonstration of physiologic function, often simultaneously. While the former goal can be attained through plain radiographic means, the latter may be achieved only through cardiac catheterization, which permits hemodynamic measurements and injection of contrast material. As will be discussed below, recent developments in imaging technology have now made it possible to make accurate diagnoses using noninvasive techniques.

This chapter will examine the criteria for certain *categories* of diseases rather than discuss specific entities. For a complete discussion of those entities, you are referred to a comprehensive text of cardiology.

TECHNICAL CONSIDERATIONS

The advances in diagnostic imaging techniques in the past 2 decades have revolutionized cardiac imaging. Plain film radiography, cardiac series, cardiac fluoroscopy, and cardiac catheterization were the mainstays of cardiac imaging prior to 1975. However, real-time ultrasound imaging, radionuclide cardiac perfusion studies, computerized tomography (CT), and magnetic resonance imaging (MR) have all become standard evaluation tools in the hands of the cardiovascular radiologist and cardiologist in the 1990s. As the clinician, you now have a greater number of options to call on to evaluate your patient. As with any other organ system, your choice of diagnostic studies will depend on getting the most information in the safest way at the lowest cost. Therefore, consulting with your radiologist or referring cardiologist is mandatory.

The same plain film technical considerations that were discussed for pulmonary disease apply to evaluation of the cardiovascular system. You should first decide if the film was a posterior-anterior or anterior-posterior

(PA or AP) view, if the patient is lordotic, and if rotation is present. The degree of penetration on the film, the presence of motion, and the degree of inspiration are all important factors to consider. A film made with the patient in a slightly lordotic position will falsely distort and magnify the cardiac size. A film that is too light will accentuate the pulmonary vessels; a film with the patient not in maximum inspiration may result in further accentuation of pulmonary vessels and cause an appearance of cardiac enlargement and/or an erroneous diagnosis of congestive heart failure (Fig. 5.1).

It is also necessary to pay close attention to the patient's body habitus. A narrow AP diameter of the chest or a pectus excavatum deformity may result in posterior compression of the heart and a spurious appearance of cardiac enlargement (Fig. 5.2).

In the bony thorax, particular attention should be given to the undersurfaces of the ribs for any evidence of rib notching. Although the most common cause of rib notching is coarctation of the aorta, you should keep in mind that many other conditions such as tetralogy of Fallot, truncus arteriosus, Blalock-Taussig operation, or neurofibromatosis produce this abnormality.

There are eight basic techniques used for evaluation of the heart: (1) plain film radiography, (2) cardiac fluoroscopy, (3) cardiac series, (4) car-

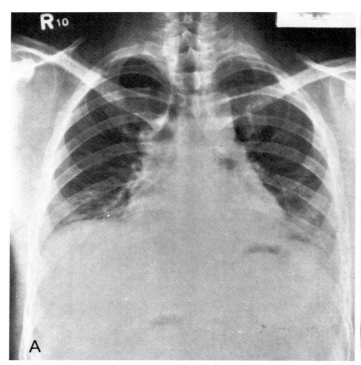
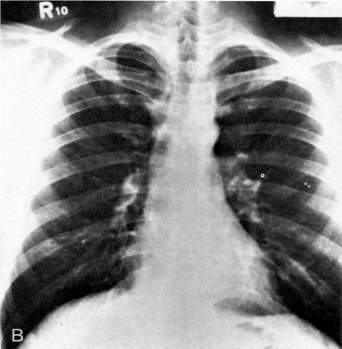

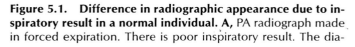

Figure 5.1. Difference in radiographic appearance due to inspiratory result in a normal individual. A, PA radiograph made in forced expiration. There is poor inspiratory result. The diaphragm is flat and the heart appears enlarged. There is prominence of the pulmonary vessels. **B,** the same individual in full inspiration. Note the differences in appearance.

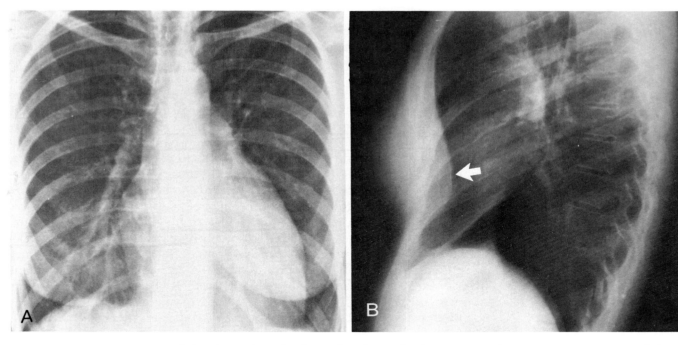

Figure 5.2. Pectus excavatum deformity. A, frontal radiograph shows apparent enlargement of the heart. The ribs are slightly more horizontal posteriorly and steeper anteriorly. **B,** lateral radiograph shows a prominent pectus excavatum deformity (*arrow*). The sternal deformity compressed the heart and gave the spurious appearance of enlargement.

diac catheterization and coronary arteriography (angiocardiography), (5) echocardiography, (6) radioisotope studies, (7) computerized tomography, and (8) magnetic resonance imaging.

Plain film radiography is a standard screening examination in patients with suspected cardiac disease. By knowing the normal anatomy portrayed on the PA and lateral films and by analyzing the sizes of pulmonary arteries and veins, you may be able to make a correct diagnosis in the majority of cases.

A popular method used to determine cardiac size is the cardiothoracic ratio: the maximum width of the cardiac shadow on the PA chest film divided by the maximum width of the thorax. This method has received criticism, since a true determination of cardiac enlargement necessitates evaluation of the cardiac silhouette on *both* the PA and lateral views. As a rule of thumb, however, the cardiac width should never exceed half the width of the thorax on the PA film.

Fluoroscopic examination of the heart and pulmonary vessels is used for (*a*) an assessment of cardiac motion, contour, and dynamics (useful for evaluation of cardiac aneurysms), (*b*) investigation of intracardiac calcifications (valvular, coronary artery, or pericardial), and (*c*) assessment of patients with suspected pericardial effusion (dampened pulsations and displaced subepicardial fat line). It has largely been replaced by echocardiography.

The cardiac series is a four-view examination consisting of PA, lateral, and right anterior oblique (RAO) views with the patient drinking barium, and a left anterior oblique (LAO) view without barium. Barium is used to determine whether or not specific chamber enlargement impinges on the esophagus. The LAO view does not use barium since that substance would obscure the aortopulmonary window. The anatomic relationships will be discussed in the next section. The cardiac series, too, has largely been replaced by echocardiography.

Cardiac catheterization and coronary arteriography are invasive procedures performed almost exclusively by cardiologists or cardiovascular radiologists. These procedures allow accurate evaluation of the size and configuration of the cardiac chambers, the great vessels, and the coronary arteries. They are also performed to evaluate patients with suspected shunt lesions. Real-time echocardiography has decreased the number of catheterizations used to determine cardiac chamber size and configuration.

Echocardiography is an ultrasound examination of the heart and great vessels using one of three techniques: M-mode, cross-sectional (two-dimensional) imaging, or Doppler technique. M-mode (motion-mode) echocardiography records echoes from cardiac structures within the ultrasonic beam and provides one-dimensional information. It is displayed on a strip chart that allows measurements to be made of the depth of the structure as well as its motion (Fig. 5.3).

Cross-sectional echocardiography provides images of the moving heart chambers. By shifting the transducer and altering the depth of penetration of the ultrasound beam, one can obtain a tomographic image of the heart and its chambers.

Figure 5.3. M-mode echocardiogram showing a pericardial effusion (eff). A, pericardium; **B,** left ventricular wall; **C,** chorda tendinea; **D,** mitral valve; **E,** septal wall; **F,** electrocardiogram; **G,** right ventricular wall; **H,** chest wall.

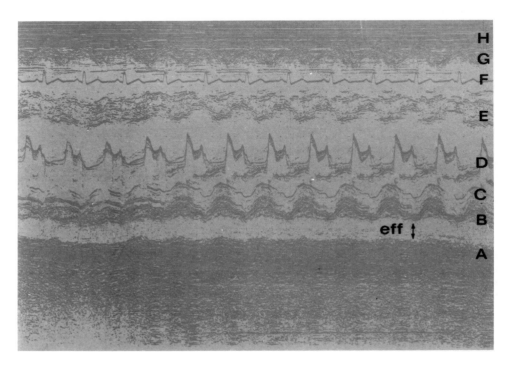

Doppler echocardiography is used primarily to assess the direction and velocity of blood flow within the heart and great vessels. It is particularly useful in evaluating the carotid vessels in patients with transient ischemic attacks.

Overall, the most common indications for echocardiography are suspected chamber enlargement, congenital heart disease, abnormalities of heart valves, abnormalities of contractility, and suspected pericardial effusions. This examination is performed primarily by cardiologists.

Radioisotope studies of the heart are performed primarily for the evaluation of cardiac perfusion. Isotopes of thallium are injected intravenously and the myocardial blood flow is recorded with the patient at rest and while exercising (thallium stress test) (Fig. 5.4). This technique is most useful for separation of patients with atypical chest pain into cardiac and noncardiac origin categories (Fig. 5.5).

Computerized tomography, performed with electrocardiographic CT gating, is used with contrast enhancement for a variety of cardiac conditions. In this technique, dynamic scanning—multiple images of one section—is performed to evaluate flow through a particular chamber or vessel. In addition, CT is used to evaluate the patency of coronary artery bypass

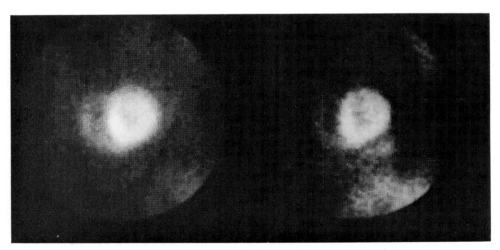

Figure 5.4. Normal thallium cardiac scan during stress testing. There is uniform distribution of blood flow over the left ventricle as evidenced by the uniform distribution of isotope.

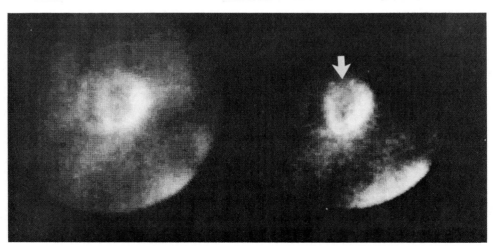

Figure 5.5. Cardiac ischemia. Ischemic disease of the anterior left ventricular wall as demonstrated by a photopenic area (*arrow*) during stress test. Compare with Figure 5.4.

Figure 5.6. Application of MRI for cardiac imaging. Parasagittal MRI showing coarctation of the aorta (*arrow*). Note the following landmarks: *A,* ascending aorta; *P,* pulmonary artery; *L,* lung; *C,* coarctation.

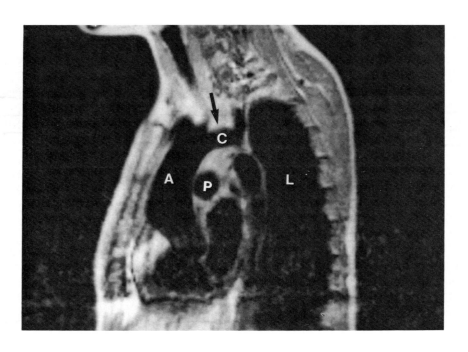

grafts, to assess the extent of myocardial infarcts, to depict the size and location of left ventricular aneurysms, to detect aneurysms of the thoracic aorta, to diagnose aortic dissections, to define certain congenital abnormalities such as coarctation of the aorta and anomalous venous connections, and to assess the pericardium for effusions. Dynamic CT is also used for determining myocardial wall thickness and dynamics, although echocardiography is used much more commonly.

Magnetic resonance imaging is employed to diagnose many of the same abnormalities that can be seen with CT. Electrocardiographic gating is used for "stop-action" images of the heart and great vessels. Magnetic resonance imaging has the advantage of portraying flowing blood as a signal void (black) so that it is easy to distinguish blood from solid structures. Magnetic resonance imaging is most useful for evaluating patients with aortic dissections and aortic coarctation (Fig. 5.6) as well as chamber abnormalities.

ANATOMIC CONSIDERATIONS

For an appreciation for the anatomic relationships of the heart and its chambers, it is necessary to think in three-dimensional terms. Let us examine the position of the cardiac chambers, the great vessels, and the aortic and mitral valves as seen in the four-view cardiac series (Fig. 5.7).

On the PA view (Fig. 5.7**A**), most of the cardiac silhouette is made up almost exclusively of the right side of the heart; the left ventricle forms the left cardiac border. The position of the anterior interventricular sulcus may be determined only on an angiocardiogram by following the course of the anterior descending branch of the left coronary artery. The right atrium forms the right border of the heart, merging imperceptibly into the image of the superior vena cava. The left atrium is not seen under normal circumstances in this view. However, a small portion of the left border of

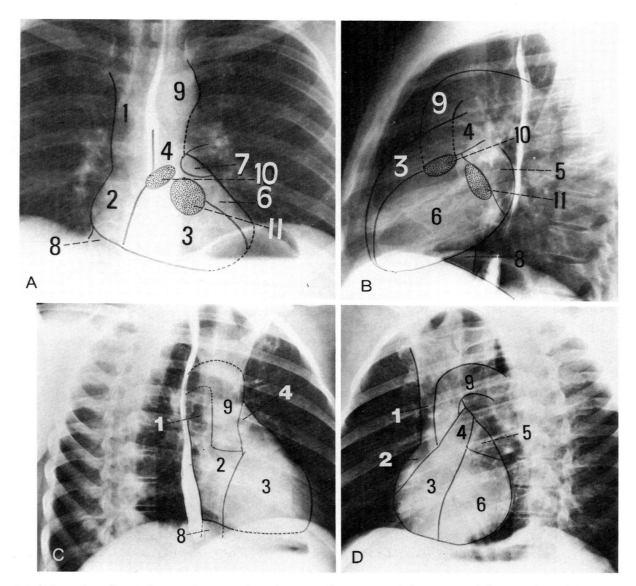

Figure 5.7. Normal cardiac series. A, PA view. **B,** lateral view. **C,** right anterior oblique. **D,** left anterior oblique. 1, superior vena cava; 2, right atrium; 3, right venticle; 4, pulmonary outflow tract; 5, left atrium; 6, left ventricle; 7, left atrial appendage; 8, inferior vena cava; 9, ascending aorta and aortic arch; 10, aortic valve; 11, mitral valve.

the heart just beneath the pulmonary trunk is represented by the left atrial appendage. In this view, the aortic valve is positioned obliquely, with its lower end oriented to the right approximately in the midline just below the waist of the cardiovascular silhouette. The mitral valve, which is oriented on a similar plane in this view, lies just below the aortic valve area and to the left.

In the normal lateral view (Fig. 5.7**B**), the anterior border of the cardiac silhouette consists of the right ventricle. The posterior and inferior cardiac border is that of the left ventricle. The image of the inferior vena cava superimposes on the posteroinferior border of the left ventricle, occasionally extending just posterior to the left ventricular outline. The left atrium forms the superoposterior border of the heart. The barium-filled esophagus courses almost immediately posterior to the cardiac silhouette. It should not be indented by the heart under normal circumstances. Occasionally, the image of the pulmonary artery may be observed arching up from the right ventricle and passing inferiorly to the arch of the aorta, which is also visible on the lateral film. In this view, the aortic valve lies almost horizontally just below the narrow waist of the cardiovascular pedicle. The mitral valve ring lies in an oblique plane, as indicated in Figure 5.7**B**, inferiorly and posterior to that of the aortic valve.

In the RAO view (Fig. 5.7**C**), the bulk of the cardiac silhouette consists of the right ventricle. The left ventricle contributes a small portion to the cardiac silhouette over the apex anteriorly. The right cardiac border consists of the right atrium inferiorly and the left atrium superiorly. In this view, the barium-filled esophagus should not be indented in any way; if this occurs, it indicates an enlarged left atrium.

In the LAO position (Fig. 5.7**D**), all the cardiac chambers contribute to the cardiac silhouette. Only a small segment of the upper portion of the right heart border is formed by the right atrial appendage; the rest is delineated by the right ventricle. On the left side, the lower border is exclusively left ventricle. The left atrium forms the upper portion of the left silhouette. Under normal circumstances the image of the left ventricle should not overlap that of the thoracic vertebrae by more than 1 cm. An overlap greater than this indicates left ventricular enlargement. A small "clear" aerated area is present just above the border of the left atrium. In patients with left atrial enlargement, this area "fills in." Barium is not used in the LAO view.

One additional useful anatomic relationship is that of the mainstem bronchi to the heart. The trachea bifurcates below the aortic arch. The bronchi continue downward and branch from this point. The left mainstem bronchus, however, has a close relationship with the left atrium. Consequently, enlargements of the left atrium may result in elevation of the left mainstem bronchus and widening the normal carinal angle above 75° in adults; greater angulation is allowed for infants and children.

The pulmonary arteries and veins constitute the lung markings seen on a chest radiograph. It is sometimes difficult to differentiate between arteries and veins on the radiograph. However, a useful method is by analyzing the *direction* of the vessels to determine whether or not they are arterial or venous. Under normal circumstances, the pulmonary arteries radiate out from the hilar region in a fairly uniform, fan-like appearance (Fig. 5.8**A**). The veins, on the other hand, follow a different course because of the lower location of the left atrium, into which they must terminate. The upper lobe veins assume an obliquely downward course, in some instances almost vertical, as they "dive" for the left atrium; the lower lobe veins assume a more horizontal course, located almost directly opposite the level of the left atrium (Fig. 5.8**B**). It is important to be able to differentiate arteries from veins, since the proposed approach for diagnosis is based on analysis of the pulmonary vasculature.

Under normal circumstances, the vascularity of the lower lobes is more prominent than that of the upper lobes. In normal individuals, this

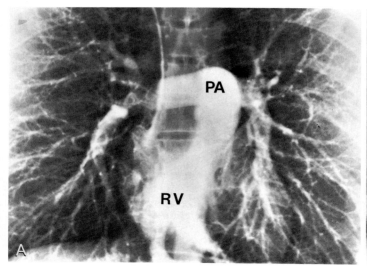

Figure 5.8.   Normal pulmonary arteriogram. A, arterial phase. Injection was made into the right ventricle (*RV*). Contrast material passes through the pulmonary outflow tract into the pulmonary arteries (*PA*). **B,** venous phase. Contrast material passes from the pulmonary veins into the left atrium (*LA*) and then into the left ventricle (*LV*). Note the difference in orientation between the pulmonary arteries and pulmonary veins.

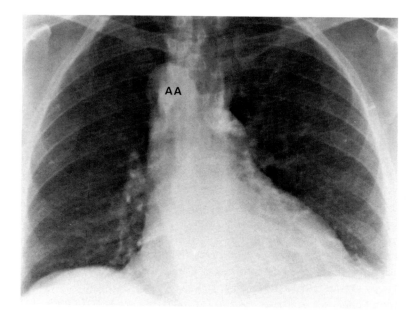

Figure 5.9.   Right aortic arch (*AA*) in an elderly individual with no evidence of heart disease.

relationship is altered in the recumbent position, where gravity results in greater flow to the cephalic regions.

Finally, it is important to observe the side on which the aortic arch is located and the position of the gastric air bubble. Under normal circumstances the aortic arch is on the left. However, there are anomalies of this vessel in which the arch is on the right (Fig. 5.9). The gastric air bubble is ordinarily on the left. However, in patients with certain forms of situs inversus and dextrocardia, the gastric bubble is on the right.

PATHOLOGIC CONSIDERATIONS

There are many ways to classify cardiac disease. A popular classification uses two large categories, *congenital* and *acquired* cardiac disease. Congenital cardiac disease is further subdivided into *cyanotic* and *acyanotic* types. Most books on cardiology prefer this method. For the non-cardiologist, a *physiologic* approach affords an understandable and useful basis for dealing with congenital and acquired heart disease. In addition to this physiologic approach, it is preferable to evaluate patients with cardiac disease on the basis of their age. This discussion will focus on the plain film evaluation of these patients, since that is the type of imaging examination you will order first and with which you will be most familiar. Once you have an idea of what kind of cardiac disease you are dealing with you can order more sophisticated imaging procedures, such as echocardiography, angiography, or MR, to make a definitive diagnosis.

Adult Patients

From a physiologic standpoint, all types of cardiac disease may be categorized into the following:

I. Obstruction
II. Volume overload
    A. Shunt (right-to-left, left-to-right)
    B. Admixture
    C. Valvular insufficiency
III. Disorders of contraction or relaxation
    A. Myocardial disease
    B. Conduction disorders (arrhythmias)
IV. Combination of the preceding

No matter what the etiology, all cardiac diseases will show evidence of one or more of these patterns.

Evaluation of the pulmonary vascularity is an important step that enables exclusion of many diseases. The *physiologic* type of disease may be inferred from the pattern of pulmonary blood flow. Pulmonary vascularity may be normal, decreased, or increased. Figure 5.10 illustrates the varying forms of pulmonary blood flow and lists some important disease processes that accompany those patterns. Normal pulmonary vessels should be about the same size as that of an accompanying airway. Any significant disparity in size is abnormal (Fig. 5.11).

Surprising as it may seem, patients with normal pulmonary vascularity may have significant cardiac disease. In these patients, the heart has compensated for the abnormality by enlarging. The pulmonary vascularity remains normal until the heart decompensates. Diseases that produce cardiac chamber enlargement without appreciable change in the pulmonary vascularity until decompensation occurs include cardiomyopathy, coronary artery disease, hypertensive cardiovascular disease, aortic stenosis, and coarctation of the aorta. All these conditions except coarctation and a form of aortic stenosis are acquired.

Decreased vascularity indicates a severe obstruction to the outflow of blood from the right ventricle, usually at the pulmonic valve or subvalvular

PATTERN

DISTRIBUTION	NORMAL Arterial and Venous	DECREASED Arterial and Venous	INCREASED Predominantly Arterial	INCREASED Predominantly Venous
NORMAL Apex less than Base	Normal	Tetralogy of Fallot or other right-sided obstructive lesion	Left-to-right shunts Systemic A-V shunts Hyperkinetic circulatory state Transposition of great vessels without pulmonary stenosis Truncus arteriosus Type I	
CEPHALIZATION Up-Shifting Apex greater than Base		Same as above with prominent bronchial collateral circulation	Same as above with left ventricular failure (PVO)	Left ventricular of any cause (PVO)
CENTRALIZATION Center greater than Periphery	Pulmonary hypertension	Severe pulmonary emphysema Chronic (diffuse) pulmonary thromboembolic disease Eisenmenger syndrome	Left-to-right shunt with pulmonary hypertension Cor pulmonale with high cardiac output	Acute pulmonary edema of any etiology
LATERALIZATION Right greater than Left or Right less than Left	Swyre-James pulmonic stenosis with intact ventricular septum Proximal interruption of one pulmonary artery without shunt	Pulmonary hypoplasia Tetralogy of Fallot after palliative shunting procedure (Blalock, Potts, Glenn, Waterston)	Multple congenital anomalies produce this pattern	Left atrial myxoma or mural thrombi causing local pulmonary edema
LOCALIZATION Local Dilatation and/or Local Constriction or Abnormal Course of Vessel	Pulmonary emboli Pulmonary stenosis of peripheral vessels	Same as normal Severe tetralogy with bronchial flow to one area	Anomalous pulmonary drainage Also multiple other types of congenital heart disease	Same as normal and decreased flow

Figure 5.10. Correlation of pulmonary vascular patterns, distribution, and diseases that produce these patterns.

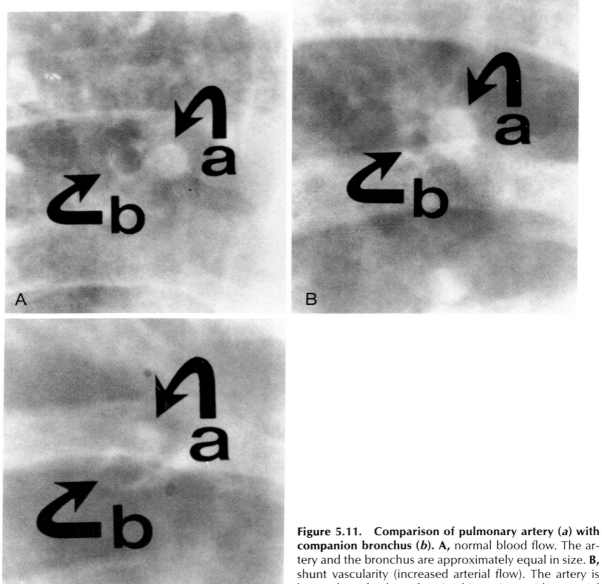

Figure 5.11.   Comparison of pulmonary artery (a) with companion bronchus (b). A, normal blood flow. The artery and the bronchus are approximately equal in size. **B,** shunt vascularity (increased arterial flow). The artery is larger than the bronchus in this patient with an atrial septal defect. **C,** diminished pulmonary arterial flow. The artery is smaller than the bronchus in this patient with tetralogy of Fallot.

level. Patients exhibiting this pattern are often visibly cyanotic. If the decreased vascularity is of a diffuse nature, a congenital anomaly is most likely. This pattern is seldom seen in the adult, since the abnormalities that produce this pattern will result in the patient's death unless corrective surgery is performed during childhood.

Decreased vascularity may be apparent locally or unilaterally. A local decrease in vascularity may be the result of pulmonary embolism (Westermark sign), emphysema (Fig. 5.12), or scarring with rearrangement of vessels in a lung. A unilateral decrease in vascularity without changes in the cardiac size may result from either hypoplasia of a lung or the Swyer-James syndrome, a rare condition caused by diffuse, unilateral bronchitis (Fig. 5.13).

Increased vascularity is of four types: (1) shunts, (2) pulmonary venous obstruction, (3) precapillary hypertension, and (4) high-output state.

Shunts represent an increased flow through the pulmonary bed. They are characterized by large vessels in the upper and lower lobes. A similar pattern may occur in high-output states. In patients with a shunt who are not in congestive heart failure, the redistribution of blood will be in the same proportion as that occurring normally: greater to the lung bases than to the upper lobes. This vascular pattern occurs most commonly in a left-to-right shunt at the cardiac or great vessel level (septal defect or patent ductus arteriosus). This pattern is uncommon in adults since the condition is usually diagnosed and treated in childhood (Fig. 5.14).

Patients with pulmonary venous obstruction (PVO) demonstrate large veins in the upper lobe as a reflection of reversal of the normal flow pattern. This indicates increased left atrial pressure. Severe PVO is manifest by pulmonary edema and prominent interlobular septal (Kerley) lines (Fig. 5.15).

Patients with precapillary hypertension (pulmonary arterial hypertension) have large central vessels that taper rapidly into small vessels peripherally. This is referred to as centralized flow and occurs in patients

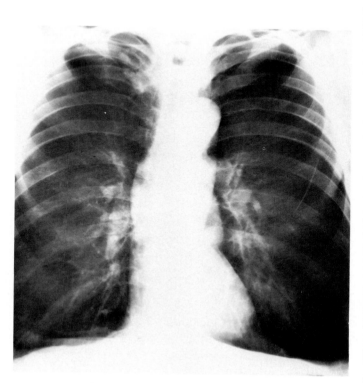

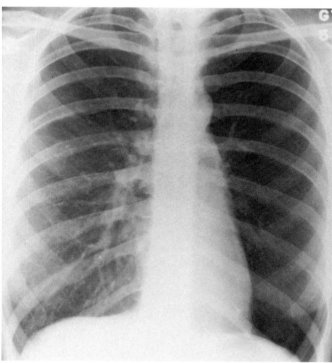

Figure 5.12.   Decrease in pulmonary vascularity in a patient with emphysema. Note the crowding of vessels centrally and paucity of peripheral vessels.

Figure 5.13.   Unilateral decrease in pulmonary vasculature in a patient with left-side unilateral hyperlucent lung (Swyer-James syndrome). Compare the vessels in this patient with normal right side to the abnormal left side.

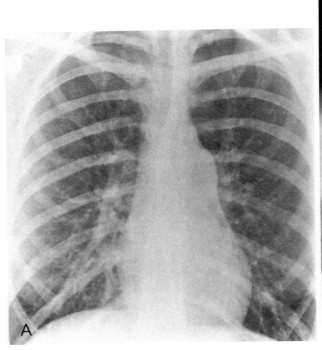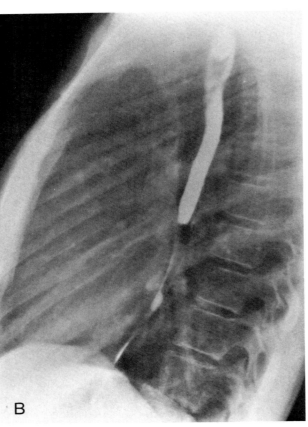

Figure 5.14. Increased pulmonary vascularity in a patient with an atrial septal defect. A, frontal view shows prominent vessels. **B,** lateral view shows right ventricular prominence in the substernal region.

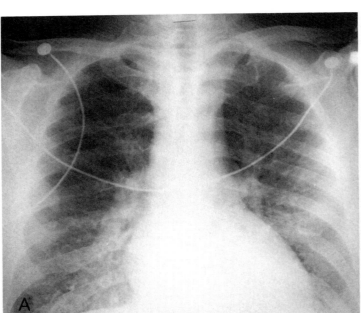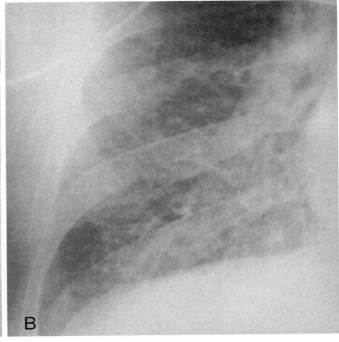

Figure 5.15. Congestive heart failure and pulmonary edema. A, frontal view shows mild pulmonary edema and pulmonary venous engorgement. **B,** detailed view shows the edema and prominent septal (Kerley) lines.

with severe pulmonary disease, recurrent pulmonary embolism (Fig. 5.16), and Eisenmenger phenomenon.

Once the pulmonary vascular pattern is decided on, look at the heart to determine if specific chamber enlargements are present. If there is evidence of left atrial enlargement (with or without PVO), rheumatic heart disease (mitral stenosis) or an obstruction at or proximal to the mitral valve is present (Fig. 5.17). If there is evidence of left ventricular enlargement with

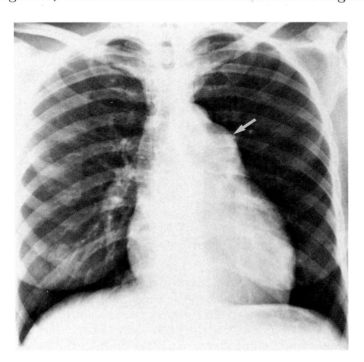

Figure 5.16. Pulmonary arterial hypertension in a patient with recurrent pulmonary emboli. There is prominence of the main pulmonary artery near the outflow tract on the left (*arrow*). The right mainstem pulmonary artery is enlarged and tapers rapidly peripherally. This is a sign of pulmonary arterial hypertension.

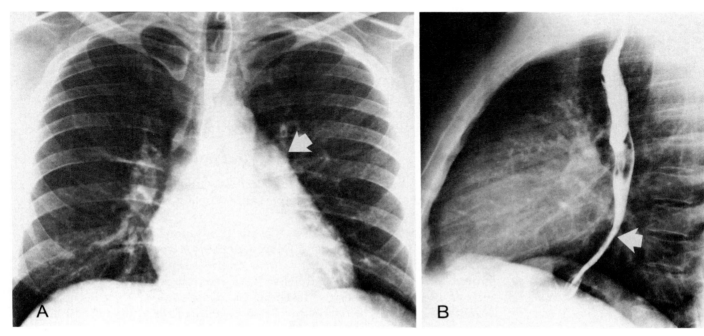

Figure 5.17. Mitral stenosis. A, frontal view shows a prominent bulge in the vicinity of the left atrium (*arrow*). **B,** lateral radiograph shows impingement of the barium-filled esophagus (*arrow*) by the enlarged left atrium.

Figure 5.18. Hypertensive cardiovascular disease. There is left ventricular prominence and a slight increase in the tortuosity of the aorta at its arch. There is calcification in the descending aorta (*arrow*).

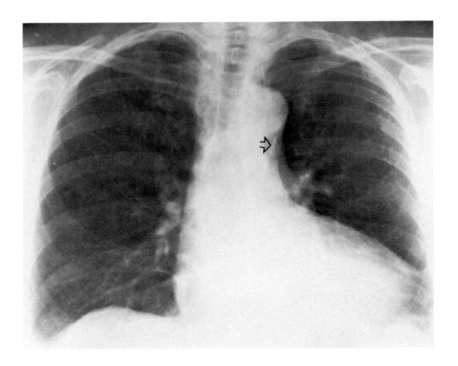

a "concavity" in the area of the main pulmonary artery, the disease is one of left ventricular stress such as hypertensive cardiovascular disease (Fig. 5.18), coronary artery disease, aortic stenosis, or coarctation of the aorta.

Pulmonary venous obstruction plus left ventricular configuration (LVC) equals left ventricular stress with failure. All the preceding conditions occur with this pattern. It is possible to further narrow the list of causes in this situation by scanning the film for evidence of rib notching and/or decreased size of the aortic knob, as in aortic coarctation (Fig. 5.19), or for calcification in or about the aortic valve (Fig. 5.20), as in calcific aortic stenosis.

A high-output state, such as severe anemia or thyrotoxicosis, may result in increased vascularity with a normal distribution as a result of the increased volume being pumped through the heart. The heart itself may be normal or slightly enlarged as a result of this increased activity.

Pediatric Patients

Cardiac disease in pediatric patients is usually congenital. However, rheumatic heart disease is an important form of acquired disease that may occur in this age group.

Before beginning an analysis of the pulmonary vascularity in pediatric patients, it is important to know whether or not they are visibly cyanotic. The presence of visible cyanosis changes the physiologic state of the patient and the category of disease. It is also important to know whether the cyanosis was present at birth (as in transposition of great vessels) or developed later (as in tetralogy of Fallot). Plain film analysis will be discussed in the acyanotic and the cyanotic patient.

Figure 5.21 is a flow sheet that summarizes the analysis necessary in the diagnosis of congenital cardiac disease.

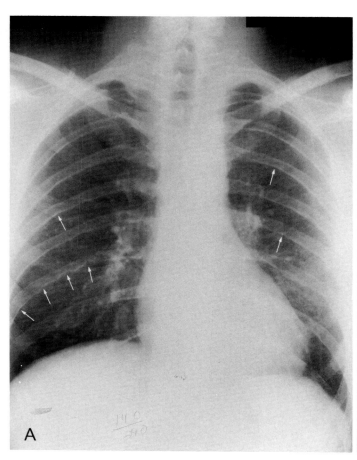

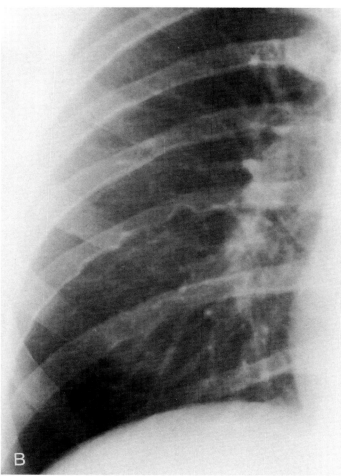

Figure 5.19.   Coarctation of the aorta. A, frontal radiograph at first glance appears normal. There is, however, slight left ventricular prominence. The aortic knob is small. Note the rib notching bilaterally (*arrows*). **B,** detailed view shows the rib notching to better advantage.

Figure 5.20.   Aortic valve calcification (*arrows*).

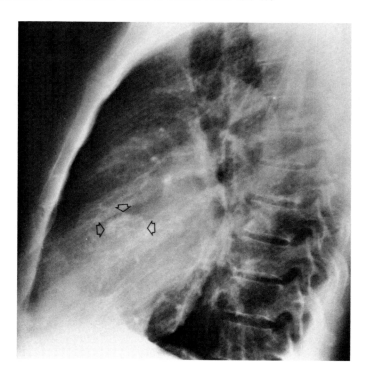

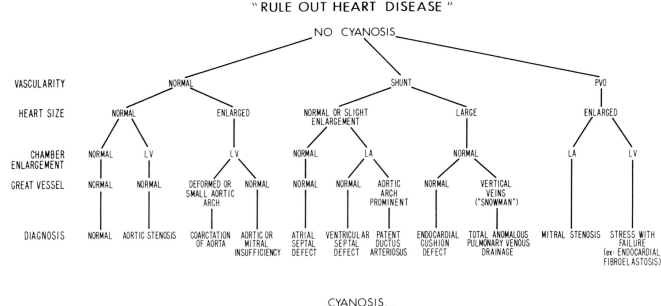

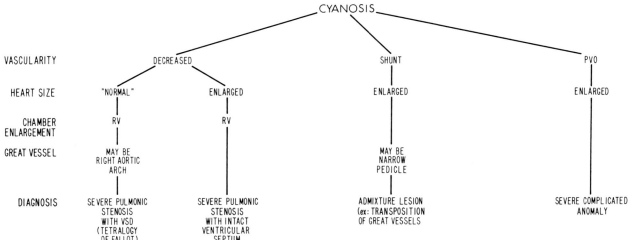

Figure 5.21.   Flow chart for a plain film radiographic diagnosis of congenital cardiac diseases. A,
acyanotic patients. **B,** cynotic patients.

ACYANOTIC PATIENTS

If the vascularity is normal, it is necessary to rely on the heart size and configuration and the appearance of the great vessels to provide clues to the etiology of the suspected cardiac disease. A normal heart size does not rule out a heart lesion. A mild or compensated lesion may be accompanied by a normal-appearing heart on plain radiographs. Furthermore, an obstructive lesion may cause hypertrophy, but not enlarge the heart enough to be detectable on the chest roentgenogram. A diagnosis of left or right ventricular *hypertrophy* is an electrocardiographic or ultrasonic, not radiographic, diagnosis. Radiography identifies chamber *enlargements*, not hypertrophy.

Left ventricular configuration in a child indicates a left-sided obstructive lesion such as aortic stenosis (Fig. 5.22) or coarctation of the aorta. The left ventricular configuration may be normal in adults, but is always abnormal in children.

A prominent main pulmonary artery or proximal left pulmonary artery segment suggests a right-sided obstructive lesion, pulmonic valvular stenosis with poststenotic dilatation (Fig. 5.23). If the peripheral vascularity is normal, the degree of stenosis is not severe.

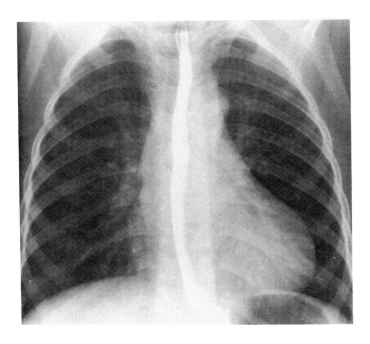

Figure 5.22. Aortic stenosis in a child. Note the left ventricular configuration.

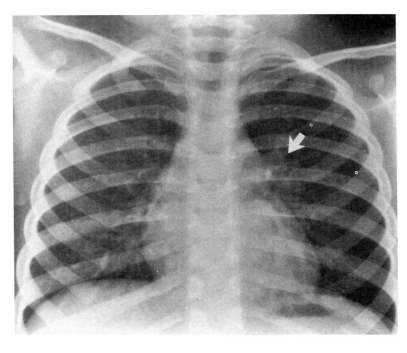

Figure 5.23. Pulmonic stenosis in a child. There is prominence of the left main pulmonary artery (*arrow*) near the outflow tract caused by the "jet phenomenon."

In patients with enlarged hearts but normal vascularity, volume overload most likely caused by valvular insufficiency may be inferred. Volume overload dilates the involved cardiac chambers without causing increased pressure until cardiac failure occurs. An LVC (indicating left ventricular stress) with an enlarged heart suggests aortic or mitral insufficiency (Fig. 5.24). In mitral insufficiency, volume overload occurs in the left atrium as well. This may be detected on plain films or on the cardiac series as (a) a bulge along the left cardiac border (indicating displacement of the left atrial appendage), (b) a double density seen on the PA film, representing the enlarged left atrium itself, (c) splaying of the carinal angle greater than 75°, and (d) impingement on the barium-filled esophagus. These findings are illustrated in Fig. 5.25 in a patient with mitral stenosis and insufficiency.

The preceding findings are summarized as follows:

1. Normal vascularity + normal heart size = normal or "mild anything."
2. Normal vascularity + left ventricular configuration (overall heart size normal) = left ventricular obstructive lesion without heart failure.

Figure 5.24. Mitral insufficiency. A, frontal radiograph shows prominence and straightening of the left cardiac border due to left atrial enlargement. Note the left ventricular prominence. **B,** lateral radiograph shows left ventricular enlargement (*arrow*).

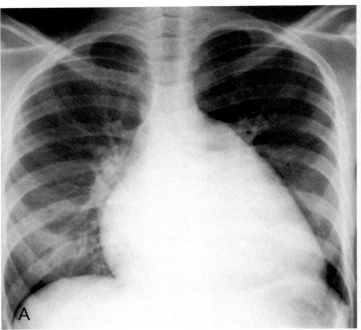
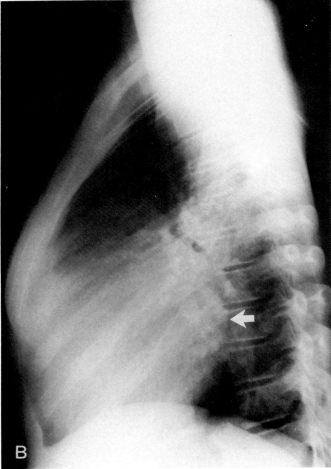

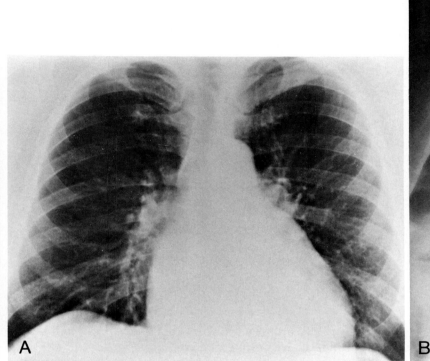

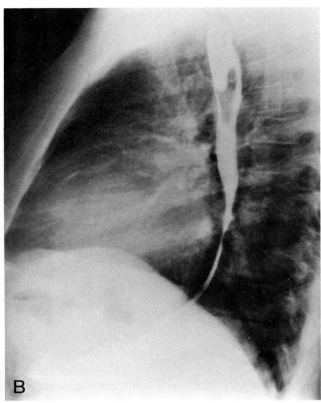

Figure 5.25. Mitral insufficiency and mitral stenosis. When these two lesions are combined, there is greater cardiomegaly than in an isolated lesion. **A,** frontal view. **B,** lateral radiograph showing impingement of the barium-filled esophagus by the enlarged left atrium.

3. Normal vascularity + prominent main pulmonary artery = right ventricular obstructive lesion.
4. Normal vascularity + big heart = volume overload lesion, valvular insufficiency type.

As mentioned previously, a general increase in the size of the pulmonary arteries throughout the lungs indicates either a left-to-right shunt or a hyperdynamic state such as thyrotoxicosis or large systemic arteriovenous (AV) fistula. In the pediatric age group, the most common congenital lesion to produce this pattern is a shunt.

Once shunt vascularity is identified, the size of the left atrium is used to determine the level of the shunt. An enlarged left atrium (LAE) indicates that the atrial septum is intact (LAE results from the increased pulmonary venous return). In this situation, the shunt must be distal to the AV valves, as in a ventricular septal defect (VSD) (Fig. 5.26) or patent ductus arteriosus.

Shunt vascularity without atrial enlargement indicates an atrial septal defect (ASD) (Fig. 5.14). In this situation, the excess blood flows immediately into the lower pressure right atrium, resulting in no net volume overload of the left atrium. In a patient with an isolated ASD, the heart is

Figure 5.26. Ventricular septal defect. Note the shunt vascularity.

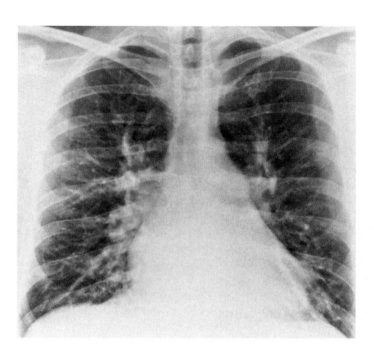

either normal in size or mildly enlarged. Shunt vascularity coupled with marked cardiomegaly indicates a complicated ASD.

These findings are summarized as follows:

1. Shunt vascularity + left atrial enlargement = shunt distal to AV valves.
2. Shunt vascularity + normal-sized left atrium = ASD.
3. Shunt vascularity + normal-sized left atrium + big heart = complicated ASD.

Severe pulmonary venous obstruction in the newborn child usually occurs in patients with cyanotic congenital heart disease. However, cardiac failure may occur in very young children in the presence of large systemic AV fistulae. Interestingly enough, because infants spend most of their hours in a recumbent position, the pulmonary blood flow is equally distributed throughout the lungs and the adult pattern of PVO—a redistribution to the upper lobes—is therefore not observed. The older a child becomes, however, the closer the appearance is to the adult pattern of PVO.

As in the adult, once a pattern of PVO is recognized, attention should be directed to the cardiac configuration to determine the level of the obstruction. If the heart is triangular in shape, i.e., having a prominent bulge along the left cardiac border, and there is evidence of LAE, the obstruction is at or proximal to the mitral valve. The most common etiology of this situation is rheumatic heart disease. Remember, however, that the failure pattern may also occur in patients with mitral insufficiency or aortic valve disease as well. These patients will have a LVC. If, however, the heart is of a pure LVC without any evidence of LAE, a primary left ventricular stress situation is present. This is similar to the case of the adult patient and results from a variety of causes.

These findings are summarized as follows:

1. PVO + LAE = obstruction at or proximal to the mitral valve (usually rheumatic).
2. PVO + LVC = primary left ventricular stress (of any cause) with failure.

CYANOTIC PATIENTS

In a cyanotic patient, the vascularity is never normal; it must be either decreased or increased. In this discussion, no attempt will be made to describe specific intracardiac lesions. The physiologic alterations produced by the lesions as manifest in the pulmonary vascularity will be stressed.

Cyanosis in the presence of decreased vascularity generally indicates the severe form of pulmonic stenosis. Once the observation of cyanosis and decreased vascularity is made, you must decide whether or not the heart size is normal. If the overall cardiac size is normal, even in the presence of evidence of specific chamber enlargement, the most likely abnormality is severe pulmonic stenosis plus VSD (tetralogy of Fallot) (Fig. 5.27).

A cyanotic patient with decreased vascularity and an enlarged heart is suffering from a complicated type of cardiac abnormality, usually severe pulmonic stenosis with an intact intraventricular septum. A shunt must be present to allow oxygenated blood to enter the circulation to permit survival.

If cyanosis is combined with shunt vascularity, an admixture lesion is present. In this situation, arterial and venous blood is mixed so that the aortic blood is oxygen desaturated. This occurs in persistent truncus arteriosus and complete transposition of the great vessels.

A cyanotic patient with a PVO pattern, particularly an infant, constitutes a medical emergency. The patient should be referred for immediate

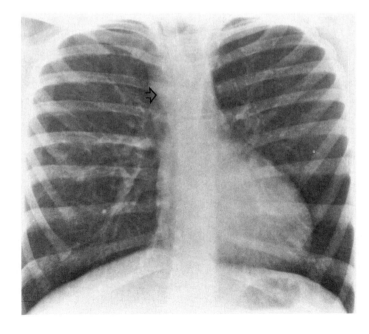

Figure 5.27. Tetralogy of Fallot. The overall heart size is normal. The pulmonary vascularity, however, is diminished. Note the right aortic arch (*arrow*).

sonography and cardiac catheterization to determine whether or not a correctable lesion is present. Most of the abnormalities found in this group of patients are complex.

The cyanotic patient is summarized as follows:

1. Cyanosis + decreased vascularity + "normal" heart size = severe pulmonic stenosis + VSD (tetralogy of Fallot).
2. Cyanosis + decreased vascularity + enlarged heart = severe pulmonic stenosis + intact ventricular septum.
3. Cyanosis + shunt vascularity = admixture lesion.
4. Cyanosis + severe PVO = severe complex abnormality—patient should be referred for emergency sonography and catheterization.

Chamber and Great Vessel Enlargements

The preceding sections considered the analysis of vascular patterns as the key to diagnosing congenital and acquired cardiac disease. At this point the radiographic appearance of specific chamber enlargements will be discussed briefly.

Left ventricular enlargement produces a downward and left bulge of the cardiac apex on the frontal film. In the lateral view, the image of the enlarged left ventricle is seen posterior to that off the inferior vena cava. Conditions that produce pure left ventricular enlargement were discussed in the previous section (Figs. 5.18 and 5.19).

Enlarged left atrium was also discussed previously (Figs. 5.17, 5.24, and 5.25). Right ventricular enlargement, when marked, may elevate the apex of the left ventricle. This produces the so-called "boot-shaped" heart (Fig. 5.27) on the frontal radiograph. On the lateral film, there is a loss of the retrosternal clear space.

Right atrial enlargement as an isolated finding is rare. It usually accompanies enlargement of the right ventricle and pulmonary arteries. Right atrial enlargement is suggested by prominence of the right cardiac border; the heart often has a box-like appearance as in the Ebstein anomaly (Fig. 5.28).

Main pulmonary artery enlargement produces bulging of the main pulmonary artery segment along the left cardiac border (Fig. 5.29). In addition, prominent right and left main pulmonary arteries may also be observed. Peripheral enlargements were discussed in the previous section.

Various portions of the aorta may enlarge, producing a prominence of that particular image. In addition, considerable tortuosity may occur in the descending aorta (Fig. 5.30).

Congestive Heart Failure

The vascular changes in congestive heart failure have been discussed. To reiterate, these include dilatation of the upper lobe vessels with contraction of the lower lobe vessels. In addition, there is enlargement of the cardiac silhouette in a poorly defined pattern. Although you may presume left ventricular enlargement, it is hard to specifically identify this in view of the "flabbiness" and poor contractility of cardiac muscles.

Associated findings of heart failure include interstitial and intraalveolar edema. Interstitial edema occurs when the left atrial pressure in-

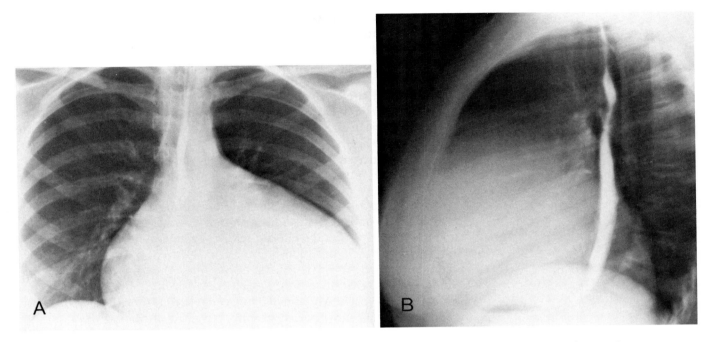

Figure 5.28. **Ebstein anomaly.** Frontal **(A)** and lateral **(B)** radiographs show massive cardiomegaly that is primarily right-sided.

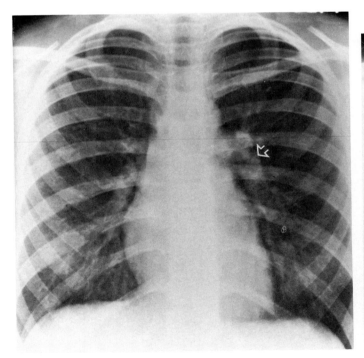

Figure 5.29. **Pulmonic stenosis in an adult.** There is prominence of the left pulmonary artery (*arrow*) secondary to the "jet phenomenon."

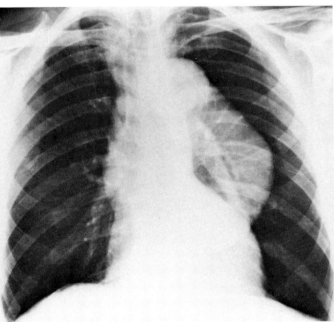

Figure 5.30. **Marked tortuosity of the descending aorta.** A subsequent arteriogram proved that the patient did not have an aneurysm.

creases and fluid transudes into the interstitial tissues, resulting in thickening of the interlobular septa. Kerley originally described these multiple linear densities and designated them according to their orientation:

1. *Kerley A lines* are long, thin, nonbranching linear densities obliquely directed toward the hilum.
2. *Kerley B lines*, the best known and most often observed, are thin, short, transverse lines best seen near the lung bases laterally at the costophrenic angle (Fig. 5.31).
3. *Kerley C lines* are in reality A and B lines oriented in an AP direction. On the frontal films, they appear as a fine reticular network.

Remember that all three types of lines represent edematous interlobular septa and not dilated lymphatic vessels.

Intraalveolar pulmonary edema results from further transudation of fluid into the air spaces, producing patchy, ill-defined, coalescent densities that radiate outward from the hilum. Sometimes this may have bat-wing- or butterfly-shaped distribution (Fig. 5.32). Air bronchograms often occur in this pattern. As with any alveolar process, the onset and clearing may be dramatic within a short period of time. Alveolar pulmonary edema may be asymmetric if the patient has been lying on one side before filming. The edema may also be mistaken for other causes of alveolar density such as pneumonia and hemorrhage. You should be careful to analyze the pulmo-

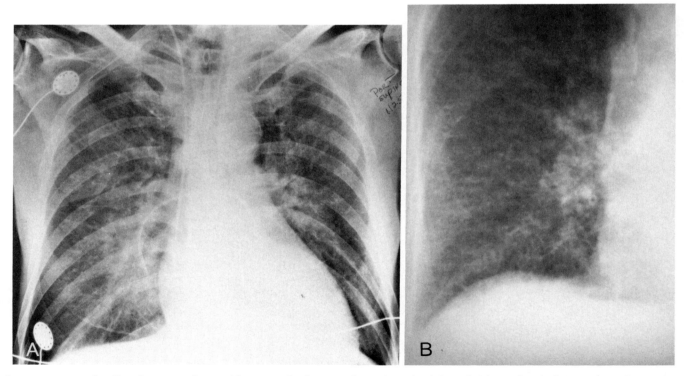

Figure 5.31.   Kerley lines in two patients with congestive heart failure. A, frontal radiograph shows pulmonary edema is present. Note the prominent intralobular septa (Kerley lines) throughout both lung fields. **B,** detailed view of another patient shows the prominent Kerly B lines.

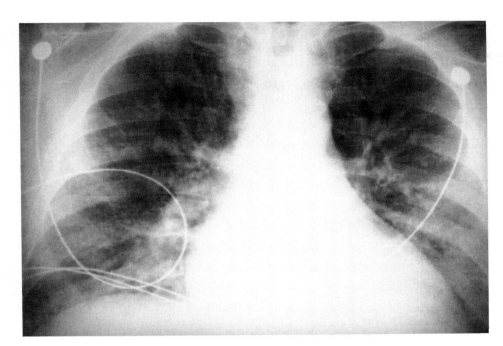

Figure 5.32. Alveolar pulmonary edema. The edema in this patient is primarily central. Note the engorgement of the pulmonary veins. There is left lower lobe consolidation as well.

nary vessels, if visible, and the cardiac size before making a diagnosis of alveolar pulmonary edema. Furthermore, edema may be present from another (noncardiac) etiology such as heroin intoxication, inhalation of noxious fumes, or drowning. In these conditions, the heart is usually normal in size.

Pleural fluid is another nonspecific finding that may be present in patients with congestive heart failure. If the fluid collects along a fissure, a *pseudotumor* (Fig. 5.33) may result. In the lateral view, the borders are generally tapering, and the collection of fluid is oriented in a slanted configuration. These densities disappear after successful therapy.

Pericardial Effusion

Pericardial effusion must always be considered when evaluating a patient with an enlarged heart. The diagnosis may be made by one or a combination of imaging studies. In general, a large heart of nonspecific configuration, particularly in the absence of pulmonary venous engorgement, should suggest a pericardial effusion (Fig. 5.34). Occasionally, the pericardium will be demonstrated in normal patients as a thin, dense line separated by layers of subepicardial and mediastinal fat. In patients with pericardial effusion, this line, which never should measure more than 2 mm, is thickened.

Cardiac fluoroscopy is a useful procedure for the diagnosis of pericardial effusion. A dampened cardiac pulse in the presence of an enlarged heart and no congestive heart failure suggests the condition. However, this is by no means pathognomonic, since a poorly contracting heart in a patient with a cardiac arrhythmia, a scarred myocardium, or an infiltrated myocardium will produce poor pulsations. A pulsating subepicardial fat

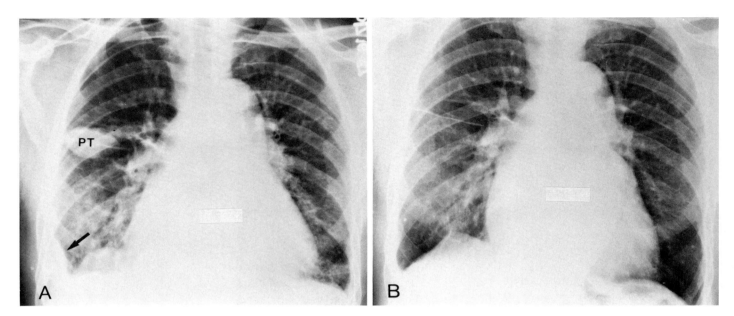

Figure 5.33. Pulmonary pseudotumor in a patient with congestive heart failure. A, frontal radiograph shows an oval density representing the pseudotumor (*PT*) along the minor fissure on the right side. There is loculation of pleural fluid in the right costophrenic angle (*arrow*). **B,** 4 days later, there has been improvement in the patient's cardiac status. The pseudotumor is no longer present. Note the change in the cardiac silhouette.

Figure 5.34. Pericardial effusion. There is massive enlargement of the patient's cardiac silhouette. An echocardiogram confirmed the presence of a large pericardial effusion.

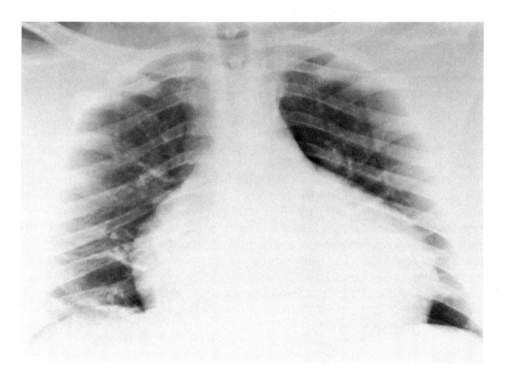

line within the immobile fluid band is, however, diagnostic of pericardial effusion.

Echocardiography is probably the most useful examination for detecting this condition and with the least risk to the patient. Ultrasonic shadows reflected off the pericardial and myocardial surfaces will demonstrate an abnormal collection of fluid in the pericardial sac (Fig. 5.3).

Computerized tomography scanning may be also used to diagnose pericardial effusion. A CT number near the density of water surrounding the heart ensures the diagnosis. This diagnosis is usually made as an incidental finding in patients studied for other reasons.

Trauma

Patients who have suffered severe thoracic trauma may have injury to the heart or great vessels. The most common mechanism for this is an accident in which the unrestrained driver of a motor vehicle strikes the steering wheel. Radiographically, the most common finding is a widened superior mediastinal shadow that is *fuzzy*. You should remember, however, that a supine radiograph in a large patient may simulate this appearance. With this in mind, you should make every effort to obtain an *erect film*. When this fails, and in the appropriate clinical setting, an aortogram should be obtained to rule out aortic injury (Fig. 5.35).

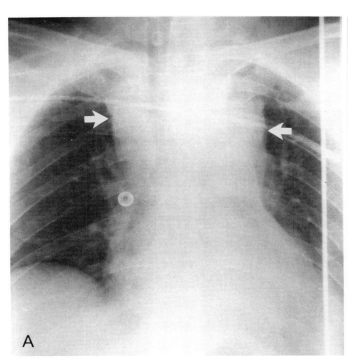
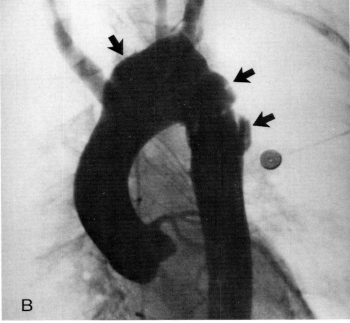

Figure 5.35. Posttraumatic aortic tear in an unrestrained driver. A, frontal view shows widening of the superior mediastinum (*arrows*). Note the tracheal deviation to the right. **B,** arteriogram shows the pseudoaneurysm (*arrows*). Note the irregular contour of the aortic arch.

Changes in the Chest with Aging

The normal aging process is reflected in visible changes on serial chest radiographs, including a change from a more horizontal to a vertical position of the heart from youth into adulthood, tortuosity of the aorta and brachiocephalic vessels, calcification within the aortic arch, and occasionally, increasing tortuosity of the descending aorta. These findings are illustrated in Figure 5.36. In addition, degenerative changes may be observed in the thoracic vertebrae. Postmenopausal women often demonstrate osteopenia and may, on occasion, show evidence of collapse of one or more

Figure 5.36. Age-related changes in cardiac silhouette in a patient with known hypertension. A, frontal radiograph shows mild left ventricular prominence. **B,** radiograph made 20 years later shows an increase in the size of the left ventricle. There is increased tortuosity of the descending aorta. There is also calcification of the descending aorta (*arrow*).

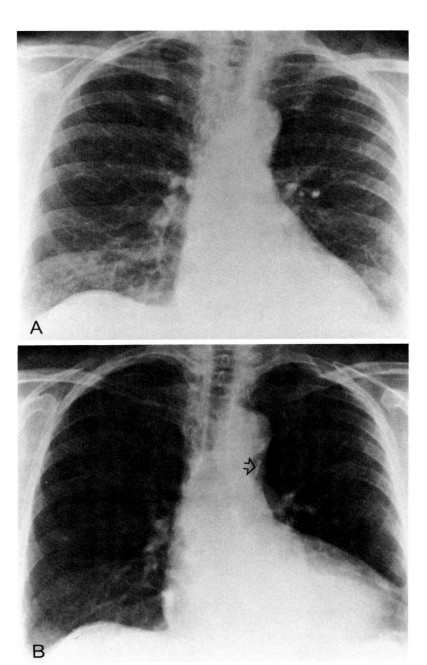

thoracic vertebrae. The lungs themselves may show little change with age. Hyperinflation, so-called senile emphysema, may sometimes occur. Scarring from subclinical pulmonary infections may be seen over both apices.

Summary

This chapter has attempted to analyze cardiac diseases based on the physiologic alterations they produce on chest radiographs. A logical analysis may be made by first observing the pulmonary vasculature. Combining the vascular findings with those of specific chamber enlargements allows the diagnosis of specific diseases. Specific attention was directed to chamber enlargement, congestive heart failure, pericardial effusion, trauma, and age-related changes in the chest.

Suggested Additional Reading

Chen JTT, Capp MP, Johnsrude IS, et al. Roentgen appearance of pulmonary vascularity in the diagnosis of heart disease. AJR 1971;112:559–570.

Elliott LP, ed. Cardiac imaging in infants, children, and adults. Philadelphia: JB Lippincott, 1991.

Gutierrez FR, Brown JJ, Mirowitz SA. Cardiovascular magnetic resonance imaging. St. Louis: Mosby Year Book, 1991.

Higgins CB. Essentials of cardiac radiology and imaging. Philadelphia: JB Lippincott, 1991.

Chapter 6

Breast Imaging

Breast cancer is a major cause of death from malignancy in American women. The American Cancer Society estimates that 1 of every 11 women will get cancer of the breast during her lifetime. The incidence is considered so common that every 15 minutes, three women develop breast cancer and one women dies of the disease. Fortunately, breast cancer can be diagnosed radiologically by the appropriate use of mammography at an early and highly curable stage. The appropriate use of mammography in conjunction with a clinical examination and breast self-examination in asymptomatic women over the age of 35 promises to significantly increase the cure rate for breast cancer. Indeed, screening with mammography and physical examination for breast cancer has been shown to lower the death rate by 30%. The following are guidelines established by the American Cancer Society and endorsed by the American College of Radiology regarding screening for breast cancer and the appropriate use of mammography.

Asymptomatic Women

1. Women 20 years of age and older should perform breast self-examination monthly.
2. Women aged 20 to 40 should, in addition, have a physical examination of the breasts every 3 years. Women over the age of 40 should have a physical examination of the breasts yearly.
3. Women aged 35 to 39 should have a baseline mammogram. Women aged 40 to 49 should have a mammogram performed every 1 to 2 years.
4. Women 50 years of age and over should have a mammogram yearly.

Symptomatic Women

1. Symptomatic women with a dominant breast mass, persistent discomfort, or nipple discharge, should have a thorough breast examination that includes mammography and any other diagnostic study (ultrasound) to determine if cancer is present. These studies should be performed regardless of the patient's age.

Further Recommendations

1. The American Cancer Society and the American College of Radiology further recommend that the mammographic technique employed produce the greatest anatomic detail and resolution possible.
2. These tests are to be provided with the lowest possible radiation dose needed to produce high-quality images. *Mammography should be performed and interpreted by experienced, well-trained individuals using modern, carefully monitored equipment.* All practices certified by the American College of Radiology conform with these high standards. The mammographic findings should be correlated carefully with thorough physical examination. However, there are limitations of mammography and the clinician must be aware of them. They should remember that the mammogram is a complementary procedure to physical diagnosis. If the physical examination reveals sufficient findings to warrant biopsy, such a biopsy should be performed even in the presence of a "normal mammogram."

The largest breast cancer screening project was performed by the American Cancer Society in conjunction with the National Cancer Institute in the 1970s under the Breast Cancer Detection Demonstration Project (BCDDP). In this study, more than 275,000 self-elected women were evaluated by physical examination and x-ray mammography at 27 centers nationwide. The results supported the value of mammography as a screening tool as well as a diagnostic method for detecting early breast cancer. Almost immediately after the study began, controversy developed regarding the safety of mammography because of the radiation dose involved. The controversy was based on several studies of women who had received extremely high doses of radiation to the breast in early childhood and who belonged to three separate populations: those exposed to the atom bombs of Hiroshima and Nagasaki, those women with tuberculosis who received repeated chest radiographs and fluoroscopic examinations, and a group of women who were treated with radiation for postpartum mastitis. The controversy spurred the development of improved machinery and improved screen and film products (low dose) to further decrease the radiation dose. Today, mammography is a safe diagnostic procedure when used by experienced personnel. For a more in-depth discussion on aspects of breast cancer, its detection, and the issue of radiation carcinogenesis, refer to the text by Kopans listed in the recommended additional readings.

TECHNICAL CONSIDERATIONS

As previously mentioned, x-ray mammography has been proven to have the greatest efficacy for detecting occult breast cancer. X-ray mammography is also used to localize a mass for surgical excision (Fig. 6.1). Diagnostic ultrasound is also used once a smooth-walled mass is detected to determine if it is cystic or solid (Fig. 6.2).

Several other imaging procedures have been used in the past to evaluate breast lesions. These include thermography, transillumination, and magnetic resonance (MR) imaging. Of the three, MR imaging appeared to show promise in the detection of breast lesions, particularly in view of the

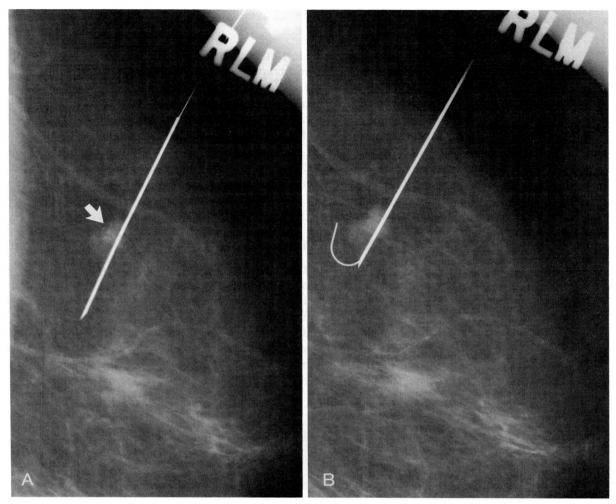

Figure 6.1. Use of mammography for needle localization. A, craniocaudad view shows a localizing needle placed through a breast mass (*arrow*). A guidewire is then placed through the needle. **B,** guidewire in place prior to needle removal. The surgeon will excise the area surrounding the end of the guidewire if the lesion cannot be palpated.

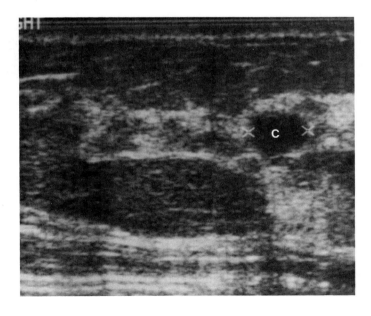

Figure 6.2. Breast sonography. There is a sonolucent area to the right of the midline representing a benign cyst (*C*). A larger area of mixed echo representing a cystic fibroadenoma is present in the middle of the figure.

cycle. The breast in the young woman is extremely dense and consists mostly of glandular tissue. This glandular tissue is even more dense in the lactating woman. The tissue also increases in density and size during the later part of the menstrual cycle. As a woman ages, the glandular tissue is slowly replaced by fat. Fortunately, breast cancer is most common in older women whose breasts contain larger amounts of fat.

PATHOLOGIC CONSIDERATIONS
Benign Lesions

There is a large variety of benign histologic changes that occur in the breast. Many of these changes likely represent variations of normal parenchyma relating to hormonal status. The term "fibrocystic disease" is a catchall category of changes that include the presence of cysts and benign fibrous solid tumors of the breast. The anatomy of the breast is such that a clinician palpating what is believed to be either a cyst or mass, in fact, may be feeling normal glandular tissue or fat surrounded by the fibrous stroma.

As a rule, benign lesions are round with smooth, well-defined margins (Figs. 6.5 and 6.6) and usually do not cause distortion of the normal

Figure 6.5. Benign fibroadenomas in a patient with advanced fibrocystic disease. Mediolateral view. A large dense lesion is present in the upper pole of the breast. A small lesion (*arrow*) is present deep to the main lesion. Note the prominent stromal pattern throughout the breast.

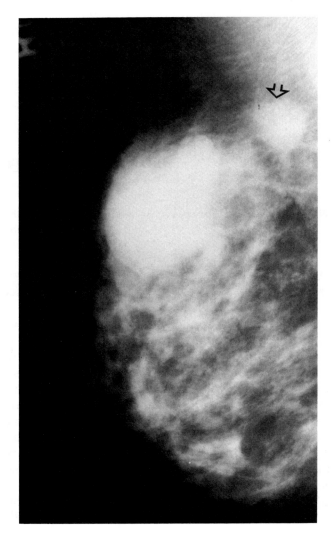

breast architecture. They are often multiple and bilateral. Calcifications, if they occur, are usually coarse and are easily detectable with the unaided eye (Fig. 6.7). Macrocysts are cystic dilatations of the lactiferous duct. The fluid contained within the cyst is of various colors. They are increasingly common in women in their mid-to-late thirties and are most commonly found in premenopausal years. They generally regress following menopause. Cysts are usually distinguishable from solid tumors by ultrasound (Fig. 6.8).

The most common solid benign tumor of the breast is the fibroadenoma. These tumors are hormonally sensitive and are found more commonly in young women. They are the solid lesions of the breast that undergo biopsy most frequently in women up to the mid-thirties. The reason for their frequent biopsy is the fact that they cannot be distinguished from well-circumscribed carcinomas, either by physical examination or

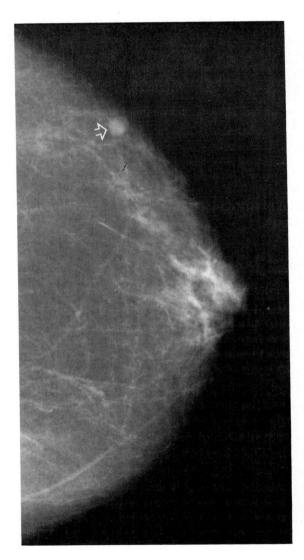

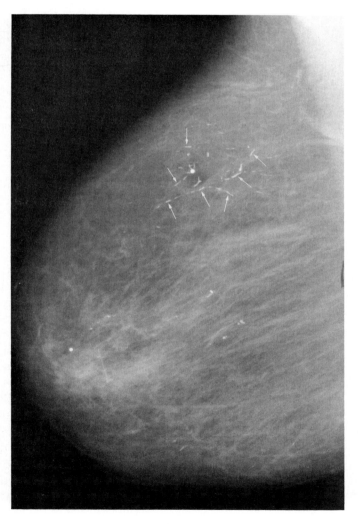

Figure 6.6.   Benign breast cyst (*arrow*). Note the smooth, well-defined margins.

Figure 6.7.   Calcified ducts (*arrows*). Fine linear calcifications are present in a branching pattern. There are more coarsened calcifications inferiorly.

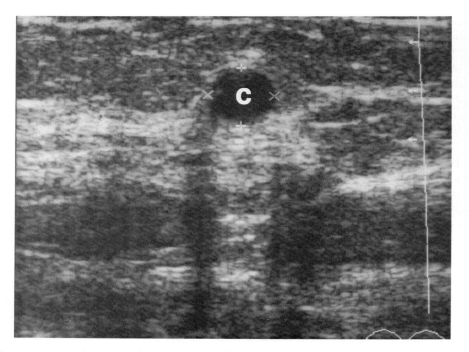

Figure 6.8.   Benign cyst (*C*) as seen on an ultrasound examination. The cyst is sonolucent and has no internal echoes.

imaging methods. Involution of fibroadenomas in postmenopausal women produces coarse calcifications.

Malignant Lesions

Ninety percent of breast cancer begins in the ductal epithelium. There is a large histologic variety of ductal carcinomas. Although the carcinoma may be confined within the ductal tissue, ultimately it will invade through the duct wall and spread via the lymphatic and vascular systems with resultant lymphatic and hematogenous metastases. The most common areas of lymphatic spread are to the axillary and substernal lymph nodes. If, at the time of detection, the axillary lymphatics are uninvolved, the 5-year survival is given as approximately 90%. This survival decreases to approximately 55% if axillary lymph nodes are involved.

The radiographic findings of malignancy are those of a mass with ill-defined or irregular margins (Fig. 6.9). Other signs include a lobulated margin (Fig. 6.10), distortion and invasion of surrounding parenchyma (Fig. 6.11), clustered microcalcifications (Fig. 6.12), asymmetric density, asymmetric dilated ducts, and nipple retraction. Skin thickening and retraction are frequently found late in the disease and result from the desmoplastic effect of the tumor on the ligamentous support of the breast. Finally, enlargement of axillary lymph nodes may also be detected in those patients in whom the carcinoma has spread beyond the breast.

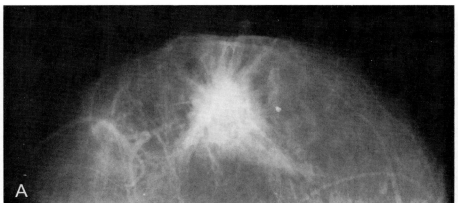
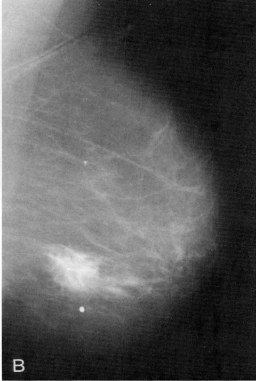

Figure 6.9. Breast carcinoma showing classic spiculated irregular margins. A, craniocaudad view shows distortion of normal breast parenchyma. **B,** mediolateral view with similar changes.

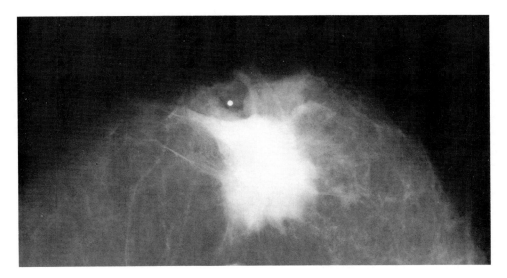

Figure 6.10. Breast carcinoma. Lobular margins and spiculated borders. Again, note the distortion of breast parenchyma anteriorly. The dense dot adjacent to the lesion is a marker placed by the technologist at the point the mass was palpated.

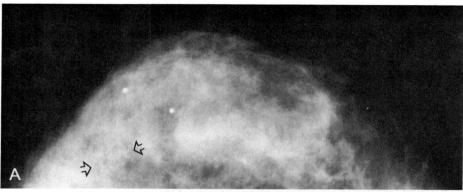

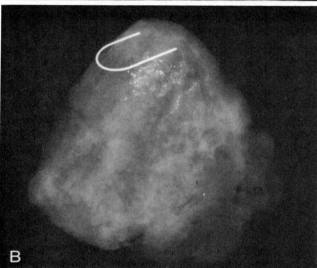

Figure 6.12.   Breast carcinoma with microcalcifications. A, craniocaudad view shows clustered microcalcifications (*arrows*). The lesion sits deeper to the palpable masses that are identified by the two small dense pieces of shot anteriorly. There is extensive fibrocystic disease present. **B,** mammogram of the surgical specimen. Localizing wire is present through the margin of the lesion. All the lesion has been excised.

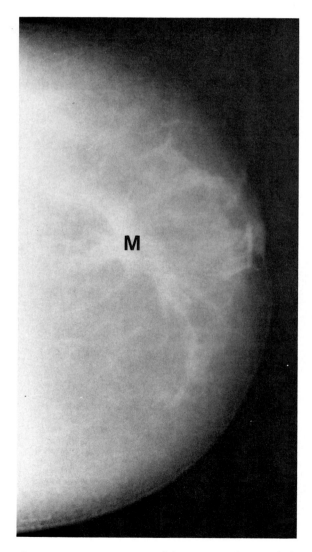

Figure 6.11.   Deep-seated breast carcinoma (*M*) with distortion of internal anatomy.

Summary

Breast cancer is one of the most common malignancies in women. The mortality may be diminished by self-examination, clinical examination, and x-ray mammography. A baseline mammogram should be obtained on all asymptomatic women aged 35 to 39. Women aged 40 to 49 should be studied every 1 to 2 years. Those women over the age of 50 should have yearly mammographic examinations. Mammography should be undertaken only by skilled technologists under the supervision of an equally qualified radiologist to produce an examination of high diagnostic quality and with a low radiation dose.

Suggested Additional Reading

Kopans DB. Breast imaging. Philadelphia: JB Lippincott, 1988.

Mitchell GW, Bassett L. The female breast and its disorders. Baltimore: Williams & Wilkins, 1990.

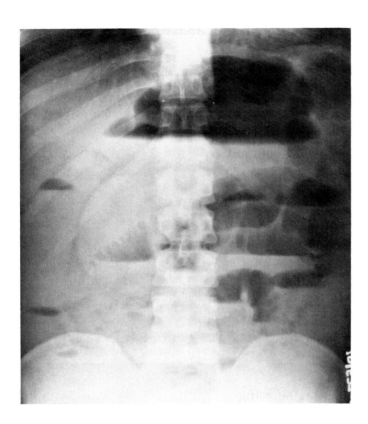

Figure 7.5.   Air-fluid levels in a patient with a small bowel obstruction. Note the dilatation of the air-filled loops.

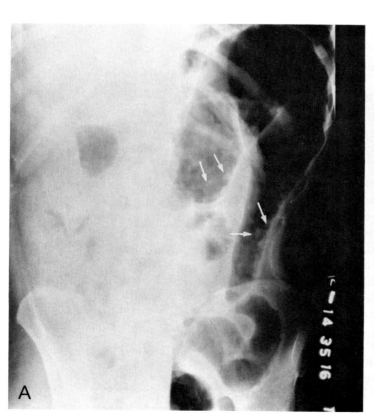

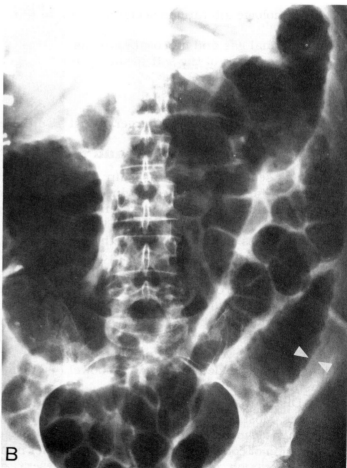

Figure 7.6.   Mucosal thickening in two patients with ulcerative colitis. A, pseudopolyps representing thickening area of pre-served mucosa are present throughout the bowel (*arrows*). **B,** note the thickened bowel wall on the left side (*arrowheads*).

tients following trauma (including surgery), with peritonitis, as a manifestation of drugs or bowel ischemia, and in chronically ill, bedridden patients.

A localized ileus seen persistently on serial films is suggestive of an adjacent area of inflammation. This occurs in pancreatitis (Figs. 7.7 and 7.8) and acute appendicitis, and is called a "sentinel loop."

Distended loops of bowel with air-fluid levels in a diffuse pattern is highly suggestive of a mechanical obstruction (Fig. 7.5). The typical pattern shows a distended cascade of loops proximal to the obstruction and an essentially gasless distal abdomen. The bowel loops frequently have a stepwise appearance or are of the hairpin (180° turn) type. *The presence of gas within the rectum does not rule out a low obstructing colonic lesion.* Gas may be introduced into the rectum by digital examination, colonoscopy, rectal temperature determination, and enemas. In an early obstruction, the characteristic pattern may not be well developed. However, serial films will show the development of the characteristic loops.

The cause of a mechanical obstruction will vary, depending on whether the patient is an adult or child. In the adult, common causes include adhesions, hernia, tumor (Fig. 7.9), and volvulus (Fig. 7.10). In infants and children, intussusception is a common cause of obstruction. In the newborn and very young infant, duodenal atresia and pyloric stenosis should be suspected.

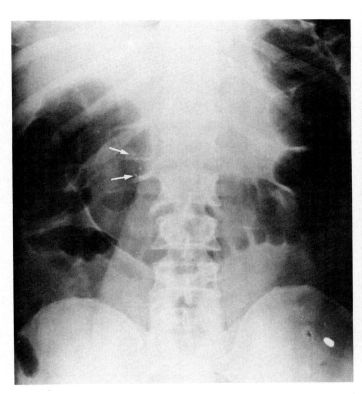

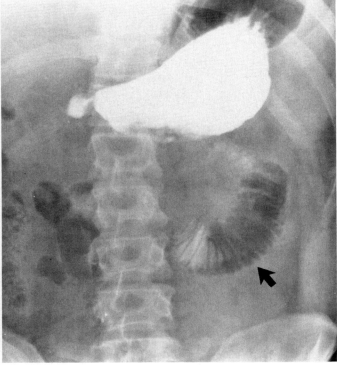

Figure 7.7. "Sentinel loop" of transverse colon in a patient with pancreatitis. Note the pancreatic calcifications (*arrows*). A bullet from a previous gunshot wound is present over the pelvis on the left side.

Figure 7.8. Small bowel "sentinel loop" in a patient with pancreatitis of the tail of the pancreas. A single dilated loop of jejunum (*arrow*) is present. Note the increased distance between the jejunum and the contrast-filled stomach as the result of pancreatic phlegmon.

Figure 7.9. Small bowel obstruction—supine view (same patient as Fig. 7.5). This supine view shows dilated air-filled loops of small intestine in a cascading pattern. This pattern is suggestive of bowel obstruction.

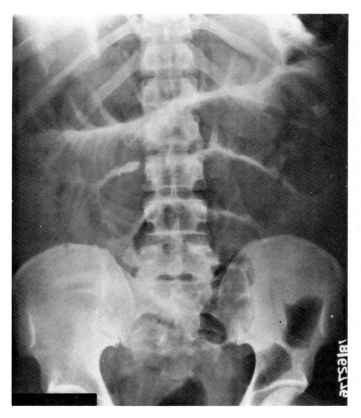

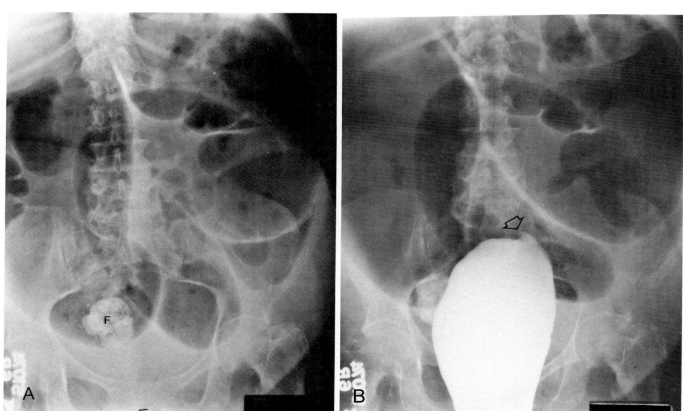

Figure 7.10. Sigmoid volvulus. A, supine abdominal film shows massive dilatation of the colon. Incidental note is made of a calcified uterine fibroid (*F*). **B,** barium enema shows the site of the volvulus (*arrow*).

The natural contrast between the soft tissues, the mucosa, and the air within the bowel allows evaluation of that bowel. A thickened bowel wall is abnormal. Mucosal thickening is generally present when the valvulae conniventes of the small intestine or the colonic haustra are thicker than 3 mm. If the bowel is distended with air, the actual (edematous) wall may be identified by air on one side and the increased soft tissue density on the other (Fig. 7.6). Thickened mucosa are most often encountered in inflammatory bowel disease (Fig. 7.6), bowel edema in hypoproteinemic and malabsorption states, submucosal hemorrhage of any cause, and ischemia. These last two conditions often produce two interesting patterns of mucosal thickening: thumb-like indentations in the gas-filled bowel ("thumbprinting") and a picket fence appearance of the valvulae in the small bowel called the "stacked coin" appearance. You cannot determine the exact etiology of the thickening without applying important history and physical examination findings. For example, a patient with a history of sudden onset of abdominal pain accompanied by blood-streaked diarrhea and dilated bowel on plain film is likely to have colitis (Fig. 7.6).

Extraluminal gas may be either free (pneumoperitoneum) or contained within an abscess cavity, the retroperitoneum, the wall of the bowel, or the portal venous or biliary systems of the liver.

Free intraperitoneal air in the absence of immediate previous surgery suggests a ruptured viscus. The most common cause is perforation of a peptic ulcer or a colonic diverticulum. Trauma is another cause. If the perforation is intraperitoneal, gas will be seen on an upright film collecting under both leaves of the diaphragm (Fig. 7.11**A**). Furthermore, decubitus positioning may demonstrate free intraperitoneal air (Fig. 7.1). However, it is possible to make the diagnosis of pneumoperitoneum based on a supine film from the "double wall sign" that results when air on both sides of the bowel outlines that structure rather distinctly (Fig. 7.11**B**). Under normal circumstances, you do not see the serosal surface of bowel because of its water density. Air within the peritoneal cavity, however, presents a change in radiographic density to outline the bowel wall.

Retroperitoneal air, particularly from a perforated duodenal ulcer or ruptured duodenum secondary to trauma, is often seen as a sharpening or enhancement of the psoas shadow. Occasionally, the renal image will be highlighted as well. This diagnosis may be difficult to make based on plain film. However, on CT scan, the presence of retroperitoneal air will be easily detected.

Gas loculated within the abdomen generally indicates the presence of an abscess. The air may be confined to a known anatomic space such as Morison's pouch beneath the liver, to an emphysematous gallbladder (Fig. 7.12), to the renal capsule, to the lesser sac, or within an organ (Fig. 7.13), or it may be free within the abdominal cavity. The gas may be a small localized collection or, more commonly, may have a mottled appearance. Frequently, it is necessary to do a contrast examination to determine the location of normal loops of bowel to rule out the presence of an aberrant loop of bowel being responsible for the abnormal shadow. The CT scan has proved quite reliable for the diagnosis of abscesses (Fig. 7.14).

Intramural air (pneumatosis intestinalis) may be seen in a variety of benign and pathologic conditions. A common cause of pneumatosis in older adults is microperforation of a diverticulum. Air appears as streaky

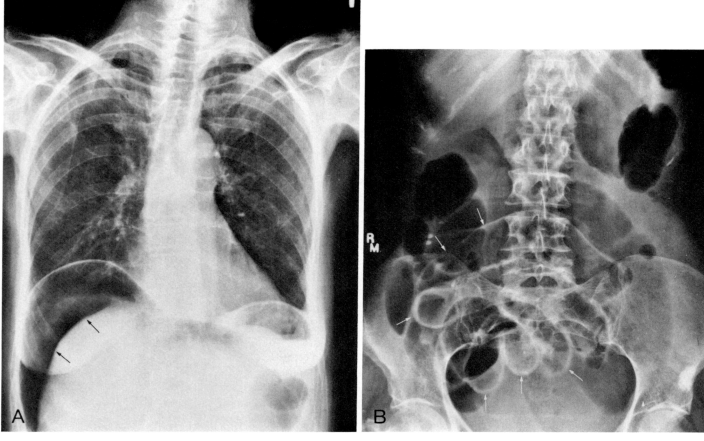

Figure 7.11.   Pneumoperitoneum. A, chest radiograph shows air beneath the diaphragm. The liver margin is outlined by air (*arrows*). **B,** a supine abdominal radiograph of this massive pneumoperitoneum shows air on both sides of the bowel wall (*arrows*).

**Figure 7.12.   Emphysematous cho-
lecystitis in a diabetic patient.** Gas outlines the gallbladder (*arrows*).

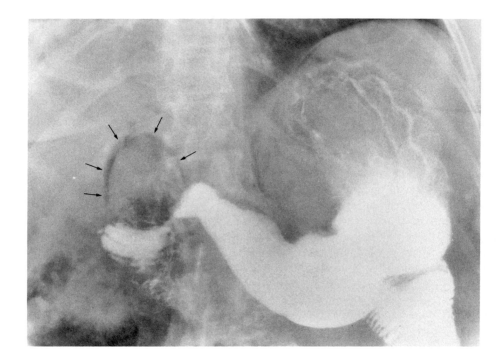

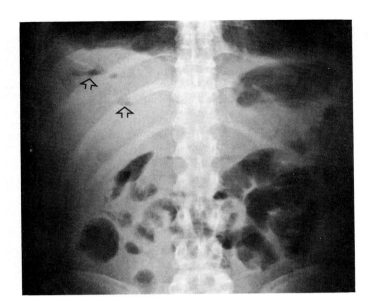

Figure 7.13. Liver abscess. There are collections of gas within the liver (*arrows*). A CT scan would be ideal for confirming the extent of the lesion.

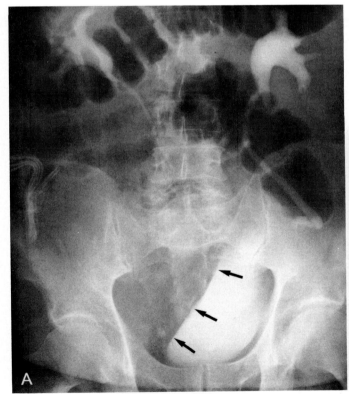

Figure 7.14. Left flank abscess. A, intravenous urogram shows displacement of the right ureter to the left by a large flank mass on the right. Note the flattening and compression of the right side of the bladder wall (*arrows*). **B,** CT scan shows the large abscess (*A*) compressing the right lateral wall of the bladder (*B*) (*arrows*).

densities surrounding the bowel (Fig. 7.15). Occasionally, a giant air cyst will occur. Intramural air may also be seen in the bowel infarction in older patients and particularly in premature newborn children with necrotizing enterocolitis (Fig. 7.16). In both these types of patients, gas may be seen in the liver within the portal system.

Air in the biliary tree may also be seen in infection or following surgery in which the common bile duct is anastomosed to the small bowel. Portal gas is usually located in the periphery, whereas biliary gas in seen more centrally. Correlation with the clinical findings is necessary for proper interpretation of this observation.

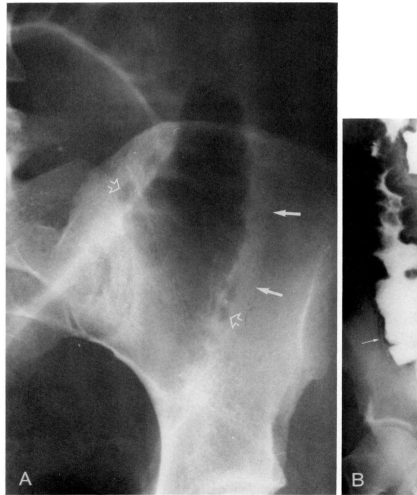

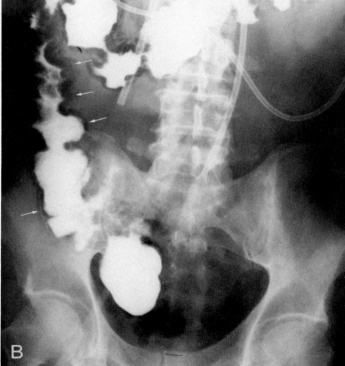

Figure 7.15. Pneumatosis intestinalis. A, detailed view of the left lower quadrant of a patient with ulcerative colitis. Note the thickening of the bowel wall (*solid arrows*). Note the gas within the bowel wall (*open arrows*). **B,** there is massive pneumatosis (*arrows*) in a patient with ischemic colitis.

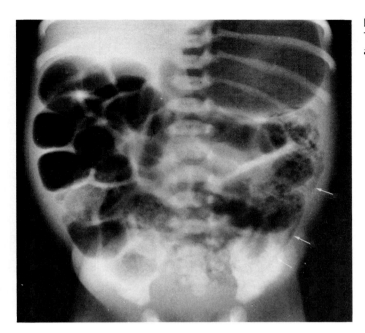

Figure 7.16. Necrotizing enterocolitis in a newborn child. There is pneumatosis intestinalis on the left side (*arrows*). The adult stool pattern is always abnormal in an infant.

Abnormalities of the Soft Tissue Shadows

Soft tissue abnormalities include displacements or misplacements, enlargement, presence of masses, and loss of margins. While CT and ultrasound examinations provide more detailed information regarding these abnormalities, the plain film can detect most of them. For example, abdominal abscesses produce plain film abnormalities in up to 70% of cases in the author's experience.

Enlargement of the abdominal organs may cause displacement of the other organs. For example, splenomegaly will displace the gastric air shadow medially (Fig. 7.17). Enlargement of the pancreas will cause anterior displacement of the stomach (demonstrated on an upper gastrointestinal series). An enlarged adrenal gland or tumor may displace the renal shadow inferiorly. Enlarged lymph nodes may displace the renal shadows laterally.

Certain congenital anomalies, particularly of the urinary tract, may result in abnormal position of the kidneys. In a patient with a horseshoe kidney, the lower poles are oriented toward the midline. A malposition of the kidney may result in the absence of the normal renal outline on the plain film, especially if the kidney is within the pelvis.

Masses within the abdomen may be seen either by themselves, or more frequently, by the displacements or distortion of normal viscera. The most common mass seen in the pelvis is a distended bladder. If you doubt the diagnosis, a repeat film should be made after the patient has successfully voided.

The loss of the margin of a soft tissue structure is a valuable sign in evaluating patients with abdominal disease. The loss of a renal outline or psoas margin (Fig. 7.18) generally indicates an inflammatory condition in

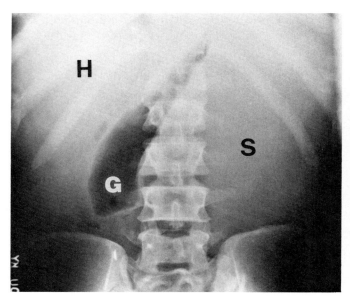

Figure 7.17.   Hepatosplenomegaly in a patient with Hodgkin's disease. Note the enlargement of the liver (*H*) and spleen (*S*). The gastric air bubble (*G*) is displaced to the right of midline.

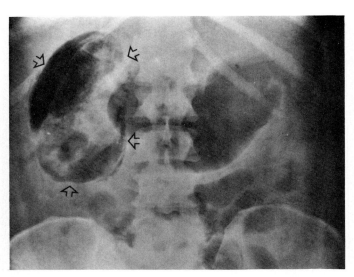

Figure 7.18.   Perinephric abscess in a diabetic patient. A large collection of air outlines the right kidney (*arrows*). The psoas margin is lost on the right.

the retroperitoneum. The loss of the psoas margin accompanied by scoliosis is a nonspecific finding that may be seen in acute appendicitis, urinary calculus, or perforated viscus. As mentioned previously, the loss of the properitoneal fat line may also be seen in several inflammatory conditions, particularly appendicitis.

Abnormal Calcifications

The list of calcifications that may be seen on abdominal plain film is quite long and beyond the scope of this text. However, there are certain benign or normal conditions that will produce calcifications frequently seen on abdominal plain films. These include the costal cartilages, vascular calcifications such as phleboliths in the pelvic venous plexus, atherosclerotic plaques of the aortoiliac vessels, prostatic calcifications, and old granulomas of spleen and lymph nodes. These are illustrated in Figure 7.19. Abnormal calcifications include biliary (Fig. 7.20) and urinary (Fig. 7.21) calculi, calcified aneurysms (Fig. 7.22), pancreatic calcifications (Fig. 7.23), calcified uterine fibroid tumors, and calcified appendiceal fecaliths (Fig. 7.24). In addition, foreign bodies may often be seen. These may include ingested foreign materials, e.g., tablets (Fig. 7.25), or traumatic foreign bodies, for example, bullets, buckshot, or shrapnel. You may, on occasion, see a patient with a self-introduced rectal foreign body (Fig. 7.26).

Abnormal Fluid: Ascites

The classic appearance of ascites has been described as diffuse, ground glass density of the abdomen. Generally by the time this has occurred, ascites is clinically apparent and need not be diagnosed by radio-

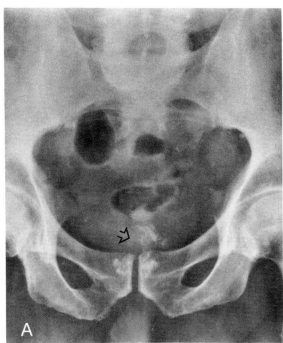

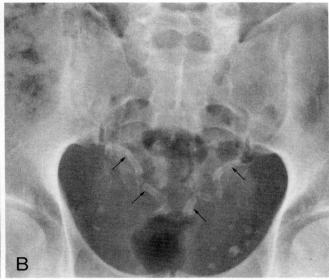

Figure 7.19. Physiologic calcifications. A, prostate (*arrow*). **B,** vasa deferentiae (*arrows*) in a diabetic man. **C,** abdominal aortic aneurysm (*arrows*).

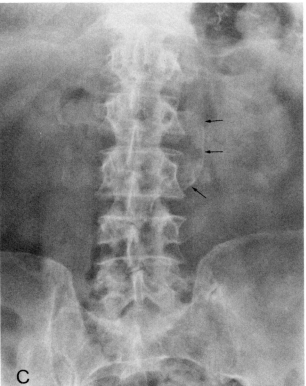

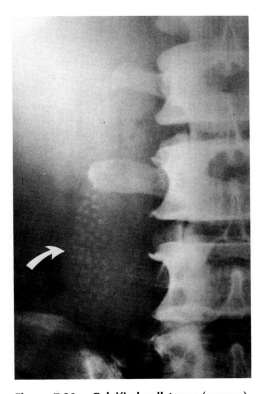

Figure 7.20. Calcified gallstones (*arrows*).

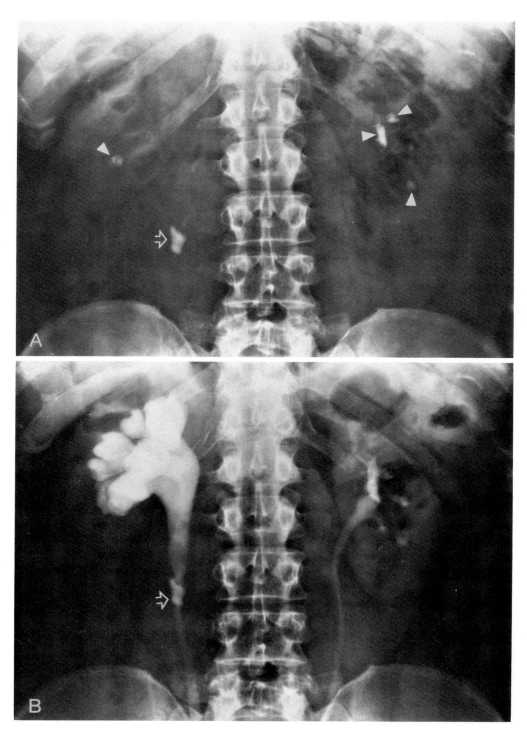

Figure 7.21.   Calcified urinary stones. A, plain film shows multiple intrarenal calculi (*arrows*). A large calculus adjacent to the transverse process of L-3 on the right (*open arrow*) is in the ureter. **B,** an intravenous urogram shows this calculus (*arrow*) to be partly obstructing the kidney and proximal ureter. Note the dilatation of the renal calycles, pelvis, and ureter on the right.

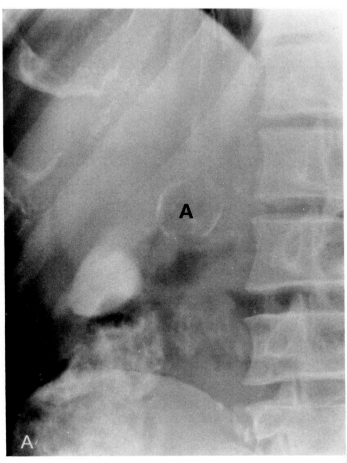

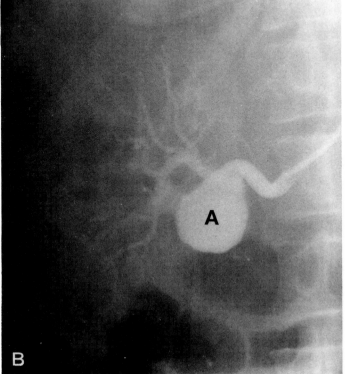

Figure 7.22.   Renal artery aneurysm. A, scout film from a cholecystogram shows the calcified aneurysm (*A*). **B,** a renal arteriogram shows the aneurysm to better advantage.

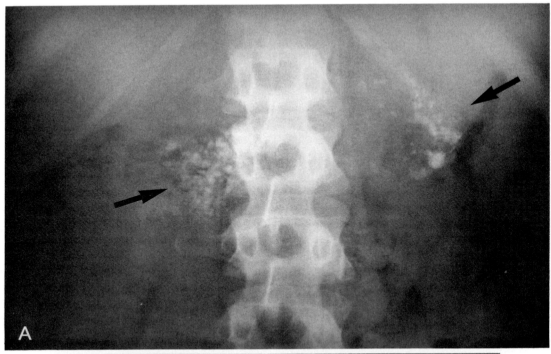

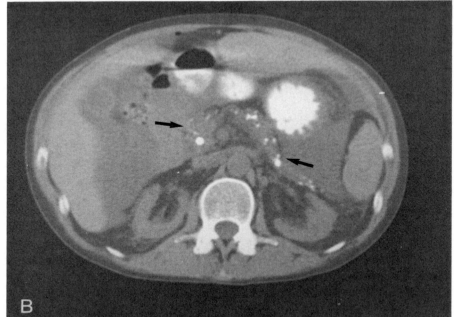

Figure 7.23.   Pancreatic calcifications (*arrows*). A, detail of a plain film. **B,** CT scan.

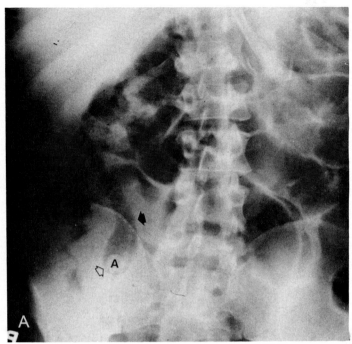

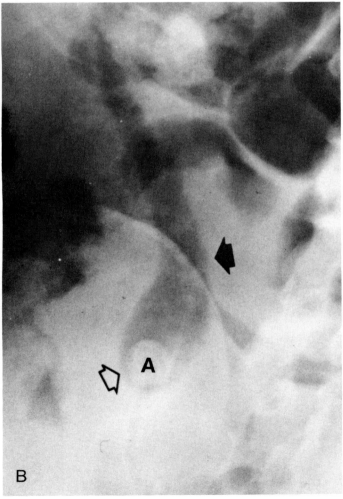

Figure 7.24. Appendicolith (*A*) (*open arrow*); in a gas-filled appendix (*closed arrow*). **A,** abdominal film. **B,** detailed view.

Figure 7.25. Ferrous sulfate tablets in the stomach (*arrow*).

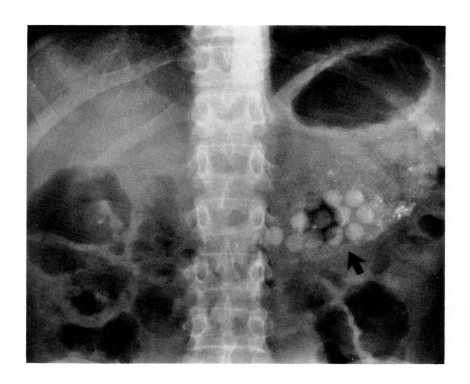

Figure 7.26. Rectal foreign body. The patient was "de-lighted" upon its removal.

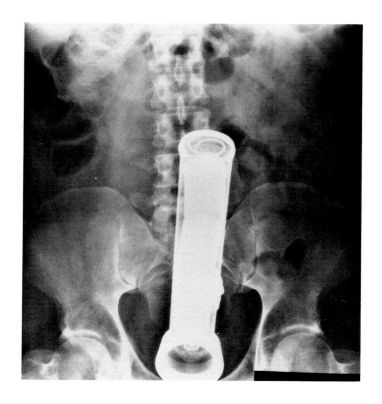

graphic means. However, small amounts of peritoneal fluid (ascites or blood) may appear in a subtle manner.

The accumulation of several hundred milliliters of ascitic fluid may be apparent on the supine film as a collection of water-density material overlying the sacrum above the bladder. This occurs because the fluid collects posteriorly in the pelvis. With increasing volume, however, the ascites extends superolaterally out of the pelvis, producing bilateral collections on either side of the main fluid bulk giving the appearance of "dog ears." Further increase in the amount of fluid (to over 500 ml) will extend up along the lateral gutters, displacing the colon medially from the radiolucent flank stripes (Fig. 7.27). As the amount of fluid increases, there is displacement of liver and spleen from the body wall. Finally, floating loops of bowel may be seen in the "sea of ascites." Computerized tomography and ultrasound are more useful in diagnosing ascites.

Postoperative Appearance of the Abdomen

It is important to recognize the signs of previous surgery in the abdomen. Wire sutures in the abdomen are one such indication. The position of the sutures or staples frequently can give an idea of what surgery was performed. For example, wire sutures extending obliquely from the midline toward the right flank may indicate that the patient has had biliary surgery. Other indications of surgery include metallic clips in the region of the esophagogastric junction from previous vagotomy or around blood vessels. If an organ has been removed, its image will no longer be present. Ostomy devices are easily demonstrated.

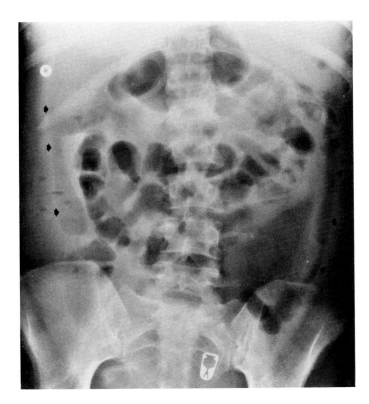

Figure 7.27. Ascites. Note the displacement of gas-filled bowel (*arrows*) from the flank stripe and clustering centrally.

Metallic clips in the abdomen or pelvis form valuable landmarks for evaluation of some diseases. In patients with known lymphomas the displacement of clips is an important indication of lymph node enlargement. Furthermore, displacement of clips or of a foreign body such as a bullet may provide clues to the diagnosis of an intraabdominal abscess.

Summary

The analysis of the abdominal plain film has been briefly discussed regarding normal appearances and pathologic alterations of those appearances. Recognition of the changes in the abdominal gas pattern and mucosal images are keys to proper diagnosis. Common conditions that manifest themselves on the plain film of the abdomen were discussed. The follow-up of suspected lesions with contrast examinations of both the gastrointestinal and urinary tract will be discussed in the following chapters.

Suggested Additional Reading

Frimann-Dahl J. Roentgen examinations in acute abdominal diseases. 3rd ed. Springfield, IL: Charles C Thomas, 1974.

Margulis AR, Burhenne HJ, eds. Alimentary tract radiology. 4th ed. St. Louis: Mosby Year Book, 1989.

Chapter 8

Gastrointestinal Imaging

Gastroenterology, like radiology, has undergone significant technical and therapeutic changes in the past 20 years. As often happens, technical advances in one specialty radically change another. Three such developments have changed the way physicians evaluate the gastrointestinal (GI) system.

The first of these developments was the perfection of and improvements in flexible fiberoptic endoscopy. Endoscopic evaluation of the stomach, duodenum, and colon has resulted in a significant decrease in the number of contrast studies of the GI tract. However, improvements in double contrast techniques themselves have improved radiologic diagnostic accuracy.

The second advance was the emergence of computerized tomography (CT). This allowed noninvasive detection of hepatic and pancreatic (Fig. 8.1) abnormalities as well as detection of traumatic solid visceral rupture. Furthermore, CT made guided-needle biopsy possible.

The third advance was the improvement in diagnostic ultrasound technology. The use of ultrasound resulted in a decrease in the number of oral cholecystograms performed and eliminated intravenous cholecystography completely. Furthermore, ultrasound is now a vital component for biliary lithotripsy, the fragmentation of gallstones using sound waves.

The real impact of these newer imaging forms can be best appreciated when one considers how we evaluated many intraabdominal lesions 20 years ago. Although intrinsic lesions of the GI tract have always been evaluated by contrast examinations and subsequently by endoscopy, the evaluation of suspected masses within the abdomen was also evaluated by studies that would show *the effect of the mass* on surrounding organs by detecting their displacement when filled with barium or some other contrast. Furthermore, once a mass was detected, angiography was then employed to determine if there were any parameters that suggested malignancy. Diagnostic ultrasound and CT as well as magnetic resonance (MR) in the last decade have afforded us an opportunity to identify the masses themselves rather than their secondary effects.

Figure 8.1.   Pancreatic pseudocyst. A CT scan shows the pseudocyst in the tail of the pancreas (*arrows*) adjacent to the spleen.

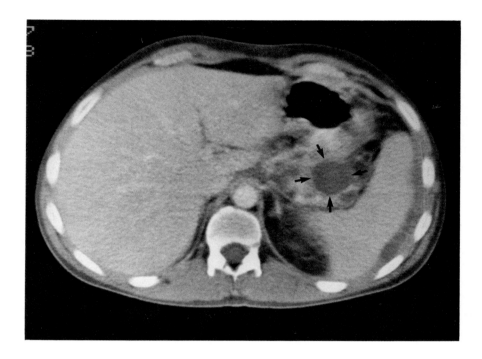

Although plain films of the abdomen are a valuable preliminary diagnostic study, it is necessary to opacify the gastrointestinal tract with contrast material to determine the presence of intrinsic abnormalities. There are four examinations used for primary evaluation of the gastrointestinal tract: upper gastrointestinal (upper GI) tract examination, small bowel "follow-through," barium enema, and occasionally the oral cholecystogram. Ancillary studies such as CT scanning, ultrasound, magnetic resonance imaging, endoscopic retrograde cholangiopancreatography, and angiography are particularly useful for examining the liver and pancreas.

TECHNICAL CONSIDERATIONS

The optimal way to study any hollow viscus filled with contrast material is to have that viscus completely empty of any other contents. For examination of the upper GI tract, an overnight fast is usually sufficient to produce this effect. Food within the stomach after a documented overnight fast is abnormal and usually indicates gastric outlet obstruction (most often secondary to peptic ulcer disease). In this situation, the stomach may be studied after passing a nasogastric tube and suctioning out the remaining contents.

Obtaining a clean colon is quite a different matter. Many preparations have been used to cleanse the colon of most of its contents. These include laxatives, enemas, and flushing by ingestion of massive quantities of fluids. In most patients, the use of laxatives the night prior to study and a cleansing enema the morning of the study will produce the desired results. These measures may have to be more vigorous during hot summer months when fluid loss through the skin hampers osmotic effects of many types of bowel preparation. Furthermore, any barium left from a previous examination should be removed. The degree of bowel cleanliness can be determined by a scout (plain) film of the abdomen. *Patients who are suspected of having toxic megacolon, acute ulcerative colitis, or obstruction should not have cleansing enemas.*

There is a logical order in which studies of the GI tract should be performed. Oral cholecystography, barium enema, and upper GI examination may be performed on the same day, in that order. The idea is to do the study that requires the greatest amount of clarity in the abdomen prior to the introduction of any additional contrast material. An upper GI series may be performed immediately after barium enema if the patient has evacuated the colon adequately. If the patient is to have an intravenous urogram or an arteriogram, it is best done prior to a barium contrast examination.

It is important for the clinician to give as much clinical information as possible to the referring radiologist. The request should always contain pertinent information and a tentative diagnosis. The radiologist should question the patient and ask about symptoms necessitating the examination. It is remarkable, however, that many patients are sent for examination without knowledge of why they are being studied or with minimal or no complaints referable to the area for which examination has been requested!

The clinician should also inform the patient that the radiologist will send the results of the examination to him or her and that he or she (the clinician) will notify the patient of the findings. This removes the radiologist from the position of reporting serious findings to a patient he or she may not know well. Radiologists should make it a practice to inform patients when a study is normal, since most patients are apprehensive about the condition for which they are studied. Quite often, they will not see their referring physician for several hours or perhaps days or weeks following the examination. To make patients worry that they may have cancer or some other serious illness when the study is normal is simply not in their best interest.

Under normal circumstances, two modes of radiographic recording are used, fluoroscopy and radiography. Fluoroscopic examination is important to determine the motility of the GI tract (peristalsis) as well as to position the patient so that all parts of the organs being studied are examined. Spot films are usually taken of strategic areas using direct fluoroscopic control: esophagogastric junction, duodenal bulb area, flexures of the colon, ileocecal area, and rectosigmoid colon. The exact number and variety of spot films will vary from examiner to examiner. Furthermore, if an abnormality is found at fluoroscopy, addition spot films are taken. Occasionally, the fluoroscopic portion of the examination is recorded on videotape for later playback and evaluation. Following the fluoroscopic portion of the study, overhead films are taken with the patient in various positions for further delineation of whole organs such as the stomach or colon.

The preferred method for routine study is to use a thicker preparation of barium and to distend the colon or stomach with gas (air-contrast study). In the first situation, air is introduced through the rectal tube. In the second, a gas-releasing preparation is ingested with the oral barium. The resulting study gives very fine detail, which is often sufficient to reveal subtle abnormalities. Often these studies are performed following pharmacologic enhancement, using glucagon to stop peristalsis and to relax spastic bowel.

Oral cholecystography is performed in much the same way, the morning after the patient ingests the contrast material. Spot films are made of the gallbladder with the patient in the upright and recumbent positions to look for the presence of gallstones. This technique is often repeated after the patient has ingested a fatty meal or has been injected with a cholecystokinin-like drug (Sincalide) to produce contraction of the gallbladder.

Ultrasound is used frequently to evaluate patients with suspected biliary and pancreatic disease. The examination is a reliable noninvasive method with a high degree of accuracy. Furthermore, the study may be performed following cholecystokinin enhancement. It has largely replaced oral cholecystography.

Similarly, abdominal CT examinations are commonly used in studying patients with jaundice, pancreatic disease, and suspected hepatic metastases. Many studies have shown the complementary nature of CT with ultrasound in evaluating patients suspected of having pancreatic or biliary disease (Fig. 8.1). Ultrasound is the less expensive screening procedure. A

Figure 8.2. Mesenteric arteriogram in a patient with lower gastrointestinal bleeding. Delayed film shows a "stain" of contrast (*arrow*) at the site of a bleeding diverticulum in the descending colon.

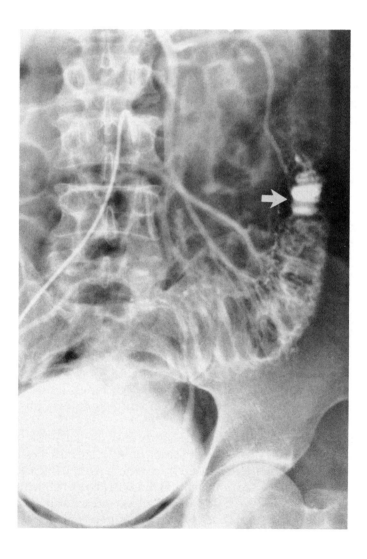

CT scan provides more definitive information, particularly in pancreatic disease. Intravenous contrast enhancement is a common adjunct to CT.

Angiography is used to evaluate the gastrointestinal tract primarily for diagnosis and therapy in patients with acute gastrointestinal hemorrhage wherein a bleeding site may be localized by selective catheterization of celiac or mesenteric branches and vasopressor infused to control or stop the bleeding (Fig. 8.2). Angiography is also used to evaluate patients with portal hypertension prior to contemplated shunt surgery and in mapping hepatic metastases if partial hepatectomy is considered.

Percutaneous cholangiography with the thin-walled (Chiba) needle is used by radiologists to study patients with obstructive jaundice. Contrast material injected through the needle, which has been placed in a dilated biliary duct, is used to localize the site of the obstruction (Fig. 8.3). Following this, a catheter may be inserted for percutaneous decompression and drainage.

Endoscopic retrograde cholangiopancreatography (ERCP) is a procedure in which ampulla of Vater is cannulated under direct endoscopic control. The examination takes a skilled endoscopist and is of some discomfort to the patient. Following cannulation, contrast material is injected into the ductal system, and fluoroscopic spot films and overhead films are made. Following this procedure, a stent or drainage catheter may be left in place. The endoscopist also can perform a papillotomy. An endoscopic retrograde cholangiopancreatography is usually performed by a gastroenterologist.

There are two types of nuclear imaging studies used to investigate abnormalities of the gastrointestinal tract: biliary scans and scans for bleeding Meckel's diverticulum. The biliary scan uses ^{99m}Tc-labeled imidodiacetic acid to investigate obstruction to the biliary tract. The agent is

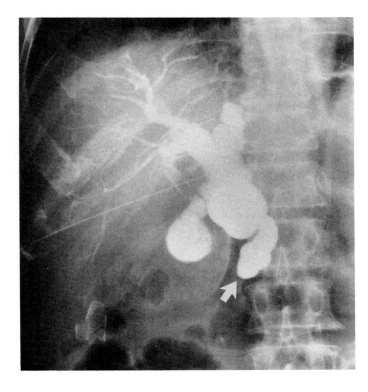

Figure 8.3. Percutaneous transheaptic cholangiogram shows massive dilation of the common bile duct and hepatic ducts in this patient with obstruction near the distal common bile duct (*arrow*). This was subsequently percutaneously decompressed with a catheter.

administered intravenously, thence is removed by the liver from the blood and concentrated in bile. Under normal circumstances, the agent can be detected in the gallbladder within 10 to 60 minutes of administration (Fig. 8.4). It is excreted through the common bile duct into the duodenum within 45 minutes. Any obstruction of the cystic duct will prevent the agent from entering the gallbladder (Fig. 8.5). It is also useful for diagnosing bile leaks following biliary surgery and for differentiating acute calculous obstruction from chronic obstruction due to neoplasm. In acute cholecystitis it has a 95% positive and negative predictive value.

^{99m}Sodium-pertechnetate-labeled red cells are used to investigate bleeding Meckel's diverticulum, a common congenital malformation of the ileocecal region. Although the majority of these diverticula are asymptomatic, most contain gastric mucosa that results in occasional bleeding. The isotope-labeled red cells are injected intravenously and the lower abdomen is scanned to find concentrated areas of activity that would represent the bleeding site (Fig. 8.6). This method will detect bleeding of as little as 0.1 ml/min flow.

Magnetic resonance imaging has limited applications for evaluation of the GI tract. It is used primarily to evaluate the liver and, to a lesser extent, the pancreas. The reason MR is not used more frequently is that motion artifacts from respiration, aortic pulsations, and peristalsis adversely affect the image. The MR studies may be augmented by intravenous use of gadolinium-DTPA, a paramagnetic contrast agent.

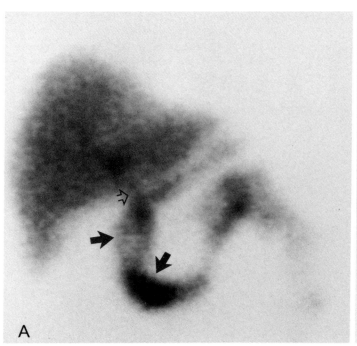

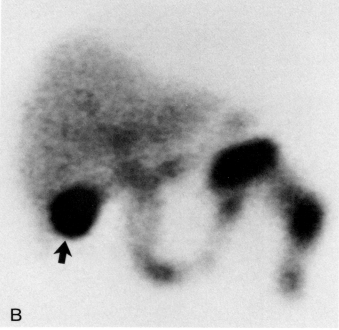

Figure 8.4.   Normal ^{99m}Tc-labeled imidodiacetic acid biliary scan. A, 30 minutes following injection, the isotope is being excreted by the liver through the common bile duct (*open arrow*) into the duodenum (*closed arrows*). **B,** at 60 minutes, the isotope is seen in the gallbladder (*arrow*).

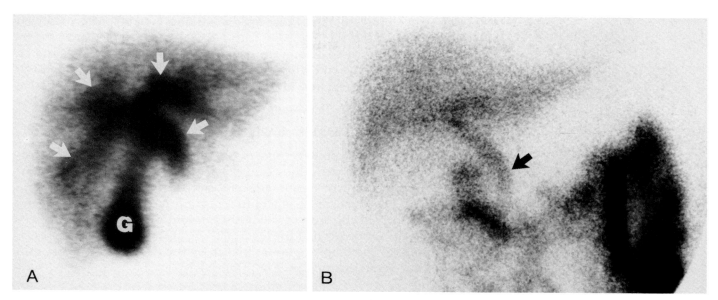

Figure 8.5.   Abnormal ⁹⁹ᵐTc-labeled imidodiacetic acid biliary scans. A, common duct stone. Ninety minutes following injection, the isotope is in the liver and gallbladder (*G*). There is no excretion into the duodenum. Note the dilated biliary tree (*ar-* *rows*). **B,** acute cholecystitis from cystic duct stone. There is no gallbladder filling at 60 minutes. The isotope passes freely into the duodenum through the common bile duct (*arrow*).

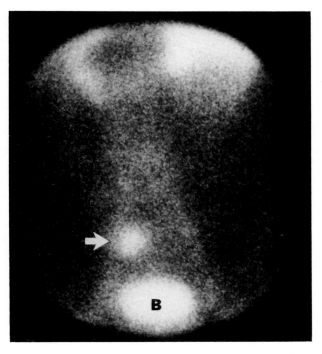

Figure 8.6.   Bleeding Meckel's diverticulum. There is increased isotope concentration in the ileocecal region (*arrow*) due to bleeding. *B,* bladder.

Before deciding which of these special studies is to be performed, you should thoroughly discuss the case with a diagnostic radiologist to determine the optimal study to do and the order in which the studies should be performed. In this way, you will save time between making the diagnosis and beginning treatment and eliminate more costly and less productive studies.

ANATOMIC CONSIDERATIONS

It is important for you to recognize the normal anatomy of the gastrointestinal tract and the variations that may occur. For example, six indentations may be seen on the esophagus as it courses from the pharynx into the abdomen. The uppermost is the indentation of the cricopharyngeus muscle posteriorly at the level of C-6. Other indentations occur at the thoracic inlet, at the aortic arch at the level of T4-5, at the left mainstem bronchus, proximal to the diaphragmatic hiatus by the descending aorta, and at the esophagogastric junction (Fig. 8.7).

Figure 8.7. Normal esophagus. There is a small amount of air present in the upper esophagus. Note the indentation at the level of the aortic arch.

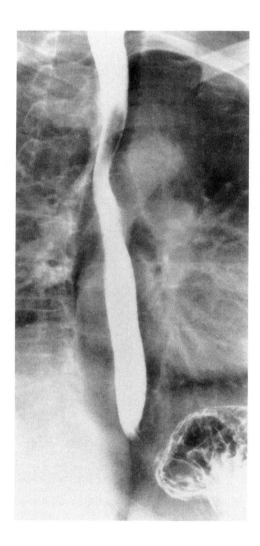

The stomach may assume a variety of positions, lying either vertically or horizontally within the abdomen. This depends mainly on the patient's body habitus. The radiologic anatomy of the stomach includes the fundus, body, antrum, prepyloric region, and pylorus (Fig. 8.8). The gastric mucosa (rugae) appears as linear parallel folds extending along the length of the stomach (Fig. 8.9). There is wide variation in the size of the rugae.

The duodenum begins at the pylorus. The first portion is the bulb, which appears as a triangular-shaped structure with the base toward the pylorus. The duodenum then sweeps downward (the second or descending portion), curves medially (third portion), and twists back upward (fourth portion), terminating at the ligament of Treitz. Occasionally, on a normal duodenal examination, a small indentation representing the ampulla of Vater may be observed along the medial border of the descending portion.

The jejunum begins at the ligament of Treitz, gradually merging with the ileum, which enters the cecum via the ileocecal valve. Usually, it is possible to differentiate jejunum from ileum by the mucosal pattern. In normal individuals, the cecum is in the right lower quadrant of the abdomen. The appendix usually projects downward from the cecum. Usually the ileocecal valve is on the medial aspect of the cecum.

The colon ascends, forming two loop-like structures in the right and left upper quadrants known as the hepatic and splenic flexures, respectively. The descending colon terminates in the sigmoid colon, which is

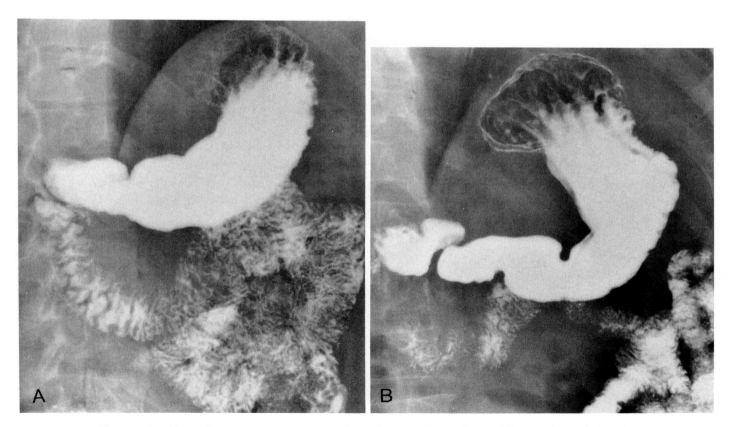

Figure 8.8. Normal stomach, duodenum, and proximal small bowel. A and **B** show the variations in normal appearance in two different patients.

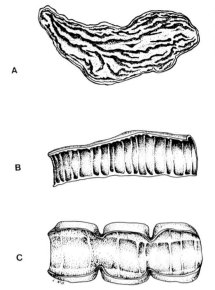

Figure 8.9. Normal mucosal patterns. A, stomach. **B,** small intestine. **C,** colon.

often quite redundant, particularly in older patients. The sigmoid colon continues on to the rectum (Fig. 8.10). Under normal circumstances, the rectum can be distended with barium greater than half the distance between the walls of the pelvis.

In addition to assessing the anatomy of the GI tract, we must also concern ourselves with its physiology, that is, the motility. The causes of motility disorders are varied and complex. It is sufficient to say here that under normal circumstances in the esophagus, one should observe a stripping wave propagating a bolus of barium in a smooth, progressive motion. Peristalsis continues in the stomach from the fundus extending down to the pylorus. In the duodenum, peristalsis is slightly different. The stripping motion found in the esophagus and stomach is not present. Instead, there is distension of the duodenal bulb, which opens at its apex and contracts forcibly as a unit moving the bolus through. Propulsive contractions are observed throughout the small intestine and colon.

In the colon there are several areas of normal or physiologic narrowing that may occur with spasm. These are found in the transverse colon near the flexures and in the descending colon.

When encountering spasm of the GI tract, particularly in the colon, it is sometimes useful to perform a pharmacologically enhanced study.

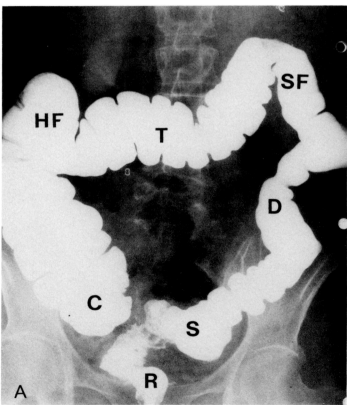
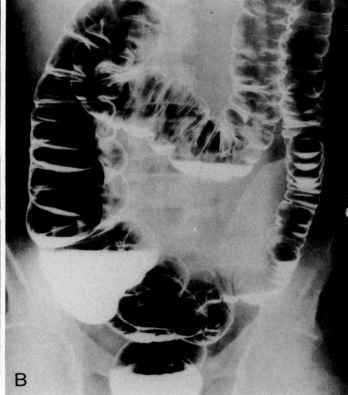

Figure 8.10. Normal barium enema. A, single contrast. *C,* cecum; *HF,* hepatic flexure; *T,* transverse colon; *SF,* splenic flexure; *D,* descending colon; *S,* sigmoid colon; *R,* rectum. **B,** double contrast.

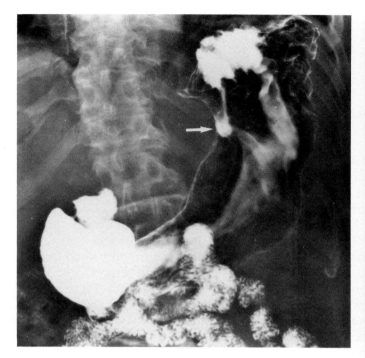

Figure 8.11. Double contrast upper GI in a patient with a lesser curvature gastric ulcer (*arrow*). Note the folds radiating into the ulcer crater.

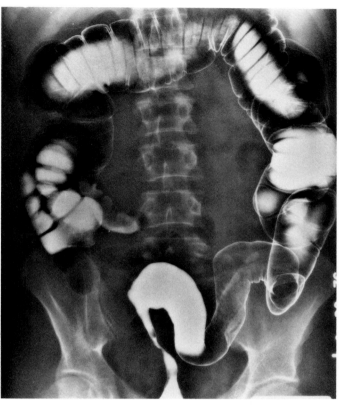

Figure 8.12. Air contrast barium enema in a patient with ulcerative colitis. Note the narrowing of the rectum and sigmoid.

Glucagon injected intravenously in 0.5 to 2 mg doses will produce relaxation of the GI tract through its antivagal action. Other drugs that have been used, although with more side effects, include atropine, 0.5 to 1 mg, and propantheline (Pro-Banthine), 15 to 60 mg. These agents may also be used to produce relaxation of the GI tract for double contrast examinations (Figs. 8.11 and 8.12), which assist in the delineation of subtle abnormalities.

PATHOLOGIC CONSIDERATIONS

Because the GI tract is a tube, pathologic alterations found in one segment will appear identical when encountered in any other segment. For example, a mucosal tumor of the esophagus has an appearance identical to a similar-sized tumor of the stomach, small intestine, or colon. The incidence of these lesions will vary from location to location, and you must learn the common locations of these lesions in the particular organs. However, do keep in mind that for practical purposes, these lesions all have similar appearances, no matter where they occur. (Using the same concept, a broad generalization may be made that similar-appearing lesions are also found in other tubular structures such as the urinary tract, bronchi, and blood vessels.)

There are six basic alterations we can recognize:

1. Polypoid lesions
2. Mucosal masses
3. Ulceration
4. Diverticula
5. Extrinsic compression
6. Benign strictures

These are illustrated in Figure 8.13.

In addition, motility disorders and dilatation may be encountered in any portion of the GI tract.

Polypoid lesions appear as small, rounded, filling defects in the lumen. They may be broad-based (sessile) (Fig. 8.14) or on a stalk (pedunculated) (Fig. 8.15). They are true mucosal lesions, and when observed end-on, their outer margins are indistinct, being obscured by surrounding barium. In contrast, diverticula profiled end-on have discernible outer margins but indistinct inner margins. This is illustrated in Figure 8.16.

Mucosal masses frequently begin as small polyps. As the polyp enlarges, its surface may become irregular. Puckering may occur near the base of the lesion. There is an abrupt change of the mucosa from normal to tumor (Fig. 8.17). Further growth will produce encasement as the tumor grows completely around the lumen, producing the classic "apple-core" appearance (Fig. 8.18).

There are two other varieties of "filling defects" that may be observed in the GI tract: mucosal hypertrophy (Fig. 8.19) and varices (Fig. 8.20). With both these entities, it is important not to misinterpret them as a tumor.

Ulceration of the GI tract results in a collection of barium being found outside the normal lumen. Quite frequently the ulcer is surrounded by an edematous ulcer collar or mound. In benign ulcers, particularly of the stomach, mucosal folds may be observed radiating into the ulcer crater.

Figure 8.13. Schematic drawing illustrating pathologic alterations affecting the gastrointestinal tract. Top row, gross appearance; bottom row, radiographic appearance.

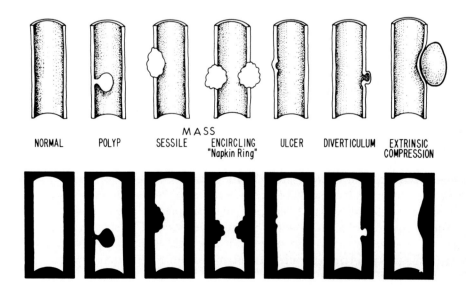

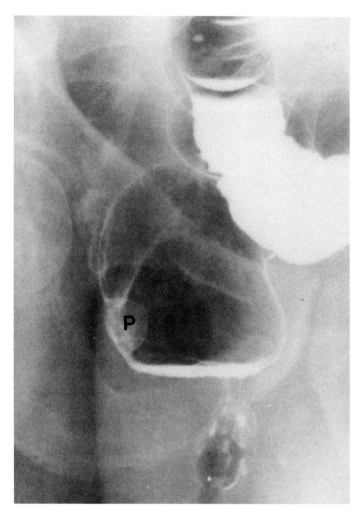

Figure 8.14. Sessile polyp (*P*) of the rectum.

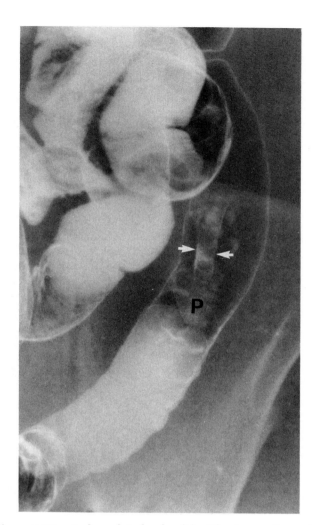

Figure 8.15. Pedunculated polyp (*P*) of the descending colon. Note the stalk of the polyp (*arrows*).

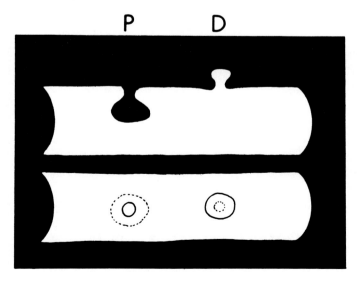

Figure 8.16. Drawing illustrating the difference between the radiographic appearances of a polyp (*P*) and a diverticulum (*D*). Top, profile view; bottom, end-on view. The mnemonic for distinguishing these two lesions when seen end-on is: "Fuzzy outside = polyp (FOP) and fuzzy inside = tic (FIT)."

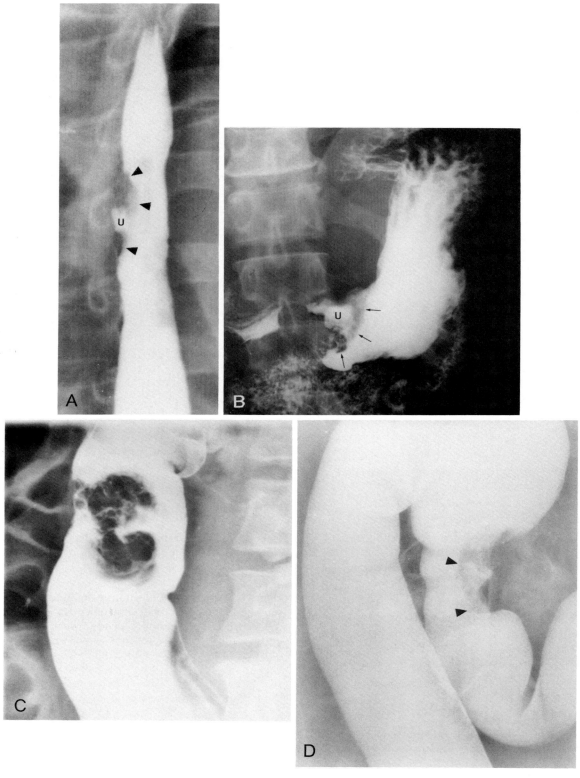

Figure 8.17. Mucosal mass lesions. A, ulcerating esophageal carcinoma. An ulcer crater (*U*) is present within the mucosal mass (*arrowheads*). **B,** ulcerating malignancy of the gastric antrum. The ulcer (*U*) is within the mucosal mass (*arrows*). **C,** polypoid colonic carcinoma presents as an irregular filling defect. **D,** sessile colon carcinoma (*arrowheads*). Note the abrupt margin between normal mucosa and tumor.

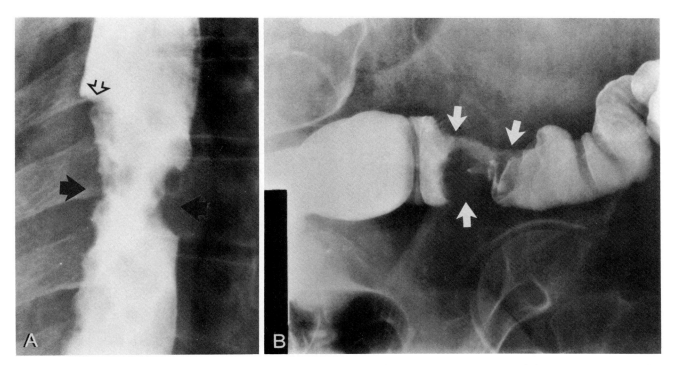

Figure 8.18. **"Napkin ring" ("apple-core") mucosal lesions.** Note the similarity of these lesions. **A,** esophageal carcinoma shows the constricting lesion (*solid arrows*). Note the abrupt mucosal margins (*open arrow*). **B,** colonic lesion (*arrows*).

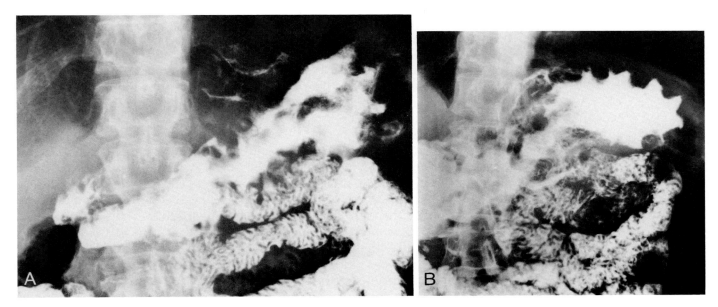

Figure 8.19. **Hypertrophic gastric mucosal folds.** Two views (**A** and **B**) show multiple filling defects in the stomach representing hypertrophic mucosa. Endoscopy was required for confirmation.

Figure 8.20. Esophageal varices. A and **B** show the multiple worm-like filling defects in two different patients with a history of chronic alcohol abuse.

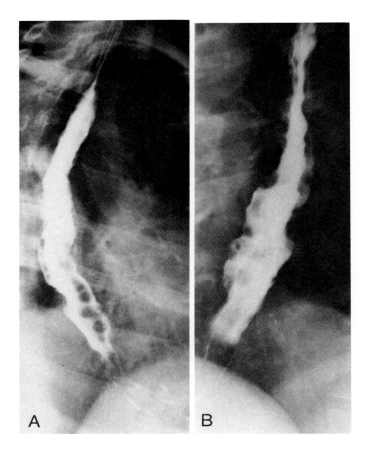

The inflammatory mass leading up to the ulcer is smooth with gradually sloping margins. Occasionally, a smooth collar of inflamed mucosa is present between the lumen and the crater (Hampton's line). This is also considered a sign of a benign ulcer since tumors do not show this feature. Penetration of the ulcer beyond the normal lumen is a sign of a benign lesion. Ulceration may also occur within masses. You should remember that there are no malignant ulcers; there are ulcerating malignancies. Several ulcers are illustrated in Figures 8.21 through 8.23. Table 8.1 lists the radiologic differential features between benign gastric ulcers and ulcerating malignancies.

Diverticula are benign outpouchings of the wall of the GI tract. Diverticula are covered by all layers of the bowel wall. They may be relatively small, as in the colon (Fig. 8.24), or quite large, as a Zenker diverticulum of the esophagus (Fig. 8.25). Occasionally, they will contain foreign material. Figures 8.26 through 8.28 show various diverticula.

Extrinsic compression (Fig. 8.29) appears as a smooth indentation of the bowel wall with gradually tapering margins. On palpation during fluoroscopy, the mucosa can be seen to be intact. It may be difficult to differentiate this from an intramural lesion causing compression.

Benign stricture formation appears as concentric or eccentric narrowing of the lumen (Fig. 8.30). The margins should be smooth and tapering. The mucosa generally should be intact. Strictures are often difficult to differentiate from carcinoma.

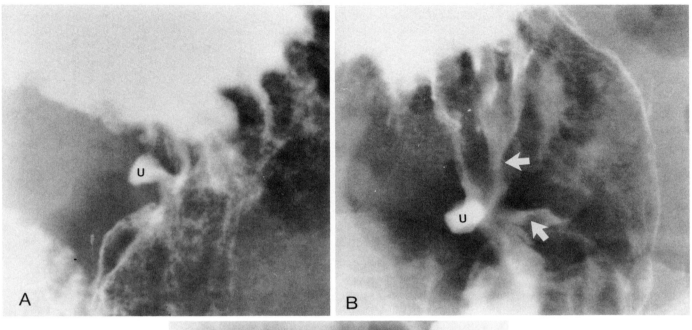

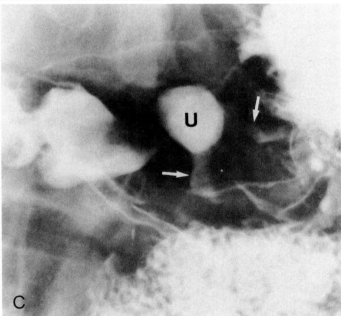

Figure 8.21. Benign gastric ulcers (*U*). A, B, and **C** show ulcers in three different patients. Note the radiation of folds into the ulcer crater in **B** and **C** (*arrows*).

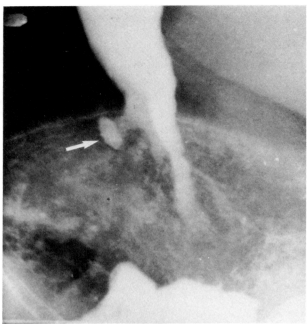

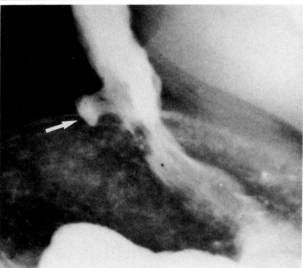

Figure 8.22. Distal esophageal ulcer (*arrow*) in a patient with gastroesophageal reflux. There is a small collar of edematous mucosa leading up to the ulcer crater.

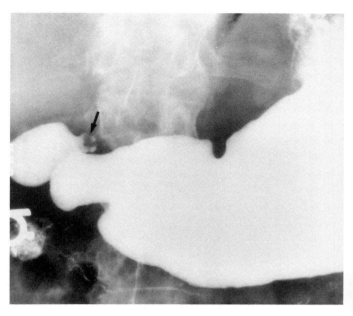

Figure 8.23. Ulcer of the duodenal bulb (*arrow*). The small filling defect within the ulcer crater represents a blood clot.

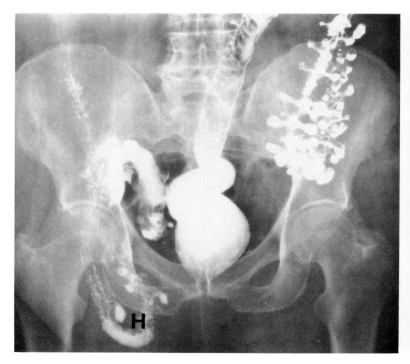

Figure 8.24. Colonic diverticulosis. The diverticulosis is worse on the left side of the colon. Note the inguinal hernia (*H*) on the right.

Table 8.1.   Comparative Features of Benign Gastric Ulcers and Ulcerating Malignancies

Benign Gastric Ulcers	Ulcerating Malignancies
Penetration beyond lumen	Intraluminal crater located between abrupt points of transition (in contrast to intraluminal crater in mound of even edematous surrounding tissue)
Mucosal folds radiate to crater edge	Crater shallow, width exceeds depth
Hampton's line	Absent Hampton's line
Ulcer collar	Ulcer irregularly shaped
Ulcer mound, gradual tapering to normal mucosa	Eccentric location of ulcer in mass
Normal distensibility and pliability	Fixation of affected area
Peristalsis transmitted through area	Peristalsis not transmitted through area
Single, centrally located blood clot in crater base	Irregular base of crater

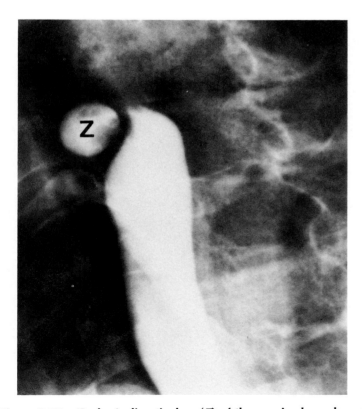

Figure 8.25.   Zenker's diverticulum (Z) of the proximal esophagus.

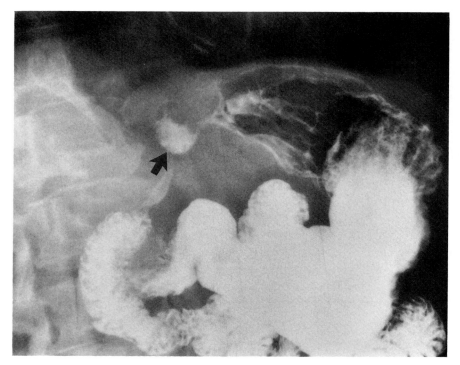

Figure 8.26. Gastric diverticulum (*arrow*).

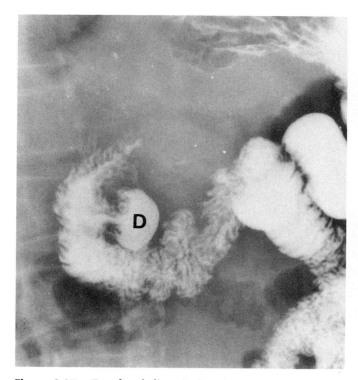

Figure 8.27. Duodenal diverticulum (*D*) in the typical location in the descending duodenum.

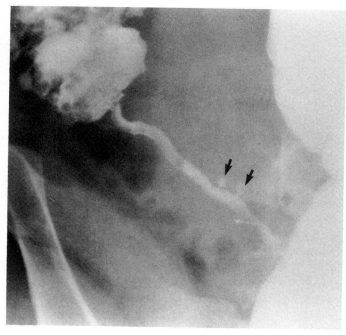

Figure 8.28. Appendiceal diverticula (*arrows*). A small lucency within the appendix is an air bubble.

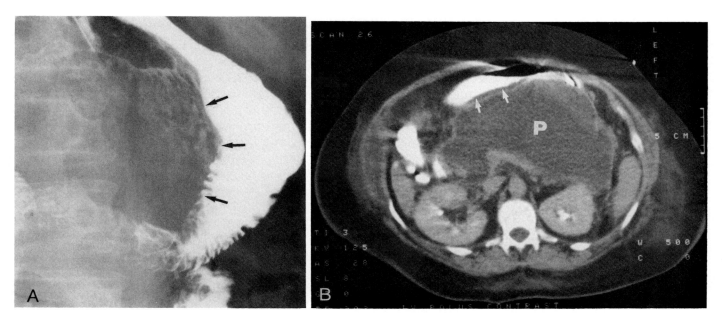

Figure 8.29. Pancreatic pseudocyst. A, spot film from an upper GI examination shows extrinsic compression of the stomach by a large pancreatic pseudocyst (*arrows*). **B,** CT scan shows the pseudocyst (*P*). Note the compression of the contrast-filled stomach (*arrows*).

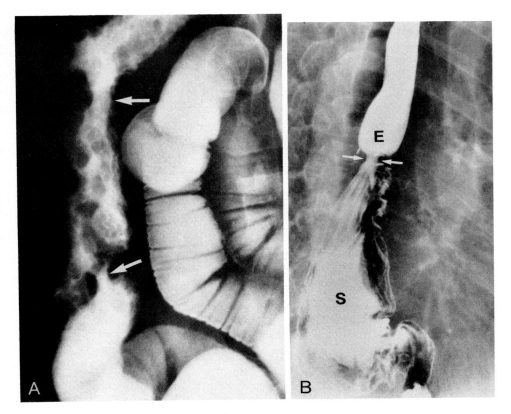

Figure 8.30. Strictures. A, small bowel strictures (*arrows*) in a patient with regional enteritis (Crohn's disease). Note the abnormal mucosa in the involved segment. **B,** stricture (*arrows*) at the site of anastomosis of esophagus (*E*) and stomach (*S*) in a patient who has undergone gastroesophagotomy.

Inflammatory Bowel Disease

Inflammatory bowel disease is a term that is applied to both ulcerative colitis and Crohn's disease (regional enteritis) of the bowel. Both diseases serve as a prototype since they produce a spectrum of radiographic changes including ulceration, pseudopolyps, stricture formation, obstruction, and fistula formation.

Both these chronic inflammatory bowel conditions are of unknown etiology. However, they share a number of clinical, epidemiologic, pathologic, radiographic, and even immunologic features. Some authorities feel that each entity represents a different pathologic response to a common cause; others believe both diseases represent different parts of the spectrum of a single disease process.

The definitive diagnosis of both these diseases is best made by endoscopy with or without biopsy. Nevertheless, classic radiographic findings have been described for each of these diseases and will be briefly contrasted here.

The typical case of *ulcerative colitis* has radiographic manifestations that directly reflect the pathologic manifestations, including exudative inflammation involving primarily the bowel mucosa and submucosa. Classically, the muscularis is spared. Edema of the bowel wall gives the impression of thickened bowel. Ulcerations are shallow and coalescent (Fig. 8.31), often isolating islands of normal mucosa that are termed "pseudopolyps" (Fig. 8.32).

In the acute stages, spasm and irritability are evident fluoroscopically. Edema results in smudging and haziness of the mucosal folds. The disease characteristically involves the entire colon. Occasionally, there is involvement of the terminal ileum; however, this more commonly occurs in Crohn's disease.

Long-standing disease results in the chronic or the "burned out" stage producing foreshortening of the colon and narrowing of the lumen. The barium enema reveals a very tubular appearance of the colon with a loss of normal haustral markings (Fig. 8.33). Carcinoma may develop in as many as 5% of patients with long-standing ulcerative colitis (Fig. 8.34).

Crohn's disease of the colon (granulomatous colitis) is identical to regional enteritis that occurs elsewhere in the gastrointestinal tract. Crohn's disease classically involves all layers of the bowel wall. This results in the development of strictures and obstruction as well as enteroenteric fistulas and enterocutaneous fistulas.

The radiographic manifestations are distinct from those of ulcerative colitis. Barium enema generally demonstrates patches of involved bowel with normal intervening mucosa—the so-called "skip areas" (Fig. 8.35). Longitudinal ulcers with transverse fissures give a typical "cobblestone" appearance (Fig. 8.36). Typically, the rectum is spared but the right colon is more severely involved. The terminal ileum is involved in almost every instance (Fig. 8.37). Fistulous tracts are often demonstrable (Fig. 8.37). Unlike ulcerative colitis, development of colon carcinoma is unusual.

Table 8.2 contrasts the two diseases.

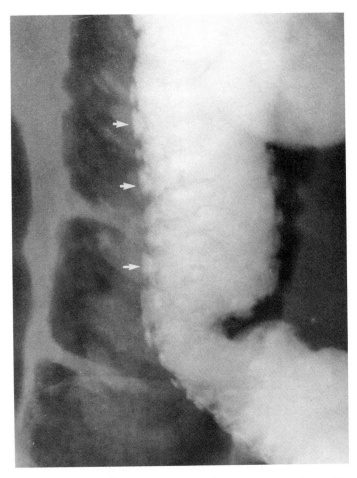

Figure 8.31. "Collar-button" ulcers (*arrows*) in a patient with ulcerative colitis.

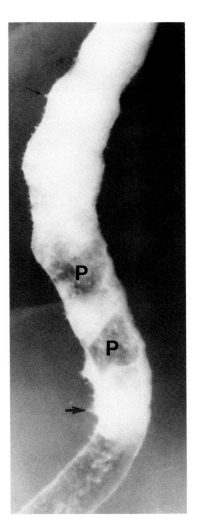

Figure 8.32. Pseudopolyps (*P*) in a patient with ulcerative colitis. Note the irregular ulcers along the colon margin (*arrows*).

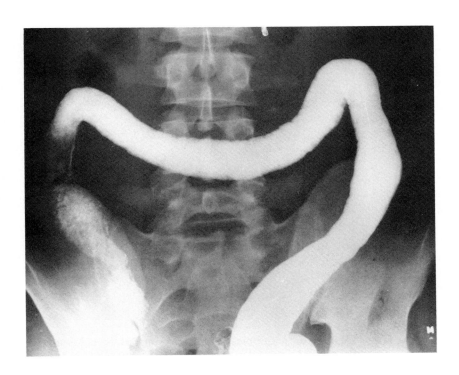

Figure 8.33. Appearance of the colon in long-standing ulcerative colitis. The colon is fairly rigid, devoid of haustral markings, and foreshortened. Compare with Figure 8.10.

Figure 8.34. Colon carcinoma in a patient with long-standing ulcerative colitis. A "napkin-ring" lesion is present in the mid transverse colon (*arrows*). This is the same patient as in Figure 8.33 7 years later.

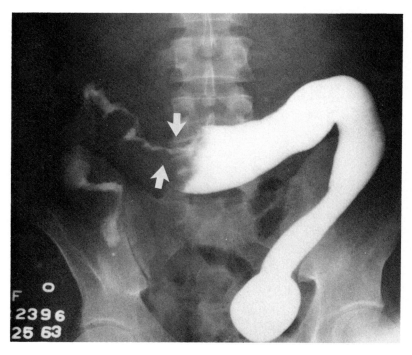

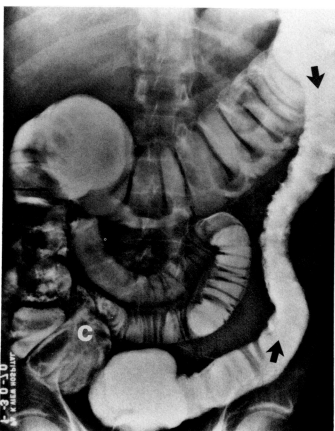

Figure 8.35. Crohn's disease of the colon demonstrating skip lesions. The involved segment of bowel is the descending colon (*arrows*). *C,* cecum.

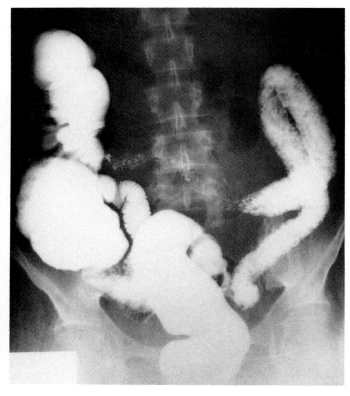

Figure 8.36. "Cobblestone" appearance of the colon in a patient with Crohn's disease. This typical pattern is best appreciated in the splenic flexure. Compare with the hepatic flexure.

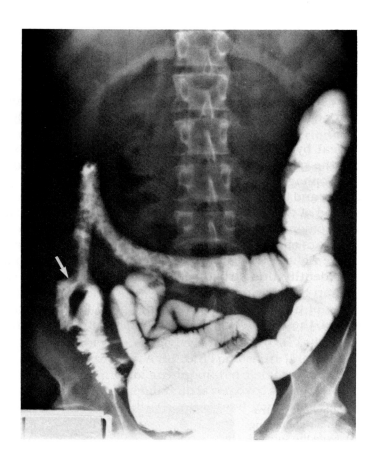

Figure 8.37. Ileal involvement and fistula formation (*arrow*) in a patient with Crohn's disease.

Table 8.2. A Comparison of Ulcerative Colitis and Crohn's Colitis

Feature	Ulcerative Colitis	Crohn's Colitis
Clinical		
Fever, malaise	+	++
Rectal bleeding	++	±
Tenderness	±	++
Diarrhea	+++	+++
Abdominal mass	–	+++
Abdominal pain	–	+++
Fistulas	–	+++
Endoscopic		
Rectal disease	+++	+
Linear ulcers	–	+
Continuous disease	+++	–
"Skip lesions"	–	+++
Radiographic		
Continuous disease	+++	–
"Skip lesions"	–	+++
Ileal involvement	+	+++
Strictures	–	+
Fistulas	–	++
Carcinoma	+++	–
"Pseudopolyps"	+++	–
"Collar button" ulcers	+++	+
"Cobblestone" pattern	–	+++

with anastomosis of the gastric stump to a loop of jejunum. An afferent loop drains the pancreatobiliary system through the duodenum. The base of the duodenal bulb usually is removed in this procedure.

In recent years there have been developed of a number of surgical procedures for the treatment of morbid obesity. These procedures involve *gastric bypasses* in which the gastric antrum is anastomosed directly to a portion of distal ileum to prevent absorption of large quantities of nutrients. Other procedures include *gastric stapling,* in which the overall volume of the stomach is made smaller by closing off a portion of the fundus and body. *Balloon implantations* have also been performed by gastroenterologists and surgeons to decrease the overall volume allowed in the stomach. These procedures may be recognized by the location of surgical staple lines at the anastomotic or operative sites. A careful history from the patient is usually sufficient to determine if the patient has had one of these procedures.

Anastomoses between the distal ileum and colon (ileocolostomy) are performed for inflammatory bowel disease or carcinoma. These are easily recognized by the filling of small bowel from a portion of colon other than the cecum. A ring of staples marks each anastomosis.

The Accessory Digestive Organs

The accessory digestive organs are the gallbladder, the liver, and the pancreas. These organs may best be evaluated by diagnostic ultrasound, CT, and occasionally by magnetic resonance imaging.

As previously mentioned, the biliary tract may be visualized either by ultrasound, biliary scintigraphy, or by oral cholecystography. The most common abnormalities encountered in the biliary tract are cholecystitis (Figs. 8.5 and 8.41) and cholelithiasis with or without obstruction (Figs. 8.42 and 8.43).

The most common abnormalities encountered in the liver are obstructive jaundice and metastases (Fig. 8.44). Both of these may be evaluated by ultrasound and CT. The CT scan, however, is particularly advantageous in evaluating metastases, and it may be used to guide percutaneous biopsy of metastatic or other masses of the liver. Magnetic resonance imaging also may be used to evaluate hepatic metastases; however, CT is much more efficient. Magnetic resonance, however, is particularly useful in evaluating patients with hemangiomas (Fig. 8.45). In these patients, the vascular lesion has extremely high signal.

The pancreas was one of the most elusive organs to image in the past. Although pancreatitis and pancreatic pseudocysts make themselves clinically apparent at a relatively early stage of the disease, pancreatic carcinoma often does not. Once the patient with pancreatic carcinoma becomes symptomatic, he or she is usually beyond cure from either surgery or radiation therapy. Direct pancreatic imaging, therefore, became one of the major advances in medical diagnosis in the last 2 decades. The pancreas lends itself readily to evaluation by either ultrasound or CT (Figs. 8.46 and 8.47).

Finally, the evaluation of intraabdominal abscess, from any cause, has been greatly facilitated by the development of CT and ultrasound.

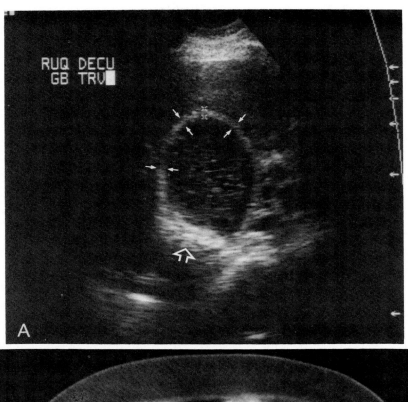

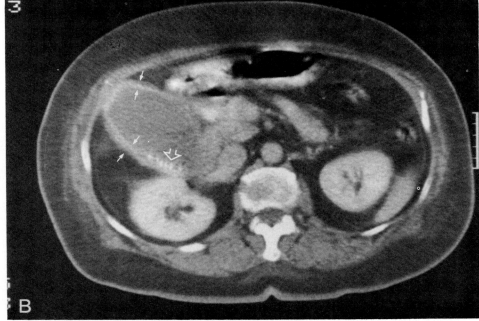

Figure 8.41. Cholecystitis. A, ultrasound shows thickening of the gallbladder wall (*small arrows*) with many internal echoes representing "sludge." Small stones layer out (*large arrow*). The obstructing calculus is not demonstrated in this study. **B,** CT scan shows the thickened gallbladder wall (*small arrows*) and the stones (*large arrow*).

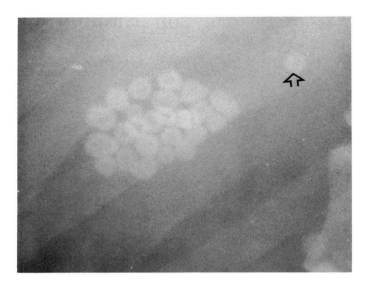

Figure 8.42. **Multiple calcified gallstones.** One of the stones (*arrow*) is near the neck of the gallbladder.

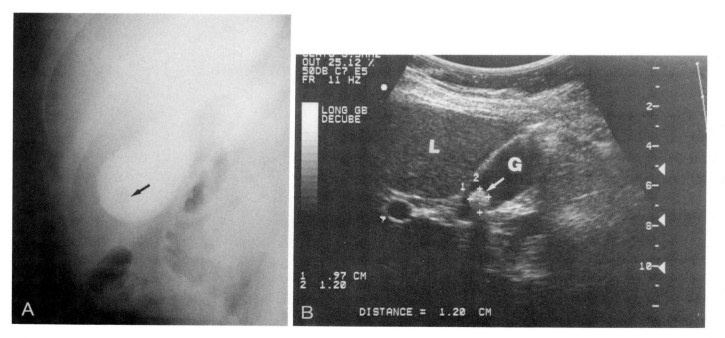

Figure 8.43. **Cholelithiasis. A,** oral cholecystogram shows a lucent stone (*arrow*) in the opacified gallbladder. **B,** ultrasound shows the stone (*arrow*) measuring 1.2 × 0.97 cm in the dependent portion of the gallbladder. *L,* liver; *G,* gallbladder

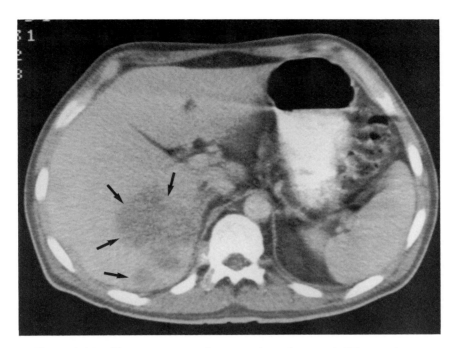

Figure 8.44. Liver metastases from renal carcinoma. A CT scan shows multiple lucent areas (*arrows*) within the liver.

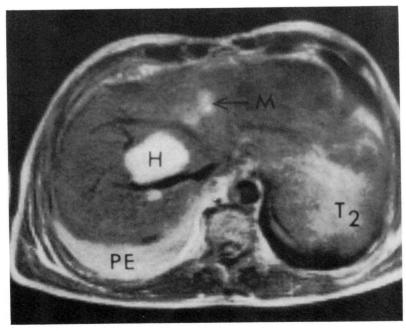

Figure 8.45. Hepatic hemangioma. This T2-weighted MR image shows the hemangioma (*H*) as a rounded area of very high (bright) signal against the darker background of the normal liver tissue. Note the coexistent metastatic lesion (*M*) and pleural effusion (*PE*) that have a lower signal than the hemangioma.

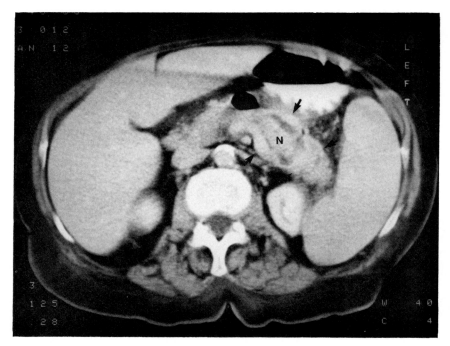

Figure 8.46. **Pancreatitis.** A CT scan shows enlargement of the pancreas (*arrows*). A necrotic focus (*N*) is present in the central portion of the pancreas.

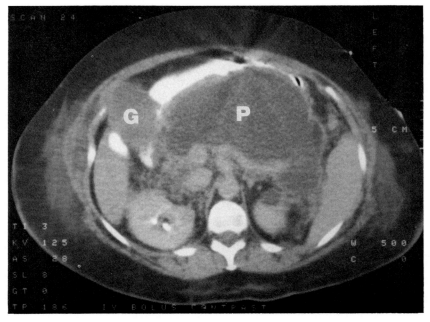

Figure 8.47. **Pancreatic pseudocyst (*P*).** A large multilocular area of lucency is present in the retrogastric region. Note the distended gallbladder (*G*).

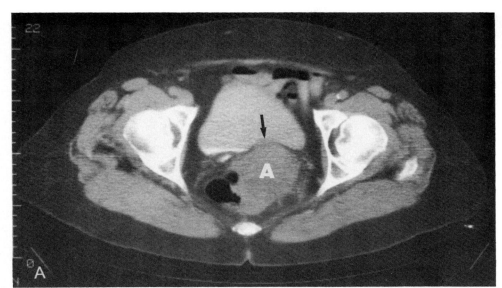

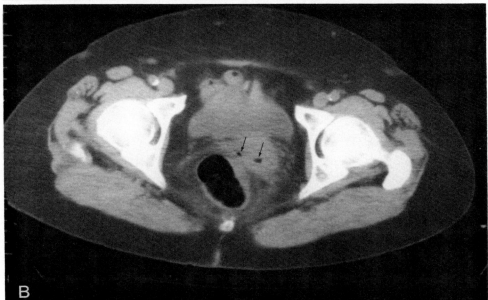

Figure 8.48. Perirectal abscess. A, A pelvic CT scan shows a large abscess (*A*) compressing the floor of the bladder (*arrow*). The air-containing rectum is displaced to the right. **B,** Slightly lower, the abscess is seen to contain gas (*arrows*).

While the majority of abdominal abscesses demonstrate abnormalities on plain films, a definitive diagnosis may be made by CT examination (Fig. 8.48). Furthermore, CT-guided drainage is now possible (Fig. 3.7).

Summary

The gastrointestinal tract is a tubular structure that allows recognition of patterns of disease that may occur in any portion. In each area, the appearance of these lesions will be quite similar. However, the incidence varies from location to location, depending on the disease. These abnormalities include polypoid lesions, mucosal tumors, ulcerations, diverticula, extrinsic compression, and benign strictures. A discussion of special imaging procedures and their application to the gastrointestinal tract was also presented.

Suggested Additional Reading

Laufer I, Levine MS. Double contrast gastrointestinal radiology. 2nd ed. Philadelphia: WB Saunders, 1991.

Margulis AR, Burhenne HJ, eds. Alimentary tract radiology. 4th ed. St. Louis: Mosby Year Book, 1989.

Chapter 9

Urinary Tract Imaging

When evaluating the urinary tract radiographically, you must keep in mind that there are basically two types of abnormalities that you may encounter, "physiologic" and morphologic. The so-called *physiologic abnormalities* include a wide variety of diseases referred to collectively as the "medical nephropathies." These include diseases of the glomeruli, tubules, and interstitial tissues. Also included are forms of tubular and cortical necrosis. In patients with these diseases, intravenous urography shows poor function or none at all; diagnosis is best determined by biopsy. Furthermore, intravenous urography may be detrimental.

The *morphologic abnormalities* constitute the other large group in which imaging is definitely of value. These will be discussed under pathologic considerations.

TECHNICAL CONSIDERATIONS

There are basically eight types of studies commonly used to evaluate the urinary tract: the intravenous urogram; the retrograde urogram; the cystogram, which is often combined with a study of the urethra as a voiding cystourethrogram; ultrasound; computerized tomography (CT) scanning; magnetic resonance (MR) imaging; renal arteriography; and isotope studies.

Since intravenous urography (IVU), often inaccurately called intravenous pyelography, is one of the more frequently performed of these examinations, the technique will be reiterated briefly. Before starting an IVU, a plain film of the abdomen should be obtained to look for calculi that may be obscured by the excretion of contrast material and to determine the degree of bowel cleanliness. As with the colon examination, preparation of the bowel is necessary to eliminate overlying gas and fecal shadows that could obscure the renal outlines.

Once you are assured that the patient's bowel has been satisfactorily prepared for the examination, you must question the patient regarding a history of allergy in general and allergy to iodinated radiopaque drugs specifically. It is very important to ask these patients if they have ever had their kidneys x-rayed before. A history of feeling warm after a contrast injection should not be considered evidence of allergy but rather abnormal physiologic reaction. This symptom may be prevented by the use of low osmolar contrast agents. If a history of a previous true reaction to contrast material is elicited, a decision must be made by the radiologist, in consultation with the referring physician, whether the study requested is absolutely necessary, or whether an alternative study such as ultrasound or noncontrasted CT can be substituted. If it is deemed that the study is needed, the patient may be "prepared" by the referring physician with 2 days of dosing of steroids and a dose of antihistamine immediately before the study. The effectiveness of this regimen has been questioned, however. There is recent evidence to suggest that some of the reactions to contrast material may be psychologically induced. The use of low osmolar contrast agents will reduce but not totally eliminate adverse reactions.

During the typical urogram, tomography of the kidneys should be used routinely to show renal outlines that may otherwise be obscured by overlying gas or bowel content (Fig. 9.1). The filming sequence employs

Figure 9.1. Use of tomography during intravenous urography. A, detailed view of kidneys shows bowel gas obscuring renal borders. **B,** tomography blurs the overlying gas and bowel content, revealing, smooth, normal-appearing renal borders.

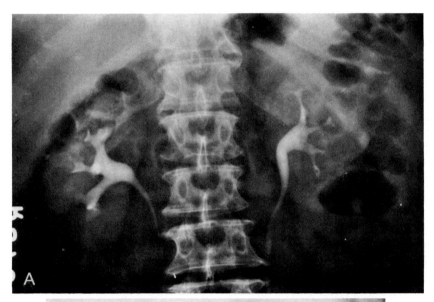

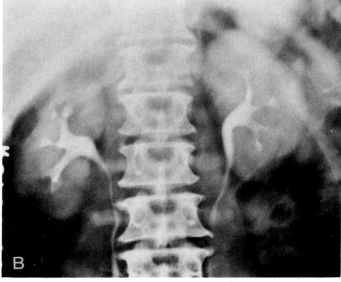

tomography during the earliest or "nephrogram" phase when contrast material is in the small vessels and nephrons. This method offers the best opportunity to evaluate the renal parenchyma as well as the renal size and shape. Two or more static films (without tomography) are obtained usually at 5-minute intervals to examine the collecting systems, the ureters, and the bladder. Additional views of the kidneys or of the bladder are taken as needed to delineate any areas still in question. Occasionally, oblique views will be obtained. In this way, the examination is "tailored" to each patient.

The urinary tract is easily studied by *real-time ultrasonography.* Renal size may be evaluated as well as renal shape. Figure 9.2 shows a longitudinal scan of the right kidney. Renal ultrasound is used primarily in assessing renal size as well as the nature of a renal mass by searching for internal echoes within the mass. Renal cysts that have only fluid within them have no internal echoes and are referred to as *sonolucent* (Fig. 9.3). Tumors, on the other hand, will frequently show internal echoes, indicating their solid nature (Fig. 9.4).

Ultrasound is also used to evaluate the prostate gland. The development of the transrectal ultrasound transducer now makes it possible to study the internal anatomy of the prostate. Preliminary reports have indicated success in differentiating carcinoma from benign prostatic hypertrophy. Furthermore, it is now possible to study by biopsy suspicious areas of the prostate utilizing a special transrectal biopsy device. The availability of these techniques holds promise to reduce the morbidity and mortality rate of prostatic carcinoma.

Abdominal CT scanning has proved to be a useful tool for the evaluation of renal mass lesions. In addition, the CT scan may be used to determine the etiology of masses that are distorting or displacing the normal urinary tract, such as enlarged abdominal lymph nodes. A CT scan is also

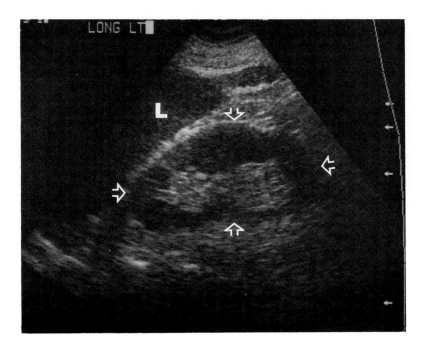

Figure 9.2. Normal renal ultrasound. The kidney has a reniform shape (*arrows*). The corticomedullary areas are relatively sonolucent. The collecting system and renal pelvis produce echoes. *L*, liver.

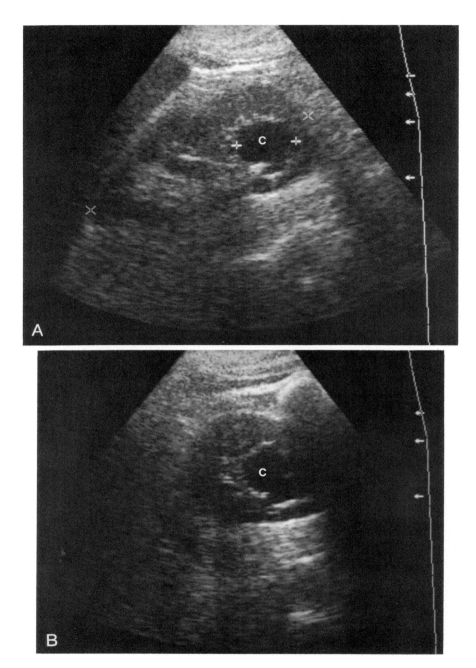

Figure 9.3. **Renal cyst. A,** longitudinal ultrasound scan shows the sonolucent cyst (*C*). Note the increased echoes beneath the cyst ("through transmission"). **B,** axial scan again shows the cyst and the "through transmission."

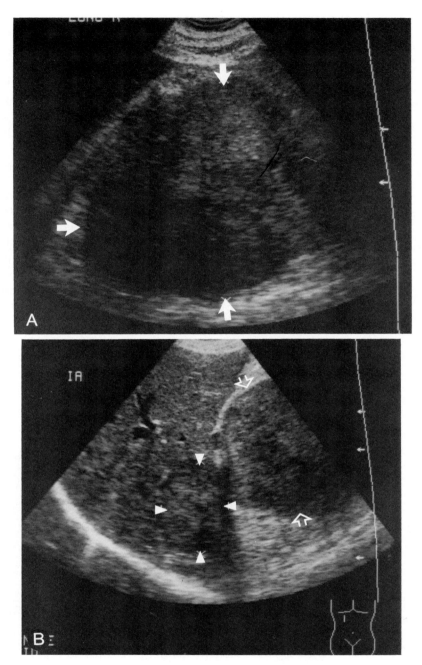

Figure 9.4.   Renal carcinoma upper pole of right kidney. A, longitudinal ultrasound scan shows gross distortion of the renal outline by a large mass (*arrows*). Note the internal echoes in the upper portion of the tumor. Contrast this with Figure 9.3. **B,** longitudinal scan slightly higher again shows the renal mass (*arrows*). Note the invasion of the right lobe of the liver (*arrowheads*). (This is the same patient as in Fig. 8.44.)

the best method of evaluating renal trauma. The CT characteristics of renal cysts show that they are of low density and of CT numbers that correspond to the numbers of urine. On intravenous injection of contrast material, there is no enhancement of the mass. Indeed, the mass stands out as a prominent "lucency" against the contrast-containing parenchyma (Fig. 9.5). Renal cell carcinoma is, on the other hand, generally isodense (density same as renal tissue) on the unenhanced scan and with enhancement may show hypervascularity, manifest by increased density of the lesion (Fig. 9.6). Contrast enhancement often aids in demonstrating necrotic areas within the mass. It is often possible to determine the extent of extrarenal involvement by tumor (Fig. 9.7), including invasion of the renal veins and the inferior vena cava.

Magnetic resonance imaging of the urinary tract is used to evaluate renal masses or the effects of pelvic neoplasms on the bladder (Fig. 9.8). The ability of MR to image in coronal and sagittal planes is also useful for evaluating the kidneys and surrounding structures. This is especially true in demonstrating invasion of the renal vein or the inferior vena cava by renal carcinoma. Most recently, MR imaging of the prostate has been performed. Preliminary results suggest the technique may be useful in differentiating benign prostatic hypertrophy from prostatic carcinoma, as well as staging known malignancies.

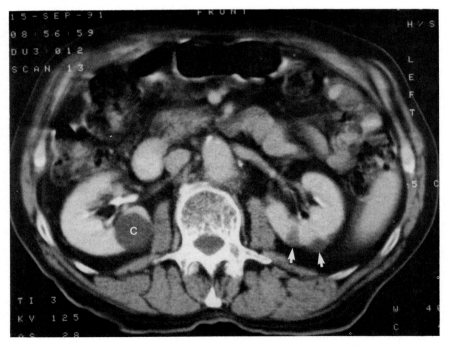

Figure 9.5.   Renal cysts. The same patient as in Figure 9.3. A CT scan shows a large cyst (*C*) in the posterior portion of the right kidney. Note the two smaller cysts (*arrows*) on the left.

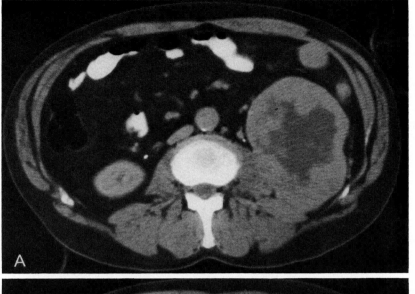

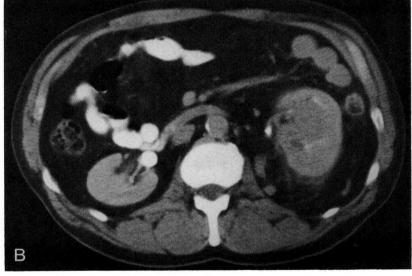

Figure 9.6. Renal carcinoma. A, CT scan shows enlargement of the left renal outline. The left kidney is devoid of normal internal markings. The low density area within the left kidney represents necrosis. **B,** a section slightly lower clearly shows difference between the two kidneys.

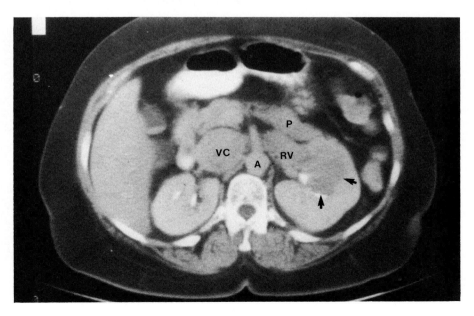

Figure 9.7. Renal carcinoma with extrarenal invasion. A CT scan shows a mass in the left kidney (*arrows*). The mass extends beyond the confines of the kidney into the renal vein (*RV*) and into the inferior vena cava (*VC*). Compare the size of the vena cava with that of the adjacent aorta (*A*). The vena cava should be the same size. Note the relationship of the pancreas (*P*) to the left kidney.

Figure 9.8. Prostatic carcinoma.
A, coronal T1-weighted MR image
shows a mass (*arrow*) invading the
floor of the bladder on the right
side. **B,** axial image shows the mass
(*arrow*) invading the bladder floor.
Note the enlarged prostate (*P*). **C,**
CT scan shows identical findings
(*arrow*).

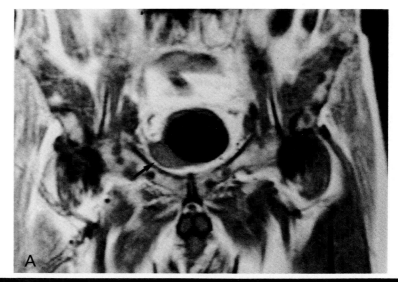

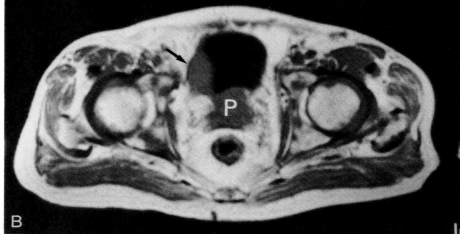

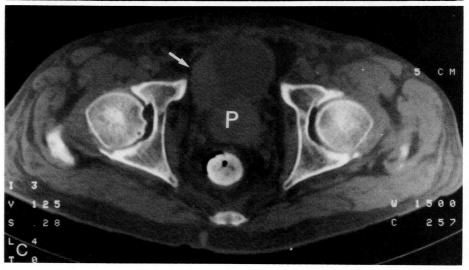

ANATOMIC CONSIDERATIONS

The kidneys in a normal adult measure 11 to 14 cm in length from pole to pole. They are invested in their own fascia, with their upper poles oriented slightly medially. There may be a normal difference in size between the right and left kidney; the left kidney is often 0.5 to 1.5 cm longer than the right.

The collecting system consists of three to five infundibula, each draining one or more calyces. The calyx forms a sharply defined "cup" around the papilla, which it drains (Fig. 9.9). These are easily discernible on the normal urogram. The infundibula unite to form the renal pelvis, which terminates in the ureter.

The ureters course down the retroperitoneal surface on either side of the vertebral column, generally in a vertical pattern, until they reach the pelvis, where they may make a slight lateral deviation before turning medially to enter the posterior aspect of the bladder at the trigone. The ureters are not bound down by fascia and are relatively free to move, a fact that is useful in the evaluation of retroperitoneal disease.

The urinary bladder should be smooth and ovoid. There are normal variations in the shape of the bladder that occasionally result in a lobular configuration.

The prostate lies immediately inferior to the bladder, and when enlarged, may indent and elevate the floor of the bladder (Fig. 9.10). The ure-

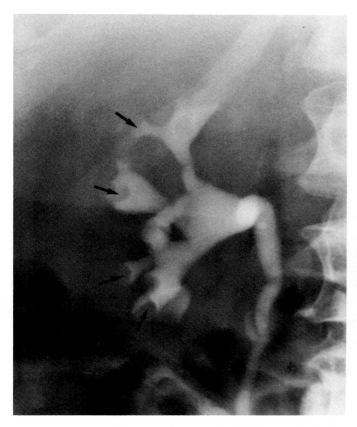

Figure 9.9.   Detailed view of a normal right kidney during intravenous urography. Note the delicate cupping of the calyces (*arrows*).

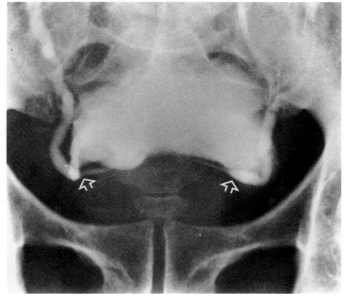

Figure 9.10.   Prostatic enlargement. The floor of the bladder is elevated by the enlarged prostate. Note the "fishhooking" of the distal ureters (*arrows*) as they enter the bladder.

thra courses through the prostate. The membranous portion of the urethra between the prostatic and bulbous urethra is fixed in the urogenital diaphragm. This area is subject to laceration from trauma to the pelvis.

The vascular supply to the kidney generally consists of a single pair of renal arteries. However, occasionally two or more arteries to each kidney are present. A single renal vein drains each kidney. On the right, the vein drains directly into the inferior vena cava without anastomosis with other veins. On the left, there is communication of the renal vein with the left adrenal and gonadal veins. These two communications form a collateral pathway for blood to drain the kidney in the event of renal vein thrombosis. There are collateral channels in the arterial system, as well, that may enlarge when there are stenotic lesions of the renal artery. The foremost of these is the ureteric artery.

PATHOLOGIC CONSIDERATIONS

As previously mentioned, the so-called physiologic abnormalities will uniformly result in a decrease or absence of renal function. The only morphologic change that may be discerned is a decrease in the size of a kidney. This discussion will concentrate on diseases that produce recognizable morphologic abnormalities, including:

1. Congenital abnormalities
2. Obstructive lesions with or without calculi
3. Infections
4. Mass lesions; cysts and tumors
5. Vascular lesions
6. Traumatic lesions
7. Extrinsic compression
8. Renal transplants

Congenital Abnormalities

Congenital anomalies of the urinary tract are not uncommon. The complex development of the genitourinary tract in embryonic life provides many opportunities for anomalous development to occur. Anomalies may be relatively benign, such as duplication of the collecting system (Fig. 9.11) or uncomplicated horseshoe kidney (Fig. 9.12), or severe, such as posterior urethral valves with secondary megacystia, hydroureter, and hydronephrosis in a newborn male infant. Other anomalies include ectopic kidneys and ectopic ureteroceles. For an in-depth discussion of these conditions consult *Clinical Urography* by Pollack.

Obstructive Lesions With or Without Calculi

Obstruction of the urinary tract may be either congenital or acquired. The acquired variety is more common and is usually the result of urinary calculi (Fig. 9.13). Other causes are tumor (Fig. 9.14) and operative manipulation. Whatever the etiology, obstruction produces a series of pathophysiologic changes that result in characteristic radiographic appearances. These changes will determine the radiographic appearance, depending on the degree of renal parenchymal destruction.

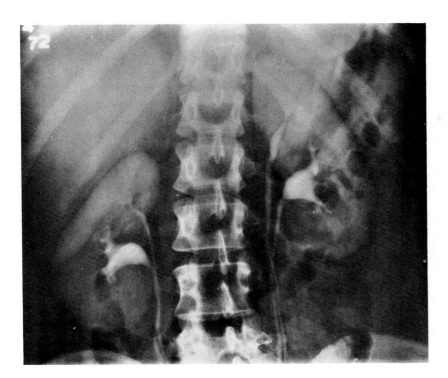

Figure 9.11. Duplication of the upper collecting system. Note the double renal pelvis from the upper pole of each kidney and the duplicated ureter. This duplication extended to the ureterovesical junction (not shown on this film).

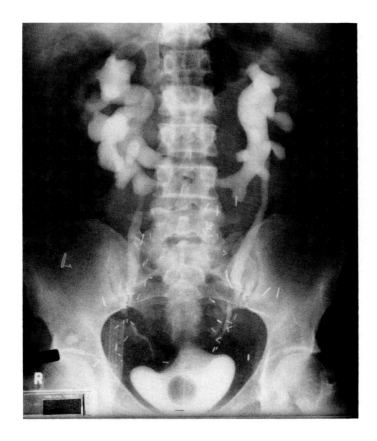

Figure 9.12. Horseshoe kidney. Intravenous urogram shows dilatation of the urinary collecting system bilaterally. Note the alteration of orientation of both renal poles. A pair of kidneys orientated in this manner should suggest the diagnosis.

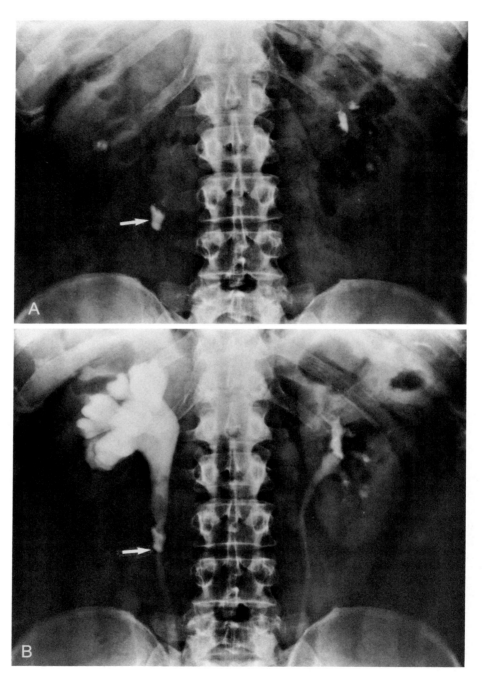

Figure 9.13. Obstructive uropathy due to urinary calculus. A, plain film shows multiple calculi overlying the renal shadows. Note the large calculus adjacent to the L-3 interspace on the right (*arrow*). **B,** intravenous urogram demonstrates partial obstruction on the right secondary to the ureteral stone (*arrow*). The left kidney is not obstructed.

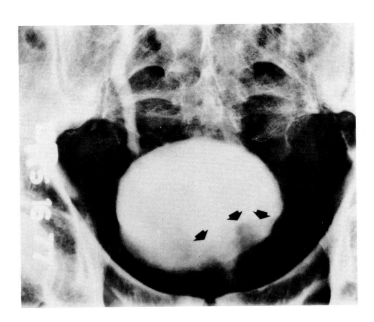

Figure 9.14. Complete obstruction of the left ureter due to bladder carcinoma (*arrows*). The right ureter was not affected.

Radiographic changes of acute obstruction include initial nonvisualization, with subsequent delayed visualization on the abnormal side, or prompt visualization, with evidence of dilation (caliectasis) of the collecting system (Fig. 9.13**B**). Frank hydronephrosis usually indicates a longstanding obstruction. If the obstruction is caused by a stone, very frequently that stone will be demonstrated. It is occasionally necessary to obtain oblique films to be certain that a calcification seen on the abdominal film is indeed present within the urinary tract.

Ultrasonography and CT are useful techniques for diagnosing hydronephrosis. Ultrasound is also particularly useful in evaluating newborns and infants with palpable abdominal masses, since many of these are due to urinary abnormalities.

Urinary calculi are the most common causes of obstruction. They may be opaque or nonopaque. Populations of certain areas, such as the southeast and southwest, have a high incidence of urinary stones. Interestingly, the composition of stones varies with the locale. In the so-called "stone belt" of North Carolina, 85% of the stones are formed of oxalate, whereas only 40% are of that composition in New York state.

Most stones contain a mineral deposit embedded in an inorganic matrix. This matrix has been found to be elevated in the urine of patients with hyperparathyroidism, renal infection, and patients undergoing steroid therapy in an amount that ranges from 3 to 15 times that of normal patients.

Urinary stones must be differentiated from nephrocalcinosis, a pathophysiologic condition in which calcium is deposited within renal tissue. It results from an underlying disease that elevates the serum calcium level. In most instances, the calcification is limited to the distal convoluted tubules. These calcifications appear as fine stippled deposits that should be easily differentiated from stones by their appearance and location. There are many causes of this condition, but the most common ones include

Figure 9.15. Nephrocalcinosis. Note the fine deposition of calcium within the renal pyramids of both kidneys. This is a reversible condition.

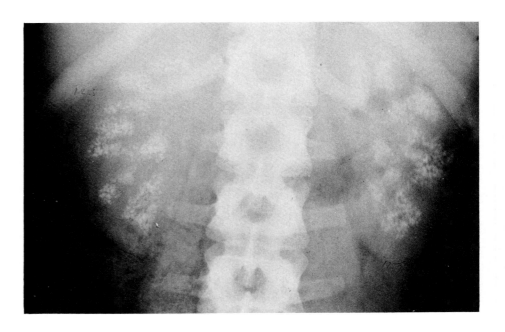

medullary sponge kidney, hyperparathyroidism, renal tubular acidosis, and milk-alkali syndrome. Nephrocalcinosis is illustrated in Figure 9.15.

Infections

Infection is a common disease of the urinary tract. It is often seen as a complication of obstruction. Acute pyelonephritis may be difficult to recognize radiographically because of the subtle changes it produces on the collecting system. Occasionally, this condition may be detected on a radiograph if it produces a large swollen kidney. More commonly, however, the effects of chronic pyelonephritis are encountered. These include marked cortical irregularity, focal cortical scarring, clubbed irregular calyces, and loss of renal volume (Fig. 9.16). Other complications of infections in the collecting system include the development of a renal carbuncle or abscess (Fig. 9.17), pyonephrosis, and papillary necrosis. This last condition results from anoxia of the renal papilla, causing sloughing of that papilla. Characteristic findings include a filling defect in a calyx, a ring of contrast surrounding a filling defect, and an abnormal blunted calyx (Fig. 9.18). There is often poor excretion of contrast medium by the abnormal kidney.

Tuberculosis of the kidney in its early stages may produce nonspecific changes such as papillary necrosis. With progression of the disease, the more characteristic findings of stricture of an infundibulum, calyceal amputation, and cavitation may occur. Tuberculosis also causes ureteral strictures. A combination of renal and ureteral abnormalities such as strictures should suggest the diagnosis. The end stage of renal tuberculosis is a small, shrunken, nonfunctioning kidney that often contains calcific debris ("putty kidney") (Fig. 9.19). Renal tuberculosis is occurring more commonly today in patients with acquired immune deficiency syndrome (AIDS).

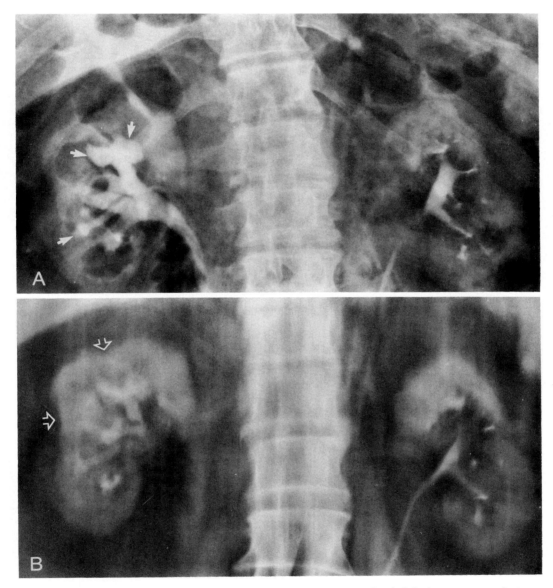

Figure 9.16.   Chronic pyelonephritis with scarring. A, detailed film shows blunting and clubbing of the calyces in the right kidney (*arrows*). The left kidney is normal. **B,** tomogram shows marked cortical irregularity (*arrows*).

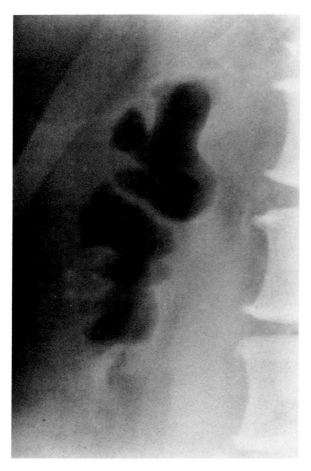

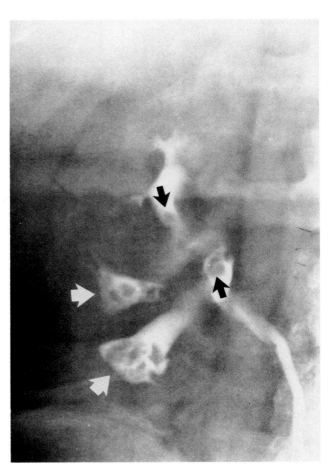

Figure 9.17. Renal gas infection. Detailed view of the right kidney in a diabetic patient reveals gas outlining the collecting system of the upper pole of the kidney.

Figure 9.18. Renal papillary necrosis. There are multiple filling defects (*arrows*) representing sloughed papillae within the collecting system.

Figure 9.19. Renal tuberculosis. A small nonfunctioning right kidney containing calcific debris ("putty kidney") is present.

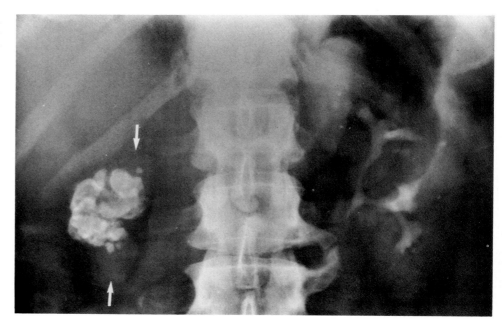

Changes of chronic inflammation of the bladder include thickening and irregularity of the wall secondary to muscular and mucosal hypertrophy.

Obstructive disease and ureterovesical reflux in association with chronic inflammatory disease may be evaluated by diuretic renal scintigraphy and radionuclide voiding cystourethrography.

Mass Lesions: Cysts and Tumors

Mass lesions in the kidneys represent either cysts, tumors, or inflammatory lesions. Filling defects elsewhere in the urinary tract generally are tumors. Renal cysts are extremely common in older individuals and are found in a high percentage of these patients undergoing autopsy. They are frequently incidental findings on abdominal CT scans. In the kidney, renal cysts appear as bulges along the cortical margin (Fig. 9.20) or as rounded absent portions of the renal parenchyma (Fig. 9.21). Quite frequently on the tomogram a thin, beak-like collection of contrast material representing compressed parenchyma may be seen along the margin (Fig. 9.20). A cyst may also displace the intrarenal collecting system.

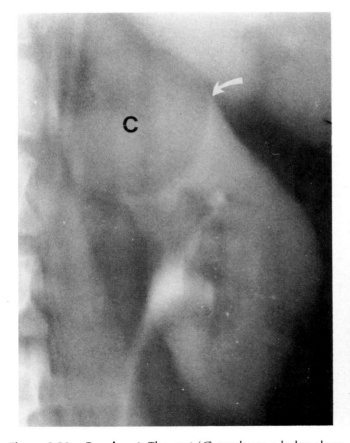

Figure 9.20. Renal cyst. The cyst (*C*) produces a bulge along the upper pole of this kidney. Note the beak-like appearance along the parenchymal margin of the cyst (*arrow*).

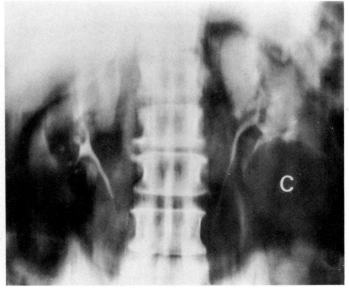

Figure 9.21. Large renal cyst (*C*) in the lower pole of the left kidney.

Once a renal mass lesion is detected on a plain film on an IVU, the next logical step should be an ultrasound examination to determine whether the mass is cystic or solid (Fig. 9.22). However, if the patient has hematuria, a CT examination should be performed. The CT appearance of a benign renal cyst includes a homogenous, smooth, rounded appearance of uniform radiographic density with a low CT value. There is no enhancement of the mass following the intravenous injection of contrast material (Fig. 9.23).

Renal tumors, on the other hand, have a considerably different radiographic appearance. On the intravenous urogram, they may produce an abnormal contour to the renal outline and distortion or displacement of the calyceal system similar to those findings seen with renal cysts. However, the similarity ends here. In addition to the distortion of the calyceal system, calyces often appear amputated. Quite often on the tomogram the mass appears mottled and not lucent, as with a renal cyst. On the ultrasound examination, the mass appears as a solid lesion with many internal echoes (Fig. 9.24**A**). This is contrary to the echo-free picture found in a simple renal cyst.

Computed tomography has contributed greatly to the differentiation between renal cyst and tumor. On an unenhanced study, distortion of the renal architecture may be plainly seen (Fig. 9.24**B**). Furthermore, when the study is enhanced by the intravenous injection of contrast material, the lesion becomes more dense, indicating it is vascular. This is quite contrary to the appearance of a cyst (Fig. 9.23). Furthermore, on a CT examination, we may often see extrarenal extension of a large tumor (Fig. 9.25).

Cyst puncture is a procedure occasionally used for the evaluation of renal mass lesions. This may be performed under ultrasonic or CT guid-

Figure 9.22.   Renal cyst (*C*). Longitudinal ultrasound scan shows the sonolucent cyst with increased "through transmission" beneath. There are no internal echoes in the cyst. Compare to Figure 9.24**A**.

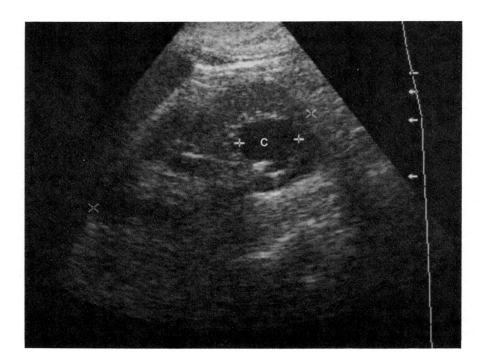

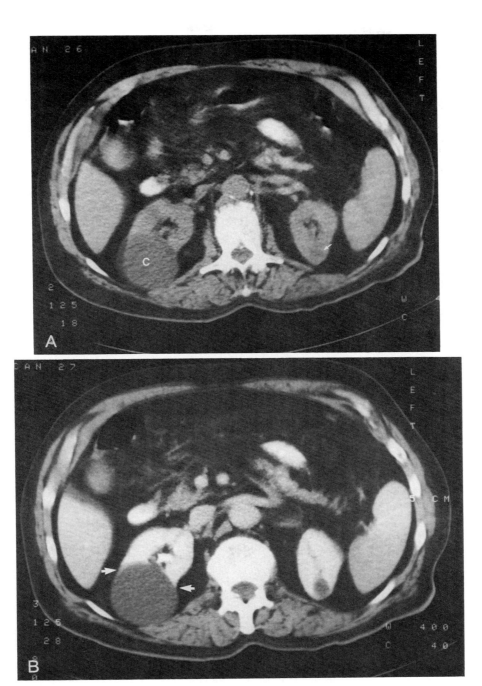

Figure 9.23. Renal cyst—CT appearance. A, unenhanced scan shows a large cyst (*C*) in the posterior aspect of the right kidney. A smaller area of lucency (*arrow*) is present in the left kidney. **B,** following intravenous contrast injection, both cysts are well-defined without evidence of enhancement. Note the beak-like appearance on the right (*arrows*).

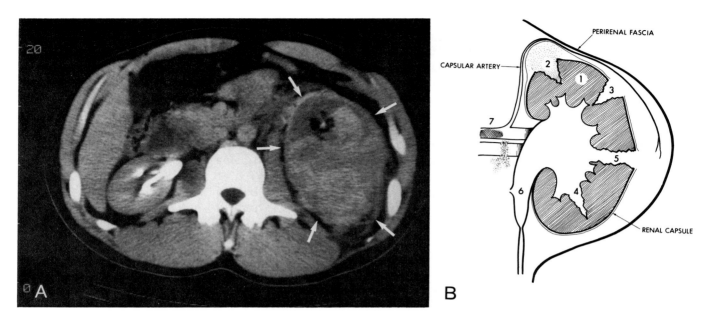

Figure 9.29. Left renal injury. A, CT scan shows enlargement of the left renal outline (*arrows*). Even though this is an enhanced scan, there is no evidence of renal function. There are, however, areas of enhancement within the renal capsule representing fragments of renal tissue. **B,** drawing of various forms of renal trauma. *1,* renal contusion; *2,* laceration with intracapsular hematoma (note the stretching of the capsular artery); *3,* laceration extending across the renal capsule; *4,* internal laceration communicating with the collecting system; *5,* renal fracture ("shattered kidney"); *6,* pelvic rupture, usually in patients with ureteropelvic obstructing lesions; *7,* vascular pedicle injury. Injuries *3* and *5* generally result in enlargement of the renal outline with extensive hemorrhage into the perirenal spaces.

Figure 9.30. Pelvic fracture with bladder rupture. The patient has suffererd a severe pelvic injury with dysraphism of the pubic symphsis (*open arrows*) and a comminuted fracture of the left acetabulum with hip dislocation. This cystogram demonstrated extraperitoneal (*white arrow*) as well as intraperitoneal (*curved arrows*) extravasation of contrast from the ruptured bladder.

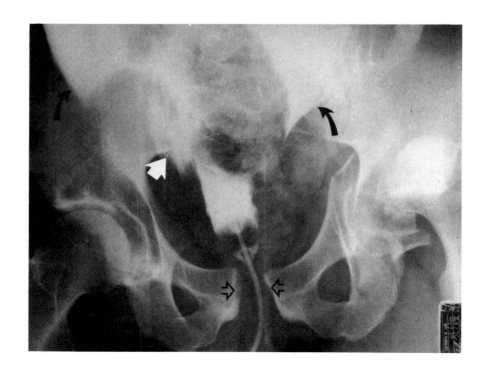

bone fragment, a foreign object (bullet, knife), instrumentation, or a biopsy; or pathologic rupture or fracture of a diseased kidney.

Trauma to the urinary tract may be very slight, such as a renal contusion, or catastrophic, such as a shattered kidney (Fig. 9.29) or ruptured bladder (Fig. 9.30). As previously mentioned, these entities occur as a result of major trauma to the abdomen and pelvis. Urethrocystography and CT are the preferred methods of evaluating bladder and urethral injury and renal trauma, respectively.

Extrinsic Diseases

Diseases in organs adjacent to the urinary tract often produce morphologic alterations of the intravenous urogram. These include displacement of a kidney by a suprarenal mass, displacement of a ureter by enlarged lymph nodes, compression of a ureter with obstructive uropathy secondary to abdominal or pelvic masses, compression of the bladder by pelvic masses, and elevation of the bladder floor by an enlarged prostate (Fig. 9.31). Abdominal CT scanning and ultrasound are the preferred methods of diagnostic imaging (Fig. 9.32).

Renal Transplants

Renal transplantation is now common in most large medical centers. You will undoubtedly treat many of these patients at some time in your medical career. Imaging studies are used to evaluate transplants and to determine their function as well as whether or not rejection is taking place.

There are three critical conditions that may affect the function of a transplanted kidney. The first of these is the rejection process itself. This will ultimately lead to a decrease in or absence of function in the trans-

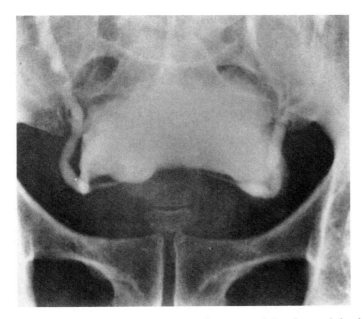

Figure 9.31. Prostatic enlargement. There is elevation of the floor of the bladder and "fishhooking" of the distal ureters by the enlarged prostate.

Figure 9.32. Retroperitoneal lymph nodes in a patient with lymphoma. A CT scan shows multiple enlarged lymph nodes (*N*) in the vicinity of the right renal pelvis. Note the vena cava (*V*) and abdominal aorta (*A*).

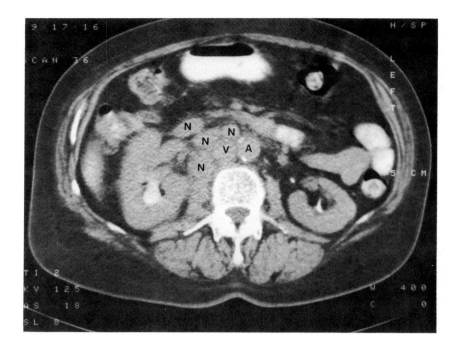

Figure 9.33. Normal renal transplant. The transplanted kidney is placed in the left iliac fossa.

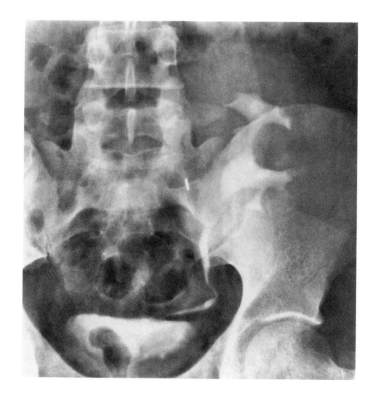

planted kidney. Obstruction at the site of ureteric reanastomosis is a second cause of decreased function. Third, a vascular abnormality at the site of grafting may adversely affect the function of a transplant. A normal renal transplant is shown in Figure 9.33. The spectrum of diagnostic examinations performed on normal kidneys is performed on renal transplants. The one major imaging improvement in diagnosing stenosis of the vessels has been Doppler ultrasound.

Summary

The urinary tract is an area of the body where many different imaging procedures are used. The diagnostic accuracy of these studies when used in combinations is exceedingly high. The various types of pathologic abnormalities you will encounter in a daily practice have been discussed.

Suggested Additional Reading

Dunnick NR, McCallum RW, Sandler CM. Textbook of uroradiology. Baltimore: Williams & Wilkins, 1991.

Pollack H, ed. Clinical urography: an atlas and textbook of urological imaging. Philadelphia: WB Saunders, 1990.

Chapter 10

Obstetric and Gynecologic Imaging

Diagnostic imaging of the female reproductive tract may be conveniently divided into obstetric and gynecologic imaging. The former discipline relies on the almost exclusive use of highly sophisticated diagnostic ultrasound. The latter, however, employs the full diagnostic methods available to both the radiologist and the gynecologist. Because of the complexity of the studies performed and their interpretation, this chapter will review the highlights of obstetric and gynecologic imaging with the goal of informing the reader of indications for various studies and their applications to a variety of common problems.

TECHNICAL CONSIDERATIONS

Diagnostic ultrasound is the primary tool for investigation of the gravid uterus as well as a variety of conditions that may affect the female reproductive tract. Ultrasound is the procedure of choice because there is no ionizing radiation associated with its use to harm either the fetus or ovarian tissue. Furthermore, because of the normal relationships of the uterus and ovaries to the bladder, it is possible to image these organs through a distended bladder without degradation of the image by bowel gas. The development of transvaginal ultrasound now provides a new means of studying the female pelvic viscera. This is particularly useful in evaluating certain neoplasms. Other noninvasive imaging studies performed include plain film radiography, computerized tomography (CT), and magnetic resonance (MR) imaging. In the past, plain film radiography was used much more extensively, particularly for the evaluation of pelvic masses, suspected infections, fetal position, and to search for lost intrauterine devices. The development of ultrasound, however, has superseded all these examinations. The CT and MR are used primarily in the evaluation of suspected infections or neoplasms involving the ovaries or uterus. These studies are used in much the same way that they would be used to evaluate similar abnormalities elsewhere within the abdomen and pelvis.

Obstetric Imaging

The evaluation of the gravid uterus is accomplished primarily through the use of ultrasound. *Obstetric sonography is a highly complex examination that needs to be performed by a carefully trained operator and interpreted with a great degree of skill.* Early in the history of obstetric ultrasound, the primary goal was to confirm the presence of an intrauterine pregnancy, to determine the location of the placenta, to detect multiple gestation, to determine the lie of the fetus, and to estimate gestational age. Refinements and improvements in ultrasound technology have added a more important indication—that of detecting congenital anomalies and other abnormalities of the fetus. Indeed, many of the malpractice actions filed against obstetricians relate to failure to detect fetal abnormalities before birth.

Since ultrasound has no ionizing radiation, there are no adverse biologic effects upon either the mother or the fetus. However, this study, like any other, should only be performed when indicated. Table 10.1 lists the varied indications for obstetric sonography. Note that the indications change with time throughout the pregnancy. This discussion will highlight the normal sonographic changes that may be observed at various intervals during pregnancy. In addition, several common abnormalities will be discussed. For a more in-depth treatment of the subject, the reader is referred to the works listed in the Suggested Additional Reading at the end of the chapter.

Table 10.1.   Indications for Obstetric Sonography

I. General Indications
  1. Confirm presence of intrauterine pregnancy
  2. Estimate gestational age
  3. Detection of multiple gestation
  4. Location and texture of the placenta
  5. Detection of anatomic and functional abnormalities of the fetus
  6. Evaluation of other pelvic masses during pregnancy
II. First Trimester
  1. Uterine bleeding
  2. Suspected threatened, incomplete, or missed abortion
  3. Distinguish intrauterine from ectopic pregnancy
  4. Suspected molar pregnancy
  5. Suspected pregnancy associated with intrauterine contraceptive device
III. Second Trimester
  1. Localization and evaluation of placenta
  2. Polyhydramnios
  3. Evaluation of fetal growth
IV. Third Trimester
  1. Possible placenta previa
  2. Fetal maturity to plan optimal time and mode of delivery
V. Maternal abdominal disorders during pregnancy
VI. Postpartum for suspected retained products of conception

The Normal Pregnancy

FIRST TRIMESTER

The first trimester is the time between conception and the end of the 13th week of gestation. The terms "gestational age" and "menstrual age" are often used interchangeably by obstetricians. However, because of variations in ovulation, there may be a 1- to 2-week discrepancy between the sonographic assessment of menstrual age and the actual gestational age of the fetus. Gestational age as a rule is determined from the time of conception. The menstrual age relies on the 1st day of the last menses. For purposes of our discussion, we will refer only to gestational age.

A gestational sac may be detected as early as 3 weeks from conception. This consists of a round-to-oval area devoid of echoes located within the body or fundus of the uterus (Fig. 10.3). This sonolucency represents the choriodecidua that surrounds the developing embryo. The embryonic period occurs between the 3rd and 8th weeks of gestational age. Embryonic development is usually not able to be delineated in its early stages. During this period, all major body organs begin forming. Further growth and differentiation occur in the fetal period. The exact transition time between embryonic and fetal periods is arbitrary.

Once a fetus can be detected, the gestational age may be estimated by measuring the crown-rump (long axis) length of the fetus. This method is accurate to within 1 week of gestational age (Fig. 10.4). The following normal structures can also be detected at the times indicated. Arm buds, 8 weeks; leg buds, 9 to 10 weeks; fetal heart, 7 to 8 weeks; choroid plexus of

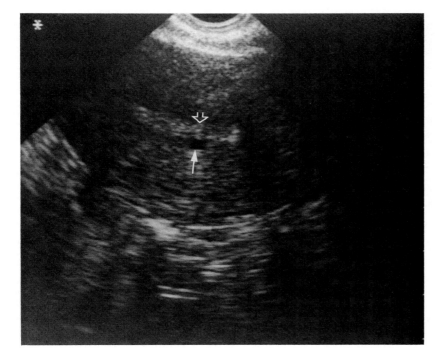

Figure 10.3. Normal 3- to 4-week gestation. Ultrasound examination shows the small gestational sac (*solid arrow*) attached to the thickened uterine wall (*open arrow*).

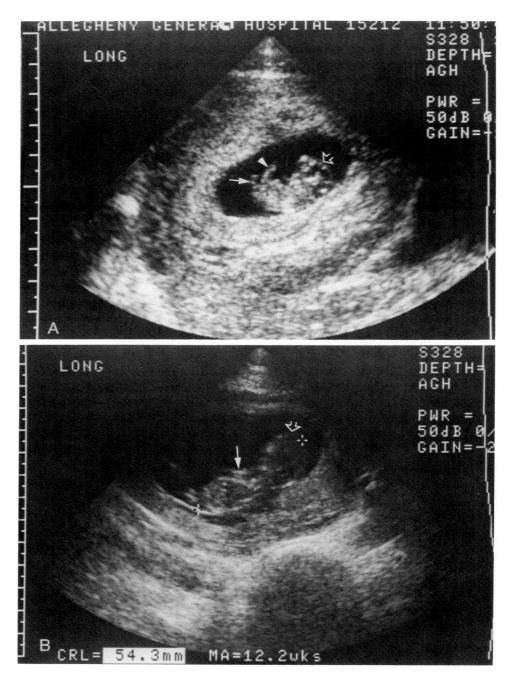

Figure 10.4.   Normal first trimester. A, fetal poles at 9.3 weeks of gestation. Note the head (*open arrow*), the foot (*solid arrow*) and umbilical cord (*arrowhead*). **B,** at 12.2 weeks of gestation, the crown-to-rump length is 54.3 mm. Note the head (*open arrow*) and upper limb (*solid arrow*).

the brain, 12 to 16 weeks. Other structures that can be detected during the first trimester include the umbilical stalk and the yolk sac.

SECOND TRIMESTER

The second trimester of pregnancy is that interval between the 14th and 26th gestational weeks. A more detailed evaluation of the fetus, uterus, and placenta is possible because of their enlargement during this time. It is during this time that amniotic fluid may be detected surrounding the fetus. As a rule, the volume of amniotic fluid should equal the volume of the fetus. The location and size of the placenta can easily be determined (Fig. 10.5). The fetal organs also enlarge and are easily detectable on sonography. It is thus possible to determine the gross morphology and function of the heart by real-time examination. In the latter portion of the second trimester, the fetal liver and kidneys can be demonstrated, and the distended fetal urinary bladder can be seen. Furthermore, it is possible to delineate the external genitalia during the latter portion of the second trimester. The extremities and their developing bones are also demonstrable. In addition, the fetal spine can also be detected. It is during the second trimester that gestational age is determined from the biparietal diameter. Tables correlating biparietal diameter with menstrual age are available in every obstetric department.

THIRD TRIMESTER

The third trimester of pregnancy is that time between the 27th week up to the time of delivery. During this time, there is continued enlargement of both the uterus and fetus as well as changes within the placenta. Sonography is clearly able to demonstrate detailed anatomy of various

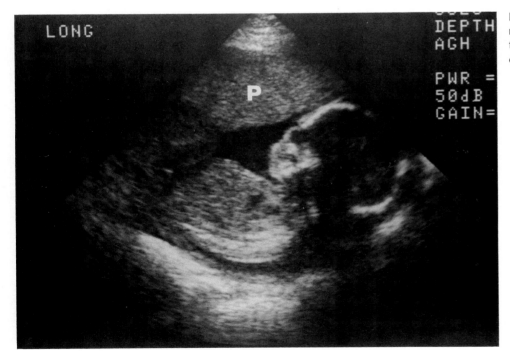

Figure 10.5. Normal second trimester fetus showing the position of the placenta (*P*). Facial features are clearly visible.

fetal organs (Fig. 10.6). In addition, fetal motion can easily be seen on real-time examination. Sonography in this period is used primarily to determine the optimal time and mode of delivery as well as to confirm or exclude the presence of a placenta previa.

PATHOLOGIC CONSIDERATIONS

A variety of abnormalities occur during pregnancy. Vaginal bleeding during the first trimester is often referred to as "threatened abortion." There are no specific sonographic findings in this condition. However, retention of products of conception is referred to as "incomplete abortion." In this situation, the sonographic findings may vary from a normal-appearing uterus to one that contains blood clots and/or fetal parts (Fig. 10.7).

Placenta previa is a condition in which a placenta is located either partially or completely across the cervical os (Fig. 10.8). This condition may result in maternal or fetal death from massive hemorrhage at the time of birth. The detection of placenta previa by the middle of the third trimester is necessary in order that the fetus be delivered by cesarean section before the onset of labor.

Abruptio placentae is the premature separation of the placenta from the wall of the uterus. This may be detected by sonography as a sonolucent area between the uterine wall and the placental shadows (Fig. 10.9).

Various fetal anomalies may be detected during the later stages of pregnancy. These include fetal hydrocephalus and anencephaly (Fig. 10.10), meningomyelocele (Fig. 10.11), and hydranencephaly. Urinary abnormalities such as urinary obstruction detected by oligohydramnios, and

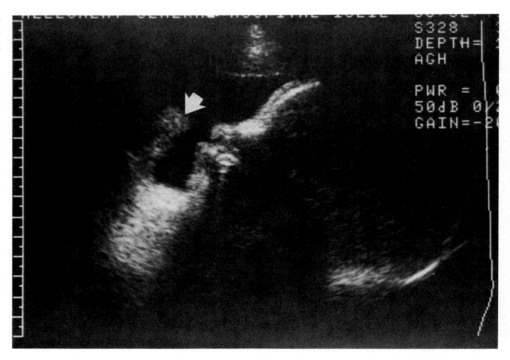

Figure 10.6. Normal third trimester fetus. Facial features are clearly visible. Is this fetus sucking its thumb (*arrow*)?

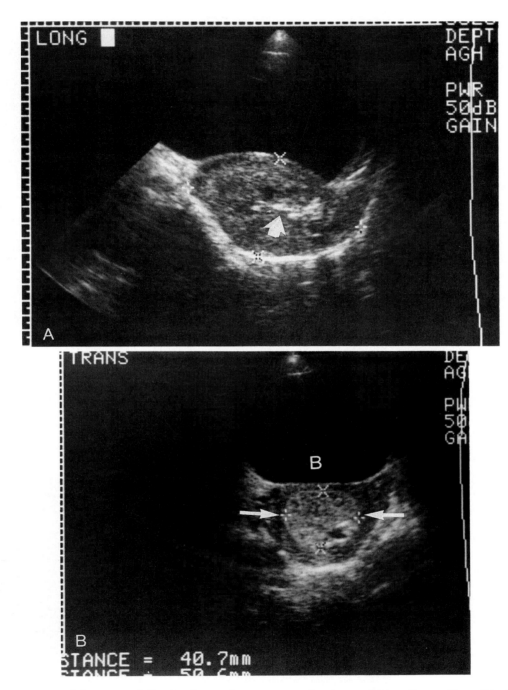

Figure 10.7. Appearance of the uterus following incomplete abortion. A, longitudinal scan shows retained placental products (*arrow*). **B,** transverse scan shows the retained products of conception (*arrows*). Note the position of the bladder (*B*) above the uterus.

Figure 10.8. Placenta previa. Longitudinal scan shows the placenta (*P*) lying just above the cervical os (*O*).

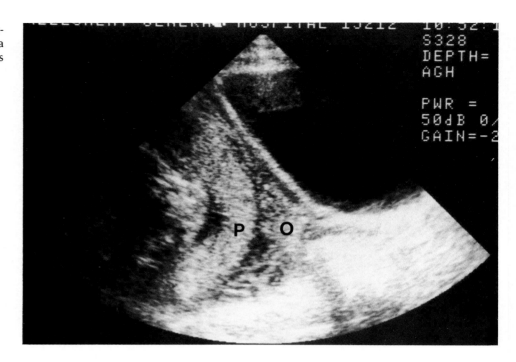

Figure 10.9. Abruptio placentae. (This is the same patient as in Figure 10.8.) Longitudinal scan made 1 week after Figure 10.8 shows separation of the placenta from the uterine wall (*arrows*).

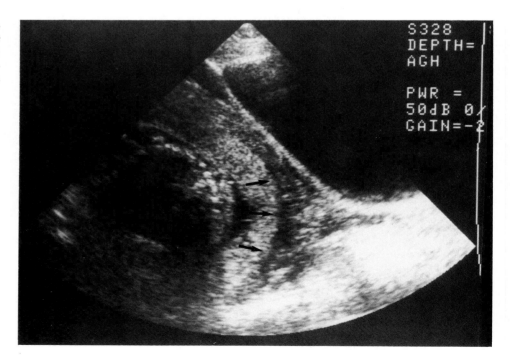

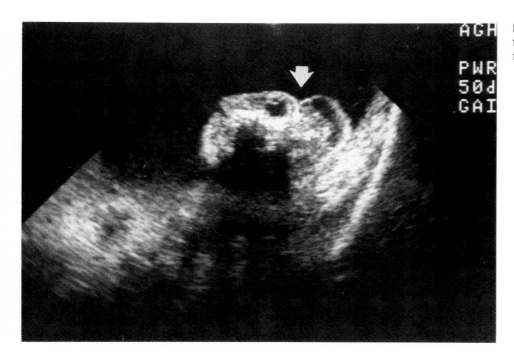

Figure 10.10.   Anencephaly. Longitudinal scan shows a grossly deformed head (*arrow*).

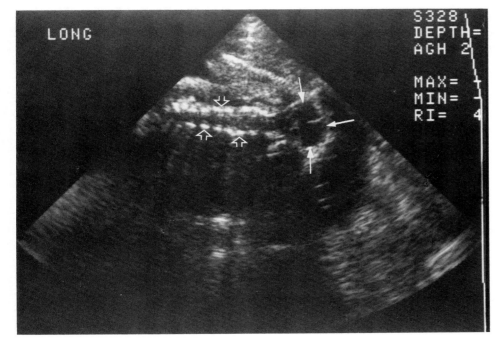

Figure 10.11.   Longitudinal fetal ultrasound showing a meningomyelocele. *Open arrows* show the individual vertebrae. *Solid arrows* show the meningomyelocele.

Figure 10.12. Ectopic pregnancy.
Transverse scan shows an irregular collection of echoes (*arrow*) behind the uterus.

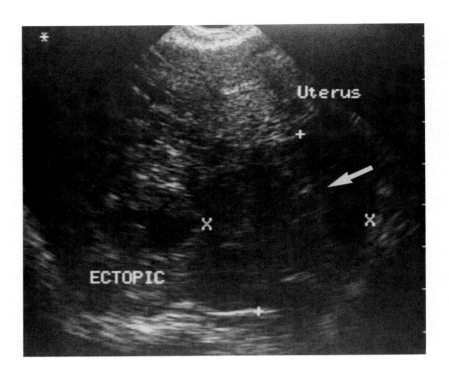

multi- or polycystic kidney disease can also be demonstrated. Abnormalities of the gastrointestinal tract that are detectable include duodenal atresia, omphalocele, and fetal ascites. Cardiac abnormalities are difficult to detect because of the cardiac motion. However, careful evaluation can result in the demonstration of certain of these anomalies. Finally, forms of dwarfism such as achondroplasia may be detected. Fractures of the fetal skeleton in utero may be the result of underlying osteogenesis imperfecta.

An ectopic pregnancy is one in which implantation occurs outside the uterine cavity. In the majority of patients, the products of conception implant in a Fallopian tube. In most cases, there has been tubal scarring as the result of previous pelvic inflammatory disease. Ectopic pregnancy is readily detectable by ultrasound (Fig. 10.12).

Gynecologic Imaging

Evaluation of abnormalities involving the female reproductive tract has benefitted greatly by the developments in body imaging. The modalities primarily used are ultrasound, computerized tomography, magnetic resonance imaging, and hysterosalpingography.

Because ultrasound is noninvasive, uses no ionizing radiation, is rapid to perform, and is relatively inexpensive, it has remained one of the initial studies to be performed in evaluation of abnormalities of the pelvis. The ability to image in both transverse and longitudinal planes give it a distinct advantage over CT, which is performed in the transverse plane only. Magnetic resonance imaging has advantages of both procedures and is particularly useful in the evaluation of pelvic neoplasms. Hysterosalpingography is the single best radiologic technique for delineating the morphology of the uterine lumen as well as the patency of the Fallopian tubes in the evaluation of patients with infertility problems (Figs. 10.13 and 10.14). Thus, the gynecologist has a large variety of imaging procedures available to diagnose abnormalities. In most instances, ultrasonography will be the first examination performed. This will be followed up by either a CT scan or MR examination.

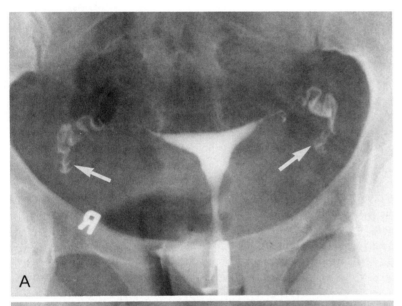

Figure 10.13. Normal hysterosalpingogram. A, following injection of contrast through the uterine os, there is spillage from both Fallopian tubes (*arrows*). **B,** delayed films shows intraperitoneal contrast outlining loops of bowel (*arrows*).

Figure 10.14. Abnormal hysterosalpingogram. There is occlusion of the left Fallopian tube near its origin (*large arrow*). There is irregularity and scarring of the right Fallopian tube (*small arrows*).

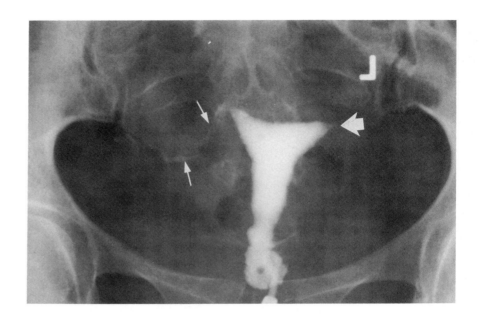

PATHOLOGIC CONSIDERATIONS

Pathologic conditions that occur within the female reproductive organs fall into four categories: congenital, physiologic, inflammatory, and neoplastic. *Congenital abnormalities* primarily appear in the uterus. As many as 0.5% of women have congenital anomalies. These may be incidental findings of no clinical significance. However, others such as bicornuate uterus may result in pregnancy disorders. Congenital uterine abnormalities are often associated with renal agenesis. For this reason, it is important to image the kidneys when a uterine abnormality is encountered.

Physiologic abnormalities include cystic diseases of the ovary and endometriosis. Because of normal physiologic functions, cysts up to 3 to 4 cm in the ovary may be simply physiologic, that is transient and changing, depending on the phase of menstrual cycle. However, a normal physiologic cyst that fails to regress or enlarges because of a hormonal imbalance or hemorrhage may form a functional or retention cyst. These are the most common pelvic masses encountered in young women (Fig. 10.15).

Endometriosis is due to the presence of endometrial tissue in extrauterine sites. The most common location for endometriosis is within the pelvic cavity. From an imaging standpoint, endometriosis produces cystic masses of various size anywhere within the pelvis (Fig. 10.16). These may implant on the colon and produce extraluminal compression defects that may be seen with a barium enema.

Pelvic inflammatory disease is the result of an ascending infection from the vagina to the endometrium, Fallopian tubes, and ultimately, pelvic peritoneum. In most instances, the etiologic organism is gonococcal. Inflammatory collections in the pelvis may be detected on either CT or

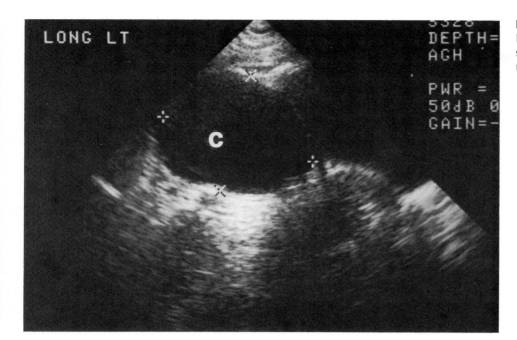

Figure 10.15. Ovarian cyst (C). Parasagittal longitudinal ultrasound shows the large cyst devoid of internal echoes.

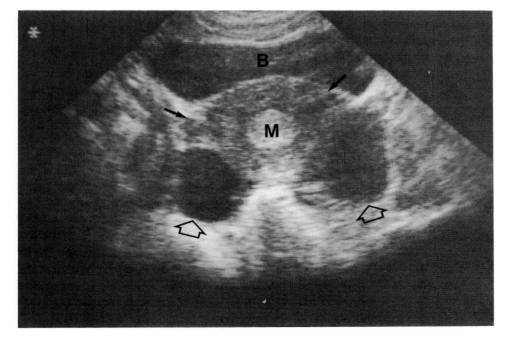

Figure 10.16. Endometriosis. Transverse ultrasound shows the bladder (*B*), the thickened uterine wall (*closed arrows*), menstrual debris (*M*), and two parauterine masses (*open arrows*) representing ectopic endometrial tissue.

ultrasound without difficulty. Occasionally, a tubo-ovarian abscess will be formed (Fig. 10.17).

Neoplasms of the female reproductive organs include both benign and malignant tumors. Common benign tumors include serous cystadenoma (Fig. 10.18), fibroid tumors, and dermoid tumors (Fig. 10.19). These latter lesions often contain fat, calcifications, and occasionally dental elements, all of which are easily demonstrable by CT. Fibroids are extremely

Figure 10.17. Bilateral tubo-ovarian abscesses. Transverse scan shows bilateral multilocular masses of mixed echogenicity (*arrows*) on either side of the uterus (*U*).

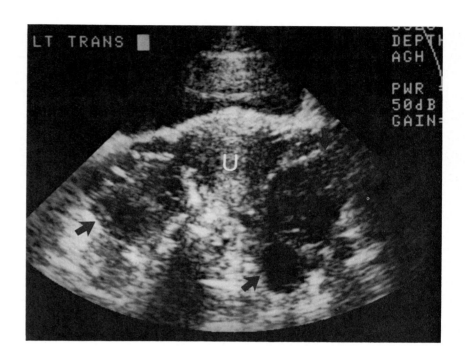

Figure 10.18. Ovarian cystadenoma. Transverse scan shows a mass of mixed echogenicity (*arrows*) beneath the bladder.

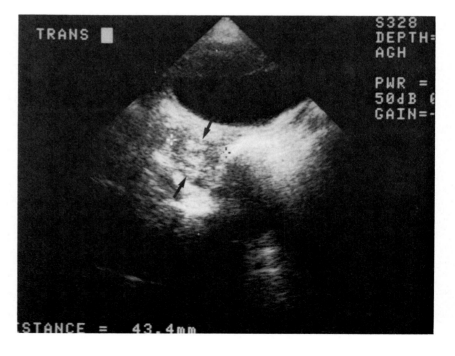

common and occur in up to 40% of women over the age of 35 years. They are often found as incidental calcifications on abdominal plain films (Fig. 10.20).

Malignant neoplasms are unfortunately common. Endometrial carcinoma is the most common invasive gynecologic malignancy. Cervical carcinoma is the second most common. It ranks sixth in cancer mortality, primarily because symptoms do not occur until late. Ovarian carcinoma is

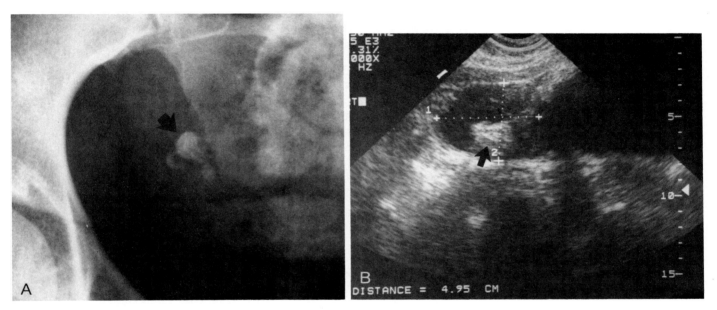

Figure 10.19. Dermoid tumor of the ovary. A, detailed view of the pelvis shows tooth-like calcifications in the right lower quadrant (*arrow*). **B,** ultrasound shows the dense calcified area (*arrow*) within the more cystic tumor.

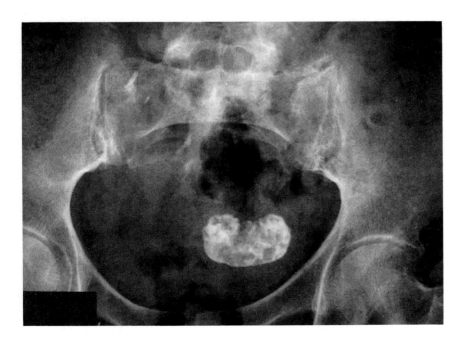

Figure 10.20. Calcified uterine fibroid in the pelvis. These calcifications are often popcorn-like in appearance.

the next most common gynecologic malignant tumor. It is responsible for 50% of the deaths from gynecologic malignancy and is the fourth most frequent cause of cancer death in women (after lung, breast, and colon). Malignancies of the vagina, vulva, and oviduct are much less common. Multimodality imaging is used in the detection, staging, and follow-up of all these neoplasms (Figs. 10.21 to 10.23). Of particular importance in the evaluation of patients with these diseases is the detection of the presence or absence of localized spread through invasion of contiguous tissues. The presence or absence of extension beyond the affected organ will determine the exact staging of the neoplasm according the standards set by the International Federation of Gynecology and Obstetrics.

Summary

This chapter has dealt with the evaluation of the female reproductive tract primarily utilizing sonography. Because of the complexity in the performance and interpretation of obstetrical sonography, the discussion has been limited to basic concepts. The reader is referred to more definitive texts or in-depth discussion of the more sophisticated aspects of this subject. The evaluation of gynecologic abnormalities utilizes a multimodality imaging approach, although sonography remains a primary tool. The evaluation of abnormalities of these structures is performed in the same manner as that of other organ systems.

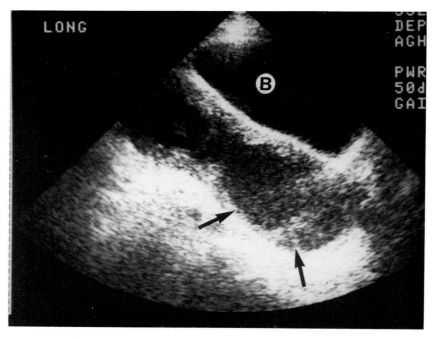

Figure 10.21. Endometrial carcinoma. Longitudinal scan shows enlargement of the uterus and echogenic material (*arrows*) immediately behind the bladder (*B*).

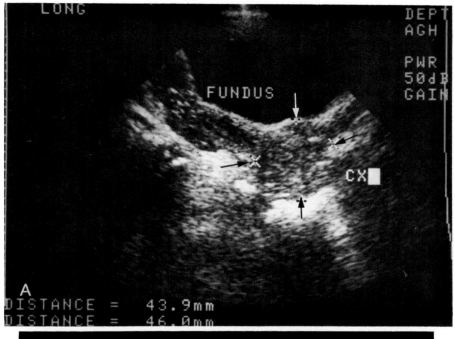

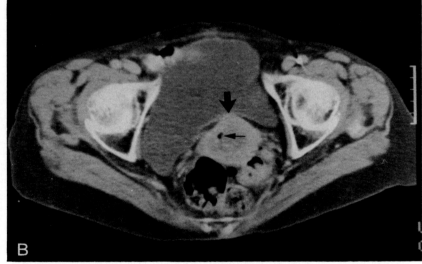

Figure 10.22.   Cervical carcinoma. A, longitudinal scan shows enlargement of the underlying cervix (*arrows*). CX, cervix. **B,** a CT scan shows the mass immediately behind the bladder (*large arrow*). A small amount of gas is present within the mass (*small arrow*) secondary to necrosis.

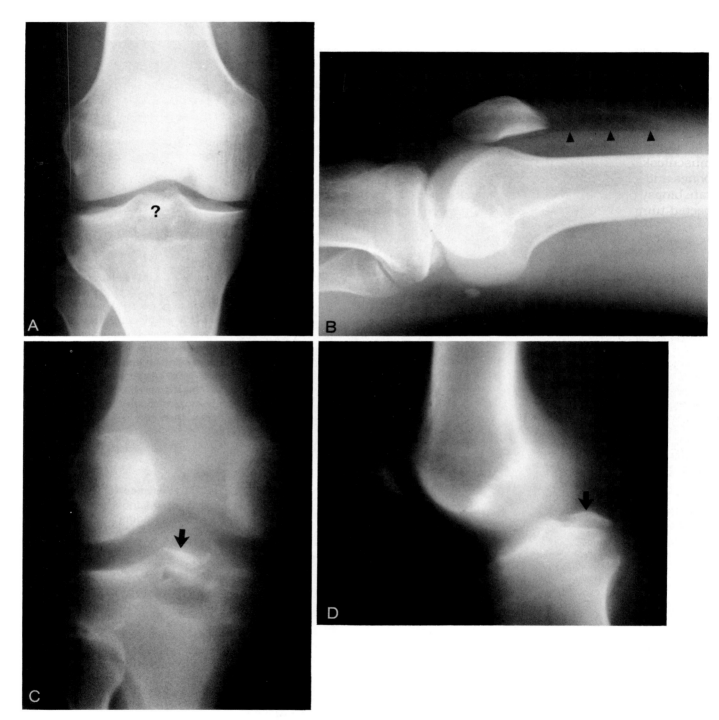

Figure 11.4. Tibial plateau fracture. A, frontal radiograph shows a vague area of irregularity involving the intercondylar spines of the tibia (*?*). **B,** a horizontal beam lateral film shows a fat-fluid level (*arrowheads*) in the suprapatellar space. This find- ing indicates that there is a fracture communicating with the synovial space. **C,** frontal tomogram shows a communited frac- ture of the intercondylar spines (*arrow*). **D,** lateral tomogram shows that one fragment is displaced posteriorly (*arrow*).

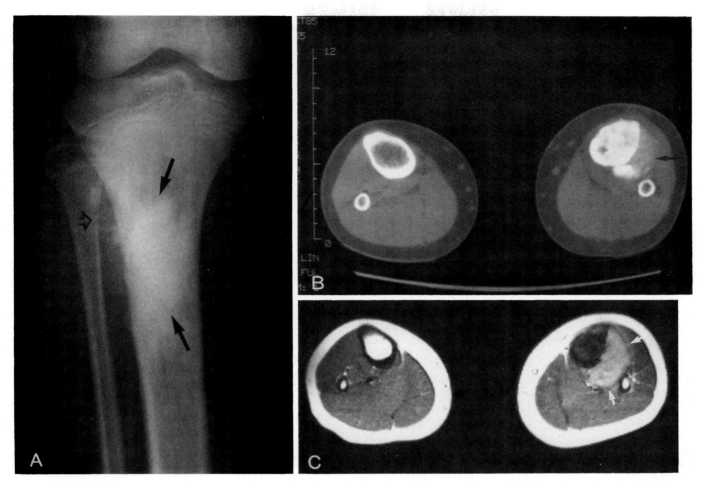

Figure 11.5. Osteosarcoma of the proximal tibia. A, frontal radiograph shows an area of bone destruction with clouds of osteoid matrix (*solid arrows*). The lesion extends beyond the margin of bone into the soft tissues (*open arrow*). **B,** CT scan shows the increased density due to this osteogenic sarcoma in the left tibia. Note the extraosseous extension into the soft tissues (*arrow*). **C,** MR image shows the extent of soft tissue involvement to better advantage (*arrows*). The dense osteoid tissue appears black on this T2-weighted image.

(Fig. 11.6), infections (Fig. 11.7), and to augment arthrograms, especially of the shoulder. Three-dimensional reconstruction of CT examinations have been found to be useful by referring surgeons.

Magnetic resonance imaging of the musculoskeletal system is the second most common use of this technique (after neuroimaging). Magnetic resonance has revolutionized musculoskeletal radiology. In addition to its ability to portray information in sagittal, coronal, and transverse planes, it can aid in the diagnosis of primary (Fig. 11.8) and metastatic tumors, infections (Fig. 11.9), vertebral trauma (Fig. 11.10), avascular necrosis (Fig. 11.11), tendon ruptures (Fig. 11.12), and internal joint derangements (Fig. 11.13). Indeed, MR has all but eliminated many types of arthrography.

Diagnostic ultrasound has been used to diagnose soft tissue lesions (Fig. 11.14). There was hope that it would be useful in assessing tears of the rotator cuff of the shoulder. However, the greater accuracy of MR as

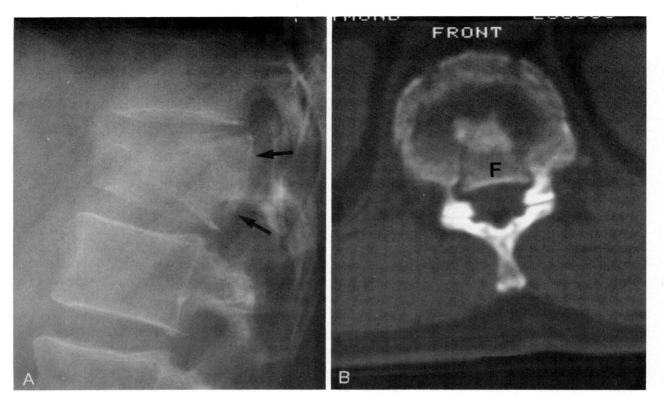

Figure 11.6. Burst fracture of T-12. A, lateral radiograph shows compression of the body of T-12 and retropulsion of the fragments from posterior vertebral body line into the vertebral canal (*arrows*). **B,** CT scan shows the displaced fragment (*F*) markedly narrowing the vertebral canal.

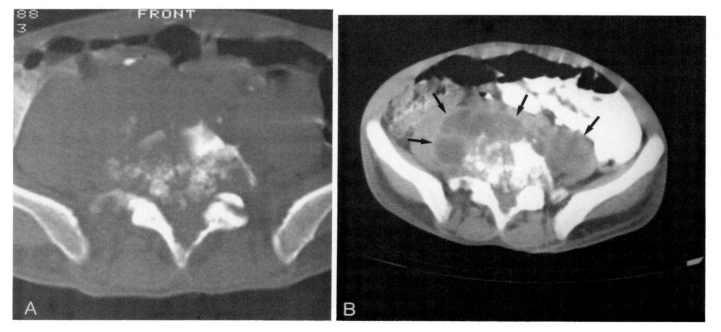

Figure 11.7. Vertebral osteomyelitis and paraspinous abscess. A, CT scan near the lumbosacral junction shows a destructive process of L-5. Note the paraspinal soft tissue mass in front of the vertebrae. **B,** CT image slightly lower made at soft tissue windows following intravenous contrast enhancement. Note the large multilocular abscess in the soft tissues (*arrows*). The rim of the abscess is enhanced.

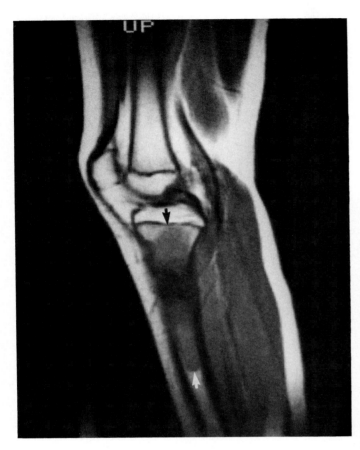

Figure 11.8.   Osteosarcoma of the tibia. Direct sagittal image of the proximal tibia shows an extensive area of marrow replacement in the proximal tibia (*arrows*). There is a suggestion of cortical breakthrough in the darkest area near the middle. (The same patient as in Fig. 11.5).

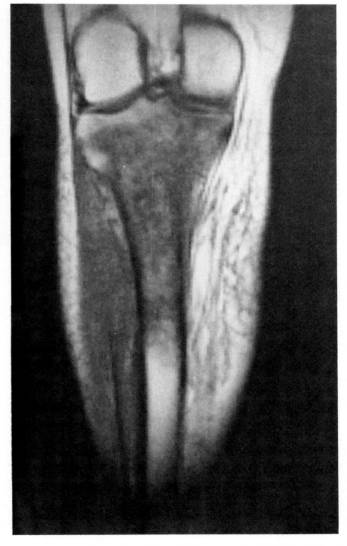

Figure 11.9.   Osteomyelitis of the proximal tibia. Direct coronal scan at T1-weighted parameters demonstrate an extensive area of low signal within the marrow space of the tibia. The process extends up to the joint line but has not yet crossed. Note that the actual extent of marrow involvement is greater than the extent of bony destruction seen on plain film. (The same patient as in Fig. 11.2.)

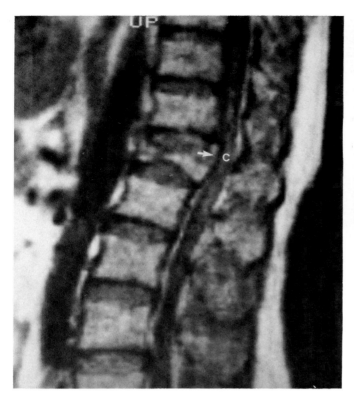

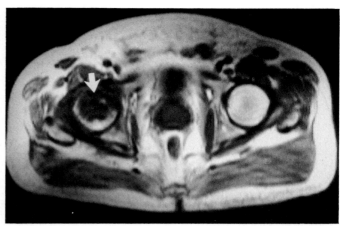

Figure 11.11. Avascular necrosis of the right hip. This T1-weighted image shows low signal within the right femoral head (*arrow*). Compare with the left.

Figure 11.10. Burst fracture of T-12. (The same patient as in Fig. 11.6.) Note the compression of the spinal cord (*C*) by the retropulsed bone fragment (*arrow*).

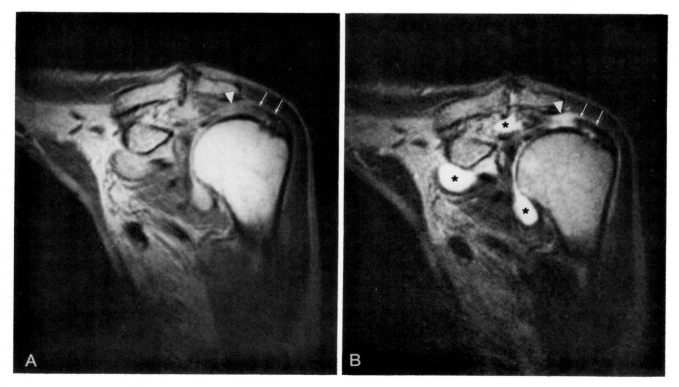

Figure 11.12. Rotator cuff tear. A, T1-weighted coronal image shows an area of interruption (*arrowhead*) of the tendon of the supraspinatus muscle (*small arrows*). **B,** gradient echo coronal image shows the findings to better advantage. The globular areas of increased signal (*) represent a joint effusion. This figure shows the difference between T1 and gradient echo imaging.

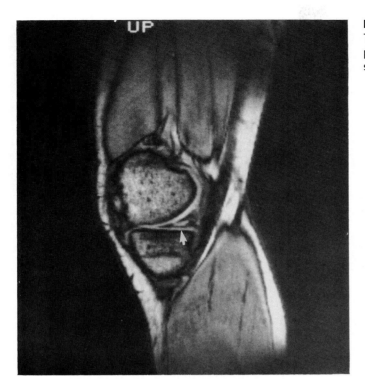

Figure 11.13. Torn posterior horn of the medial meniscus. There is an area of increased signal (brightness) (*arrow*) in the posterior horn of the medial meniscus. Normally, the meniscus should be a uniform black triangle.

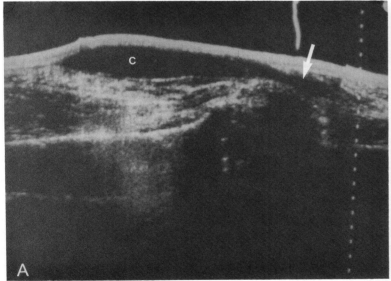

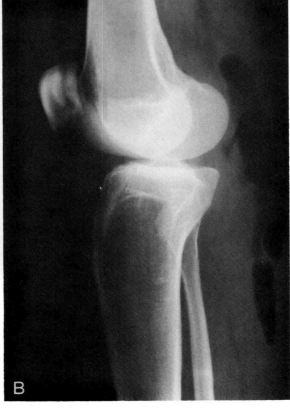

Figure 11.14. Large dissecting popliteal (Baker's cyst) in a patient with rheumatoid arthritis. A, longitudinal ultrasound shows a large sonolucent cystic area (*C*) in the proximal calf. Communication with the joint space is shown by the *arrow*. The knee joint is to the reader's right. **B,** lateral radiograph following air arthrogram shows the air dissecting in the large cyst in the calf.

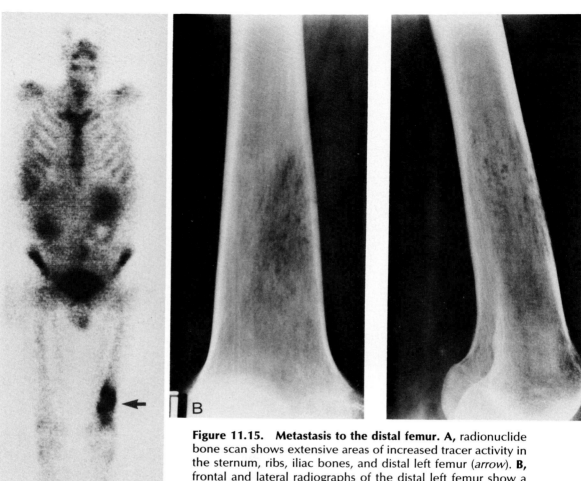

Figure 11.15. **Metastasis to the distal femur. A,** radionuclide bone scan shows extensive areas of increased tracer activity in the sternum, ribs, iliac bones, and distal left femur (*arrow*). **B,** frontal and lateral radiographs of the distal left femur show a moth-eaten-to-permeative bony destructive process.

well as its ease of performance has resulted in abandonment of this endeavor. Ultrasound is an excellent choice for diagnosing congenital hip dysplasia (CDH) in the infant whose femoral head epiphyses have not yet ossified. Ultrasound can show the unossified cartilaginous femoral head and the acetabulum without the danger of irradiation of the pelvis and gonads. Despite the availability of this study, pediatricians still order pelvic radiographs when they suspect CDH in their patients. Ultrasound is also useful for locating nonopaque foreign bodies in soft tissues.

Nuclear imaging studies of the skeletal system include the radioisotope bone scan and indium scan. The bone scan is a valuable and useful tool for detecting areas of abnormal metabolic activity within bone. With the introduction of ^{99m}technetium-labeled phosphorus compounds, a new dimension of safety and accuracy was accomplished. The phosphorus contained within the isotope is exchanged in areas of rapid bone turnover: destructive lesions such as osteomyelitis and tumors, arthritis, and areas of growing bone. Although the scan itself is not specific for a particular disease, it indicates an area of bony abnormality to which radiography, CT, and MR may be directed. The bone scan is often positive before the conventional radiograph shows any abnormality in a particular bone. It should be used as the primary screening examination for the detection of metastases (Fig. 11.15) and in suspected child abuse.

As mentioned previously, the technetium scan is often nonspecific. One area where a more specific isotope scan may be used is in suspected osteomyelitis. These studies use ^{111}indium-labeled white cells to identify areas of inflammatory activity. This is particularly useful in patients with metallic implants (plates, screws, prostheses) who are suspected of having an infection about the implant, since MR imaging often cannot be used because of the artifacts from the metal.

Arthrography is the study of joints, utilizing positive contrast material, with or without air, that is injected into the joint space. It was most often used to evaluate the knee for meniscal and ligamentous tears. Arthrography is also used in the shoulder to detect tears of the rotator cuff (Fig. 11.16), in the wrist for ligamentous tears, and in evaluating patients with painful joint prostheses (Fig. 11.17). Knee and shoulder arthrography have been replaced for the most part by MR.

Arteriography is used infrequently to evaluate patients with suspected bone tumors because MR has also largely superseded angiography for this purpose. Arteriography is also used to evaluate blood vessels in severe skeletal trauma where vascular injury is suspected (Fig. 11.18).

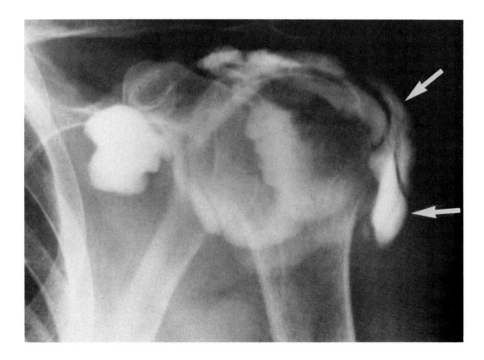

Figure 11.16. Shoulder arthrogram demonstrating a complete rotator cuff tear. Contrast injected into the glenohumeral joint has extravasated into the subacromial/subdeltoid bursa (*arrows*). An intact rotator cuff prevents this from occurring.

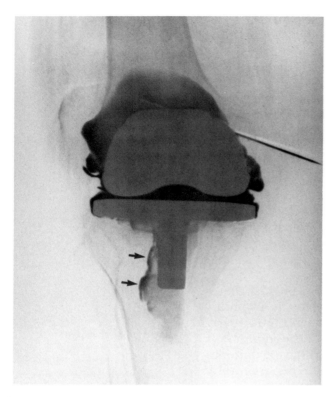

Figure 11.17. Loose total knee prosthesis. Subtraction film following intrarticular injection of a contrast shows the contrast tracking between bone and cement at the site of implantation of the tibial component (*arrows*).

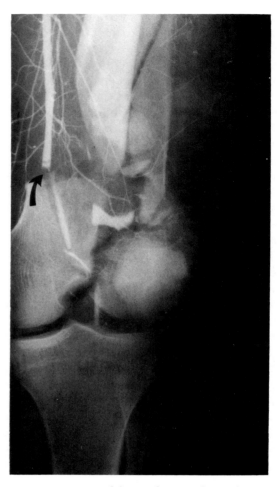

Figure 11.18. Transected femoral artery (arrow) in a patient with a severe comminuted intercondylar fracture of the distal femur.

Concern for patients with osteoporosis has led to the development of several methods for assessing bone mineral mass using imaging studies: dual photon (nuclear) absorptiometry, CT densitometry, and computer-enhanced scanning. Each of these methods has advantages and drawbacks regarding sensitivity and accuracy. If you have a patient on whom you are considering performing bone densitometry study, you should consult your radiologist.

ANATOMIC CONSIDERATIONS

The specific anatomy of each of the 206 bones in the skeleton will not be reviewed. For that purpose, consult a good textbook of anatomy. However, you should remember that, because you are dealing with three-dimensional structures in the skeleton, many bony projections may overlap and produce "strange" shadows with which you are not familiar.

The best way to avoid this confusion is to have a thorough knowledge of the anatomy of the bone being studied.

There are five types of bone, based on their shapes:

1. Long bones, which have two ends and a shaft (femur, humerus, and, interestingly, phalanges, which are miniature long bones)
2. Short bones, which are, as a rule, six-sided (carpal and tarsal bones)
3. Flat bones (calvaria, ribs, and sternum)
4. Irregular bones, which have many sides (vertebrae)
5. Sesamoid bones, which lack periosteum and develop in tendons (the largest is the patella).

Furthermore, bone may be of two architectural types: compact (dense) bone or cancellous (spongy) bone. The distribution of these types of bones depends on the stress to which each bone is subjected.

There are three locations within a bone: the epiphysis, or growth center; the metaphysis, an area that lies just beneath the physis, or growth plate; and the diaphysis, or shaft. As you will see later, these locations are of considerable importance in predicting the nature of some bone lesions.

PATHOLOGIC CONSIDERATIONS

Analysis of bone and joint lesions can be as simple as the ABCS.

A Anatomic appearance and alignment abnormalities
B Bony mineralization and texture abnormalities
C Cartilage (joint space) abnormalities
S Soft tissue abnormalities

These will be elaborated on as they apply to the analysis of bone lesions later in the discussion. Using this approach, however, you will find how adept you will be at recognizing and diagnosing many bone lesions.

There are six basic pathologic categories of skeletal disease: *congenital, inflammatory, metabolic, neoplastic, traumatic, and vascular.* A seventh category, *miscellaneous* or *other,* might be added to encompass those diseases that do not fall strictly into one of the first six.

The logical approach to musculoskeletal radiology begins by defining the distribution of a lesion and by applying a number of factors that can further narrow the diagnostic choices. These factors have been termed "predictor variables."

Distribution

The distribution of a bone or joint lesion provides important clues to the etiology of that lesion. Lesions may be monostotic or monoarticular, i.e., confined to one bone or joint; polyostotic or polyarticular, i.e., located in many bones or joints; or diffuse, that is involving virtually every bone or joint. Applying this distribution pattern to the six pathologic categories produces a scheme shown in Table 11.1. By studying Table 11.1, you can see that there are only two disease categories that may occur diffusely, neoplastic and metabolic. Metabolic disease by definition is a diffuse disease; however, occasionally monostotic or polyostotic forms occur. Examples of these lesions are shown in Table 11.2.

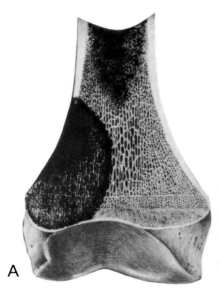

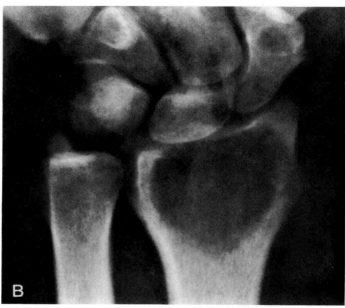

Figure 11.19. Geographic bone destruction. A, drawing shows a large destructive lesion. The lesion is easily seen with the unaided eye. **B,** giant cell tumor of the distal radius, an example of a geographic lesion.

Figure 11.20. Moth-eaten bone destruction. A, drawing showing typical appearance of moth-eaten destruction. In most instances, this may be seen with the unaided eye. **B,** osteomyelitis of the distal tibia, an example of moth-eaten bony destruction.

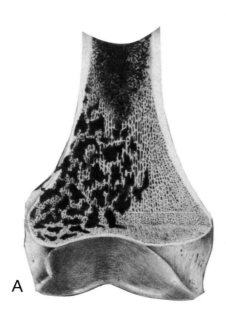

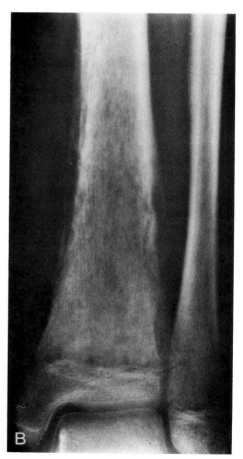

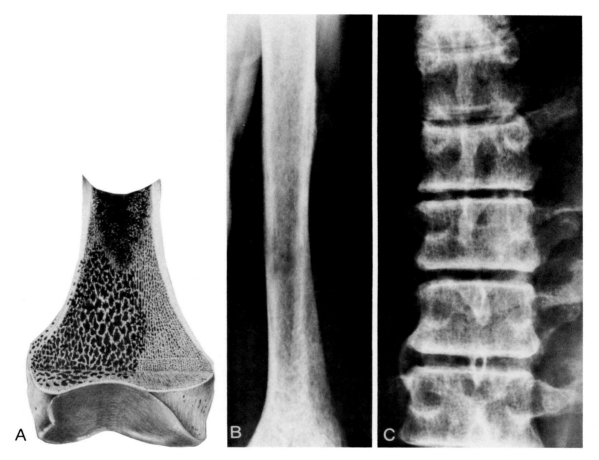

Figure 11.21. Permeative or infiltrative bone destruction. A, in this instance, the pathologic process is infiltrating the Haversian system. Magnification may be required to see the lesion. **B,** permeative bony destruction in a patient with metastatic breast carcinoma. The entire humerus is involved. Note the severe soft tissue wasting, an indication of cachexia in this patient. **C,** permeative destruction of the spine in a patient with multiple myeloma. At first glance, this appears like osteoporosis. On closer inspection, there is actual bone destruction.

BONE INVOLVED

Some diseases have a predilection for certain bones. Figure 11.22 illustrates the preferred location of many common bone lesions. This information is quite useful in diagnosing many bone lesions. For example, chondrosarcomas (Fig. 11.23) favor the pelvis, whereas enchondromas (Fig. 11.24) favor the phalanges and metacarpals; Paget's disease commonly affects the pelvis, skull, and spine, while sparing the fibula (Fig. 11.25); gout favors the bones of the hands and feet (Fig. 11.26); rheumatoid arthritis affects the hands and feet (Fig. 11.27); and hyperparathyroidism commonly affects the skull, distal clavicles, and bones of the hands and feet (Fig. 11.28).

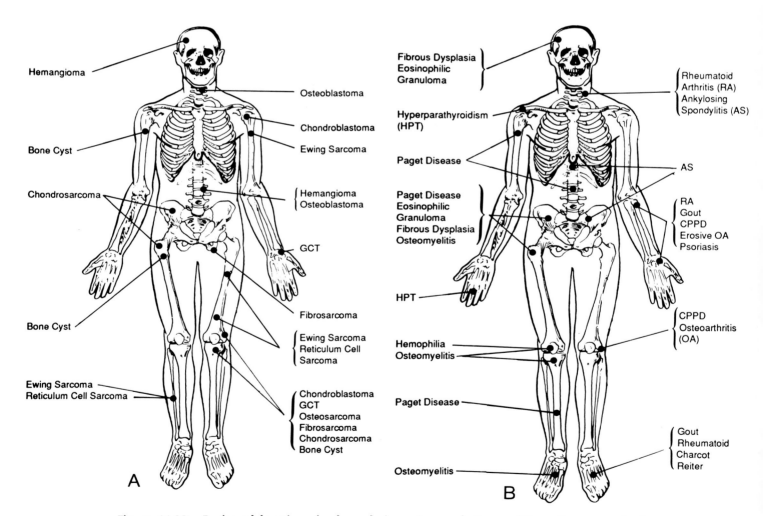

Figure 11.22. Preferred locations for bone lesions. A, neoplastic conditions. **B,** nonneoplastic conditions.

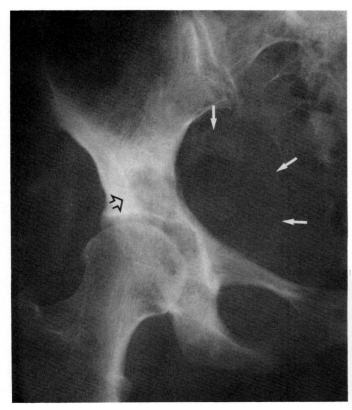

Figure 11.23. Chondrosarcoma of the pelvis. There is a large lytic lesion just above the acetabulum (*open arrow*). A soft tissue mass with flocculent calcification represents extension into the pelvis (*closed arrows*).

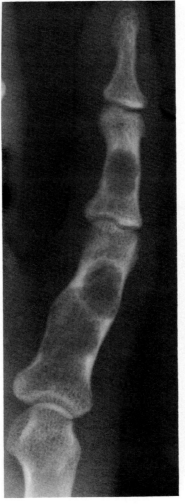

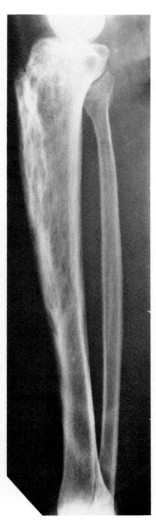

Figure 11.24. Enchondromas of the proximal and middle phalanges.

Figure 11.25. Paget's disease of the tibia. Note that the fibula is spared.

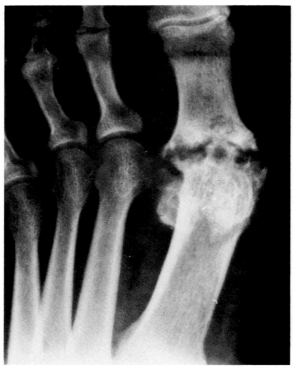

Figure 11.26. Gout. The metatarsophalangeal joint of the great toe is severely involved in this patient with long-standing gout.

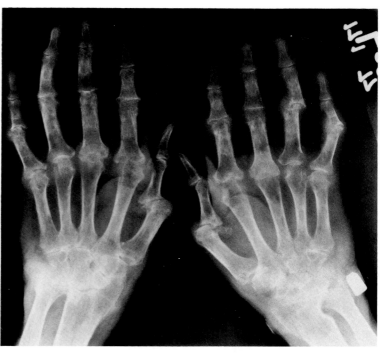

Figure 11.27. Rheumatoid arthritis of the hands and wrists. Note the involvement of the wrist joints, the metacardophalangeal joints, and interphalangeal joints.

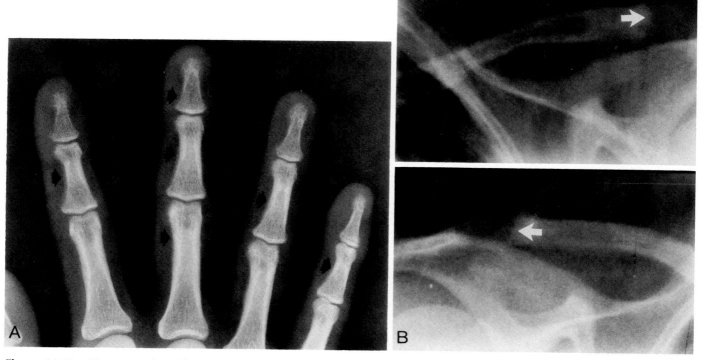

Figure 11.28. Hyperparathyroidism. A, detailed view of the hands shows subperiosteal resorption in the phalanges *(arrows).* **B,** detailed views of both distal clavicles shows subchondral resorption bilaterally *(arrows).*

LOCUS WITHIN BONE

The location of a lesion within a bone can provide an important clue to the etiology. Many lesions have a predilection for the epiphysis, metaphysis, or diaphysis. The common locations of bone tumors are shown in Figure 11.29. Nonneoplastic lesions also have a predilection for favored areas of bone; e.g., osteoarthritis prefers the weight-bearing surfaces of the large joints (Fig. 11.30), whereas rheumatoid arthritis affects the entire surface of the same joint (Fig. 11.31). Osteomyelitis favors the diametaphyseal region where red marrow is prevalent. Similarly, eosinophilic granuloma is found in areas rich in red marrow.

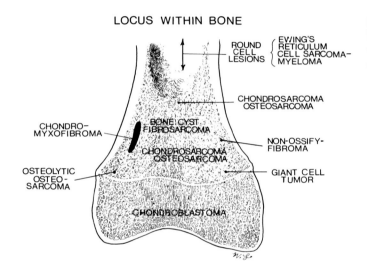

LOCUS WITHIN BONE

Figure 11.29. Common locations of bone tumors. Chondroblastoma favors the epiphysis in the skeletally immature patient. Round-cell lesions favor the diaphysis. The majority of other lesions favor the metaphysis.

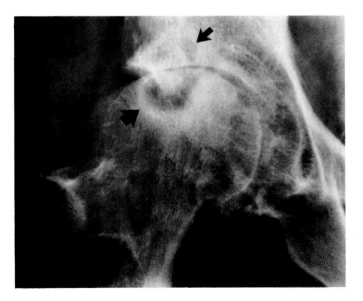

Figure 11.30. Osteoarthritis of the hip. There is narrowing of the hip joint, particularly superiorly. Large degenerative synovial cysts (geodes) are present in both the femoral head (*large arrow*) and acetabulum (*small arrow*). Note the osteophyte formation in both the acetabulum and femoral head.

Figure 11.34. Metastatic lung carcinoma demonstrating poor transition zone. It is impossible to tell where normal bone is.

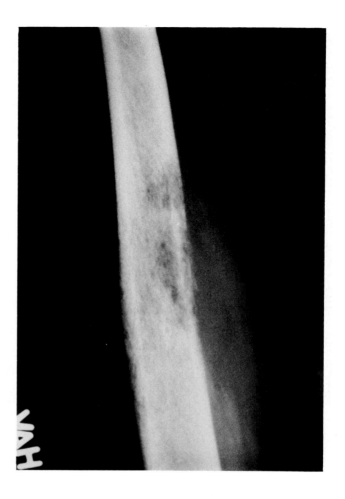

SHAPE OF LESION

The shape of a lesion helps determine its growth rate in the same way that the margin does. A lesion that is longer than it is wide, i.e., oriented with the shaft of the bone, is likely to be a nonaggressive benign process. In this situation, the lesion is growing with bone and not faster than bone. On the other hand, a lesion that is wider than the bone, has broken out of the bone and has extended into the soft tissues is a more aggressive type of lesion (Fig. 11.35). Magnetic resonance imaging is particularly useful for assessing the extraosseous extent of bone lesions.

JOINT SPACE CROSSED

If a lesion has crossed the joint space, it is most likely an inflammatory process. This is generally the case, no matter how aggressive or malignant a process may appear (Fig. 11.36). Infections will extend across a joint space, but tumors will not. Tumors that have a predilection for the ends of bones, such as chondroblastoma and giant cell tumor (Fig. 11.37), will extend to the joint but will not cross it. Furthermore, even the most malignant bone tumors respect the cartilage of the growth plate area (Fig. 11.38). Abnormalities found on both sides of a joint that has *intact cortical margins* should suggest a polyostotic disorder rather than an arthropathy.

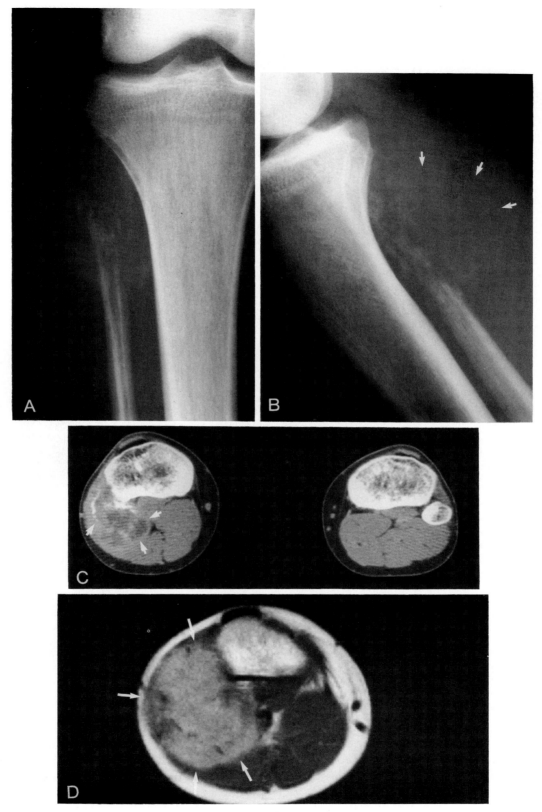

Figure 11.35.   Osteosarcoma of the proximal fibula. A, a frontal radiograph shows a poorly defined destructive lesion involving the head and proximal shaft of the fibula. The lesion has broken out of bone. **B,** lateral radiograph shows the extent into the soft tissues (*arrows*). **C,** CT scan shows the extent into soft tissues on the right side (*arrows*). **D,** T2-weighted MRI scan shows the soft tissue involvement to better advantage (*arrows*).

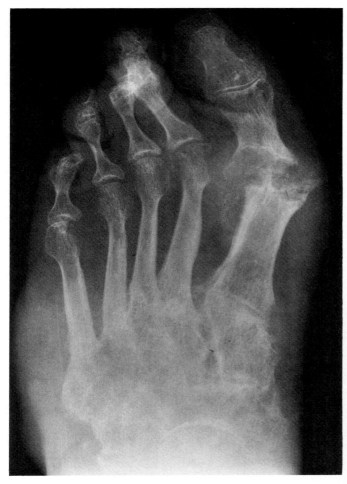

Figure 11.36. **Tophaceous gout.** This extensive destructive lesion involves both sides of the joint. This signifies that the process is either an arthropathy or an infection.

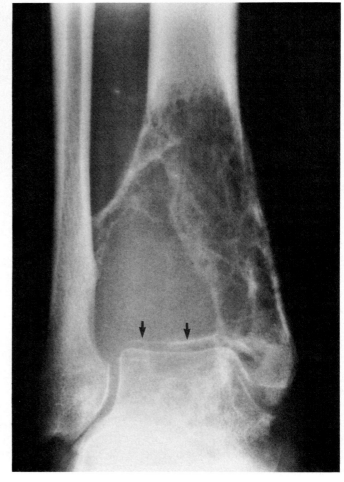

Figure 11.37. **Giant cell tumor of the distal tibia.** This large lesion extends down to the joint line (*arrows*) but has not crossed it. As a rule, tumors respect joint surfaces.

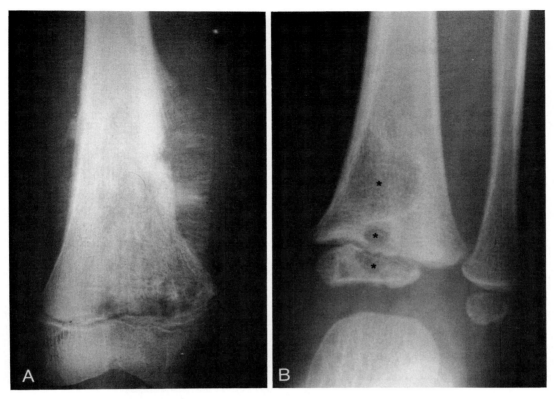

Figure 11.38. Relationship of lesions to the physis. A, osteosarcoma extends down to the physis but does not cross it. **B,** tuberculous osteomyelitis has produced cystic lesions (*) on both sides of the physis. The ankle joint is still not crossed.

BONY REACTION

Bony response to insult includes periosteal reaction, sclerosis, and buttressing. Periosteal reaction is of four varieties: solid, laminated or onionskin, spiculated (sunburst or "hair-on-end"), or Codman triangle. *Solid* periosteal reaction (greater than 2 mm) indicates a benign process. It most often occurs in osteomyelitis and fracture healing (Fig. 11.39). A *laminated* or *onionskin* type of periosteal reaction indicates repetitive injury to bone. This was previously thought to be pathognomonic of Ewing's tumor or reticulum cell sarcoma of bone. However, this type of reaction also occurs in any type of repetitive injury to bone such as in the "battered child" (Fig. 11.40). Once again, the nature of the laminated periosteal reaction may be determined by its thickness. In a Ewing's tumor, the periosteum is quite thin, irregular, and disorganized (Fig. 11.41), whereas in a benign process such as osteomyelitis or battered child, the reaction is considerably thicker and often wavy. A *spiculated, sunburst* or *hair-on-end* appearance is almost always associated with a malignant bone lesion (Fig. 11.42), most often an osteogenic sarcoma. Occasionally, this occurs in metastatic squamous cell tumors. This form of periosteal reaction is the result of the neoplastic process breaking through a layer of periosteal new bone, followed by new periosteal response and subsequent breakthrough. The *Codman triangle* represents triangular ossification of a piece of perio-

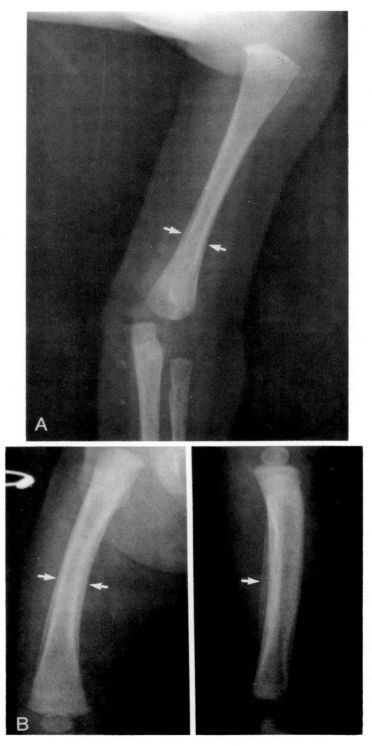

Figure 11.39. Solid periosteal reaction (*arrows*) in a patient with congenital syphilis.

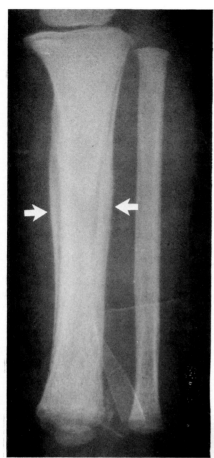

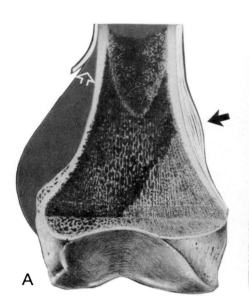

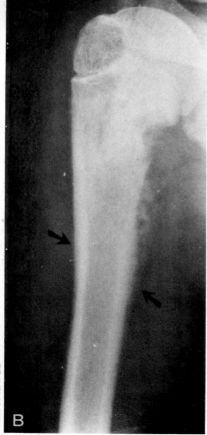

Figure 11.40. Laminated but solid periosteal reaction (*arrows*) in a battered child.

Figure 11.41. Laminated periosteal reaction. A, drawing shows laminations (*closed arrow*). A Codman triangle is demonstrated on the opposite side (*open arrow*). **B,** irregular interruped periosteal reaction (*arrows*) in a patient with a Ewing's tumor.

Figure 11.42. Spiculated-type periosteal reaction. A, drawing showing variations on spiculated periosteal reaction. **B,** osteogenic sarcoma demonstrating spiculated periosteal reaction (*straight arrow*). Note the Codman triangle (*curved arrow*).

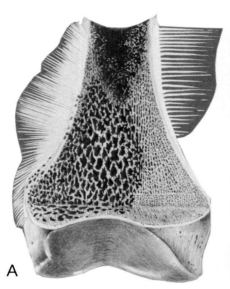

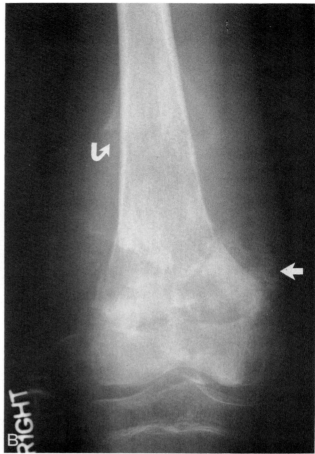

A

B

Figure 11.43. Reactive sclerosis. A, drawing showing sclerotic rim around a geographic lesion. **B,** sclerosis around a focus of fibrous dysplasia of the proximal femur.

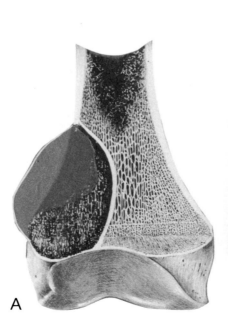

A

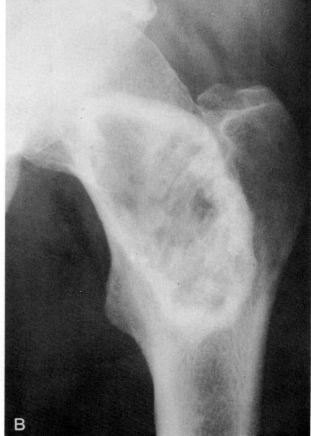

B

steum that has been elevated (Figs. 11.41**A** and 11.42**B**). In the past that was thought to be pathognomonic of tumor. However, it is seen in many benign conditions, including subperiosteal hemorrhage in scurvy and the battered child.

Sclerosis is an attempt by the bone to wall off a diseased area. It generally indicates a benign process (Fig. 11.43). *Buttressing* is an attempt by the bone to reestablish architectural integrity. The term is derived from the flying buttresses of Gothic architecture. The most common example of this is the osteophyte of degenerative arthritis (Fig. 11.44).

MATRIX PRODUCTION

Matrix is a substance produced by certain bone tumors. It may be chondroid (cartilaginous), osteoid (bony), or mixed. Chondroid matrix appears as fine, stippled calcification or multiple popcorn-like calcifications. Quite often it occurs in bulky masses of tumor within the soft tissues (Fig. 11.45). Osteoid matrix, on the other hand, is dense and usually of the same radiographic density as bone. It occurs most often in osteogenic sarcoma (Fig. 11.46,) but also may be seen in the benign ossifying condition, myositis ossificans.

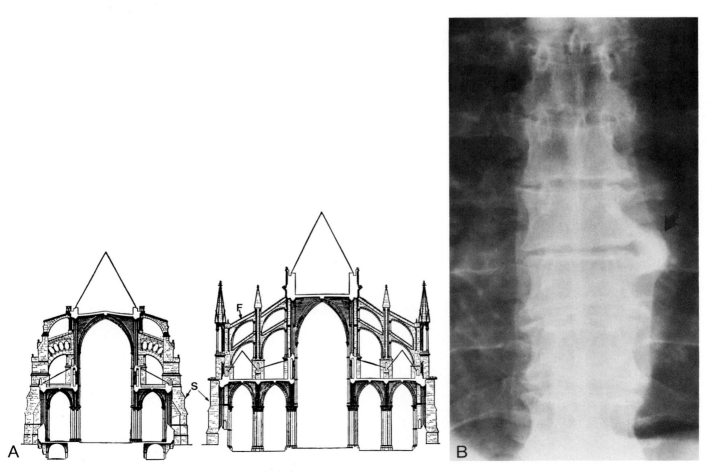

Figure 11.44. Buttressing. A, drawing illustrates flying (*F*) and standing (*S*) buttresses as used in Gothic architecture. **B,** detailed view of the thoracic vertebral column shows a large osteophyte (*arrow*) bridging two thoracic vertebrae.

Figure 11.45. Matrix formation. A, drawing showing lumpy and flocculent types of matrix. **B,** chondroid matrix in a patient with chondrosarcoma. Note the flocculent calcifications within the soft tissues adjacent to the iliac bone.

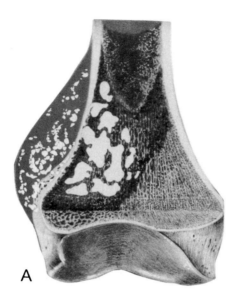

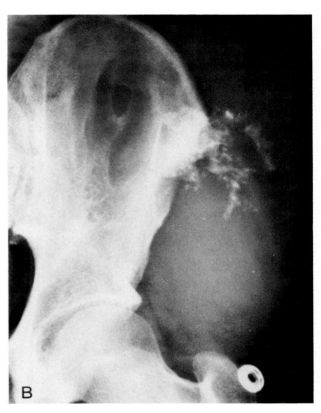

Figure 11.46. Osteosarcoma of the pelvis demonstrating osteoid matrix. Note how dense the lesion is because of the osteoid matrix formation.

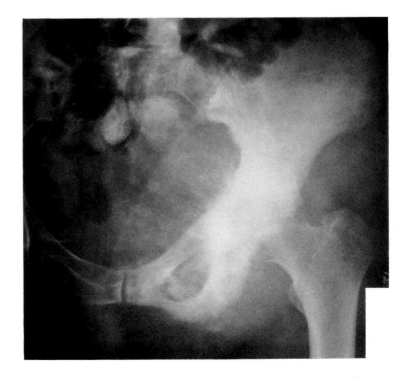

SOFT TISSUE CHANGES

By analyzing the soft tissues, you may obtain important clues regarding an underlying injury, disease process, or a specific bone lesion. For example, diffuse muscle wasting suggests a patient with paralysis, primary muscle disease, or severe inanition caused by disseminated carcinomatosis or AIDS. The presence of soft tissue swelling may be indicative of a mass (Fig. 11.47), hemorrhage, inflammation, or edema. The loss or displacement of fat lines normally found in the soft tissues is another indication of adjacent abnormality. For example, displacement or obliteration of the pronator quadratus fat line in the wrist (Fig. 11.48) usually indicates a fracture of the wrist. Elevation or displacement of the fat pads of the elbow indicates fluid within the joint space, usually the result of trauma (Fig. 11.49) but sometimes seen in an inflammatory condition such as rheumatoid arthritis. The presence of a fat-fluid level (lipohemarthrosis) on a horizontal radiograph of the knee is indicative of a fracture communicating with the joint (Fig. 11.50).

Calcifications within the soft tissues may result from old trauma or connective tissue disorders. Occasionally, old parasitic disease will be manifest by soft tissue calcifications.

Gas in the tissues indicates trauma or gas gangrene. Other soft tissue findings include the presence of foreign bodies, abdominal aortic aneurysm, or renal calculi in a patient being evaluated for back pain.

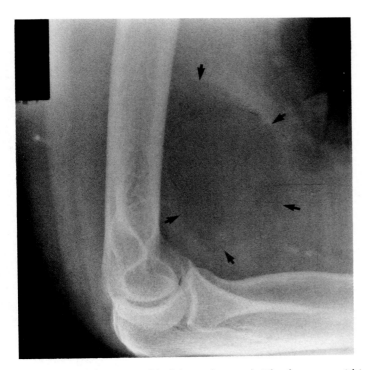

Figure 11.47. Lipoma of the antecubital fossa (*arrows*). The lucency within this large mass indicates that a major component is composed of fat.

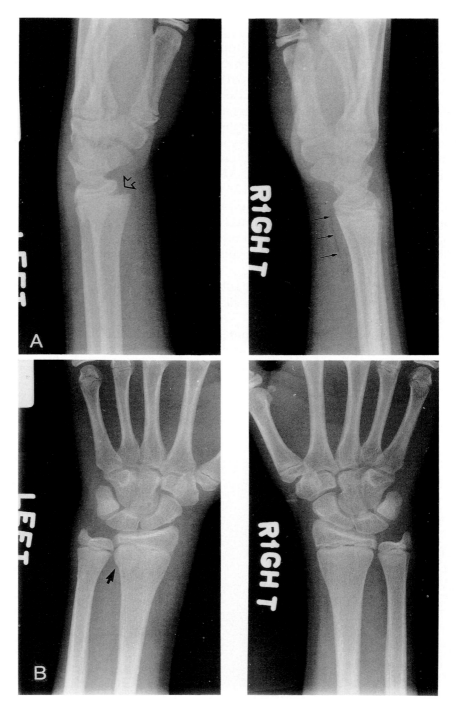

Figure 11.48. Soft tissue changes in a patient with a Salter type II fracture of the distal radius. A, lateral view shows the normal pronator quadratus fat stripe (*small arrows*) on the right. Note the obliteration of this line and overall soft tissue swelling on the left. There is widening of the epiphyseal plate on the left (*open arrow*). **B,** frontal view shows buckling of the ulnar cortex of the distal radius on the left (*arrow*). Note the differences in soft tissue when compared with the right. The changes on this frontal view are even more subtle than those on the lateral view.

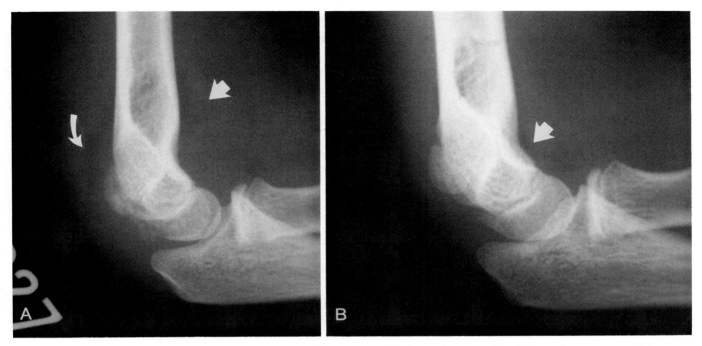

Figure 11.49.   Elbow fat pad. A, elevation of the anterior (*large arrow*) and posterior (*curved arrow*) in a patient with a subtle fracture of the distal humerus. **B,** lateral radiograph of the oppo-site side shows the normal position and appearance of the anterior fat pad (*arrow*).The posterior fat pad is never visible under normal circumstances.

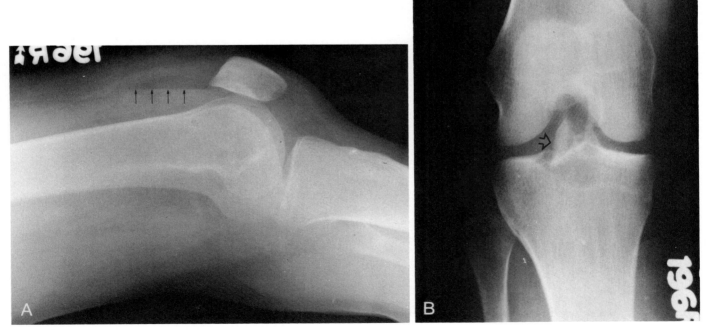

Figure 11.50,   Tibial plateau fracture. A, horizontal beam lateral film shows a fat fluid level (*arrows*) in the suprapatellar space. **B,** frontal view shows avulsion of the intercondylar spines (*arrow*).

HISTORY OF TRAUMA OR SURGERY

Since trauma constitutes the most common bone "disease" you will see, it is very important to elicit a history of trauma whenever possible. A stress fracture (Fig. 11.51) may be misdiagnosed as a malignant bone tumor unless a specific history of "trauma" (pain with an unusual activity, condition worsening with that activity, and relief achieved by rest) is obtained. Occasionally, however, a history of trauma will be deliberately withheld as in the case of the battered child or of a child or adult who, prior to injury, was doing something that was prohibited or illegal.

Similarly, it is important to know whether the patient has had surgery to a particular bone. Healing surgical sites, particularly those used for bone graft donation, may have ominous radiographic appearances; it is therefore necessary to know about any previous operations.

ADDITIONAL OBSERVATIONS

Bony Anatomy and Alignment

Deformities in bone generally indicate congenital abnormality (Fig. 11.52). However, they may also occur as a sequel of poorly treated trauma (Fig. 11.53). There are two types of malalignment that may occur in joints, subluxations and dislocations. Subluxation is a partial loss of continuity

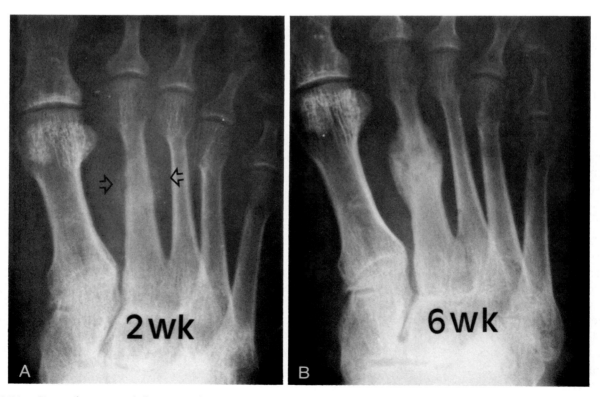

Figure 11.51. Stress fracture of the second metatarsal. A, frontal radiographs made 2 weeks after onset of symptoms shows irregular periosteal reaction along the midshaft of the second metatarsal (*arrows*). The underlying bone appears moth-eaten. **B,** 6 weeks after onset of symptoms and healing has occurred, note the solid periosteal reaction across the fracture site. There has been some bony resorption of the fracture.

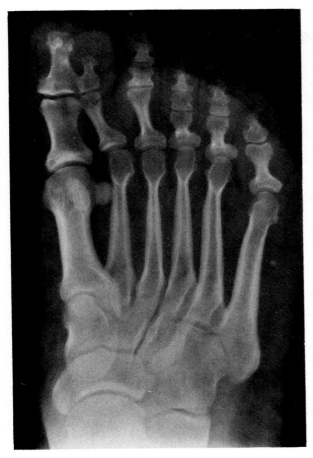

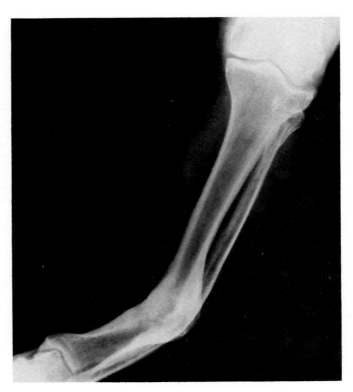

Figure 11.53. Deformity of the distal tibia and fibula secondary to poorly managed fractures.

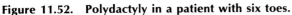

Figure 11.52. Polydactyly in a patient with six toes.

between articulating surfaces; dislocation is the complete loss of continuity at that joint space. These are illustrated in Figure 11.54. Shoulder, hip, and finger dislocations are the most commonly encountered.

Bony Mineralization and Texture

The degree of mineralization of a bone is directly related to the patient's age, the physiologic state, and the amount of activity or stress being placed on that bone. Furthermore, the texture of the trabeculae (thin, delicate, coarsened, smudged) may tell you something about the patient's state. Osteoporosis commonly occurs in the elderly patient and in postmenopausal women. However, an acute form of osteoporosis may occur following immobilization of a limb. Diminished mineralization is also a common manifestation of certain diseases such as renal osteodystrophy, scurvy, and rheumatoid arthritis (Fig. 11.55). Renal osteodystrophy is a complex of several metabolic conditions with four prominent radiographic manifestations: osteoporosis, coarsening of bony trabeculae, osteomalacia, and hyperparathyroidism. It is most often encountered in patients with chronic renal failure. The radiographic picture may feature one of the components more prominently than others or sim-

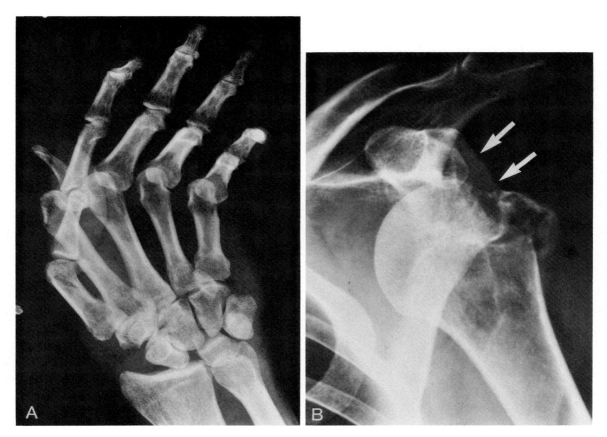

Figure 11.54. Subluxation and dislocation. A, ulnar subluxation of the carpus and metacarpophalangeal joint subluxations in a patient with systemic lupus erythematosis. **B,** anterior-inferior humeral dislocation. There is complete loss of continuity between the joint surfaces. There is a naked glenoid (*arrows*). Note the fracture of the humeral head (Hill-Sachs deformity) as well.

ply be a combination of all four. Features of osteomalacia include osteoporosis, smudged and indistinct trabeculae, resorption about the growth plates in the skeletally immature, and a curious appearance in the vertebral column of alternating horizontal bands of osteoporosis centrally with osteosclerosis along the disc termed *"rugger jersey spine"* (Fig. 11.56). Hyperparathyroidism, on the other hand, produces osteoporosis, resorption of the tufts of the distal phalanges, subperiosteal resorption along the radial borders of phalanges, resorption about the distal clavicles (Fig. 11.28) and other symphyseal joints as well as along entheses (tendinous insertion points), and a curious mixed pattern of osteoporosis and fluffy sclerosis in the skull called *"salt and pepper skull"*.

It is sometimes difficult to differentiate osteoporosis from permeative bone destruction on either plain films or CT. For this reason, we often resort to MR imaging to help make the differentiation. Osteoporosis produces a scan that shows fatty replacement of marrow that is high on T1-weighted images. Infiltrative disorders generally produce low signal in the marrow spaces on T1-weighted studies. Furthermore, osteoporotic vertebral fractures, if recent, usually have more of a linear distribution of abnormal sig-

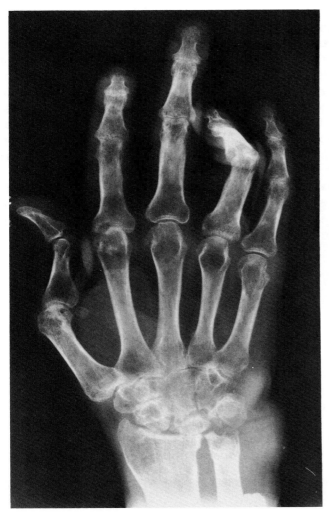

Figure 11.55. Advanced rheumatoid arthritis. This disease primarily involves the wrist joint, the metacarpophalangeal joints, and the proximal interphalangeal joints. Note the erosive changes in these locations.

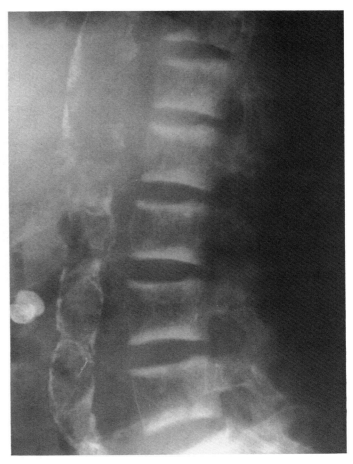

Figure 11.56. "Rugger jersey spine" in a patient with chronic renal failure and osteomalacia. Note the striped appearance due to the alternating areas of osteosclerosis along the disc plates with central osteoporosis. The relatively lucent disc spaces also contribute to the striped appearance.

nal than does that associated with infiltration. In some instances, biopsy may be necessary to establish the proper diagnosis.

For an excellent in-depth discussion of bone mineral deposition, consult Resnick's *Diagnosis of Bone and Joint Disorders*.

Joint Space Changes

The width of the joint space and the appearance of the distal ends of articulating bones are important in the diagnosis of arthritis. The distribution, location, and erosive patterns produced by the various arthritides allow considerable accuracy in radiologic diagnosis, particularly when correlated with clinical and laboratory findings. You should familiarize yourself with the changes in the three most common types of arthritis you will

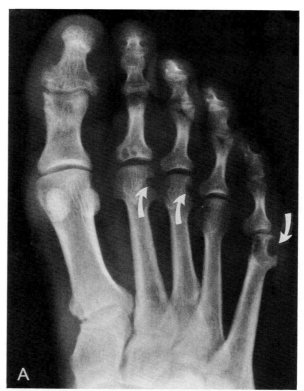

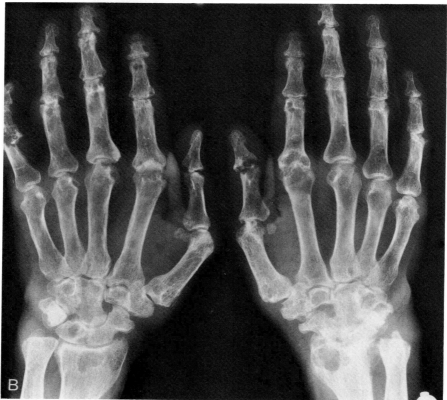

Figure 11.60. Gout. A, detailed view of a foot shows paraarticular punched out lesions in the distal metatarsals (*arrows*). Other joints are involved as well. **B,** involvement of the hands and wrists in the same patient shows multiple lesions. Note the asymmetry, predominantly paraarticular involvement and overall preservation of mineralization around the joints. Compare with Figure 11.55.

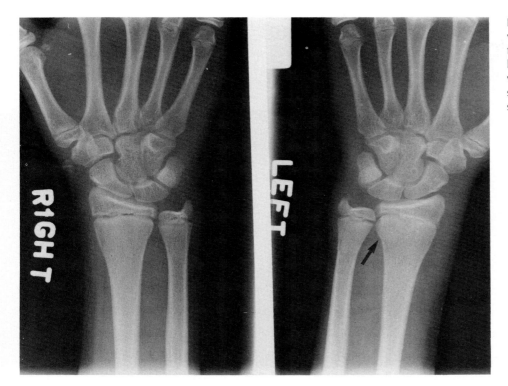

Figure 11.61. Use of comparison views in trauma. There is a subtle fracture of the distal radius on the left (*arrow*). Note the differences in width of the growth plate and in the soft tissues when comparing side to side.

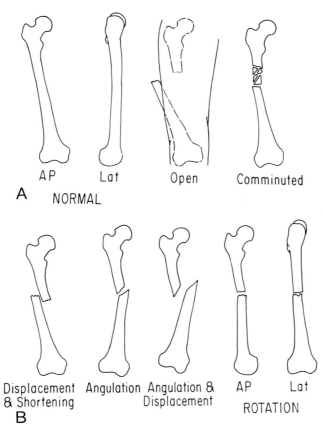

Figure 11.62. Schematic drawing of fracture terminology.

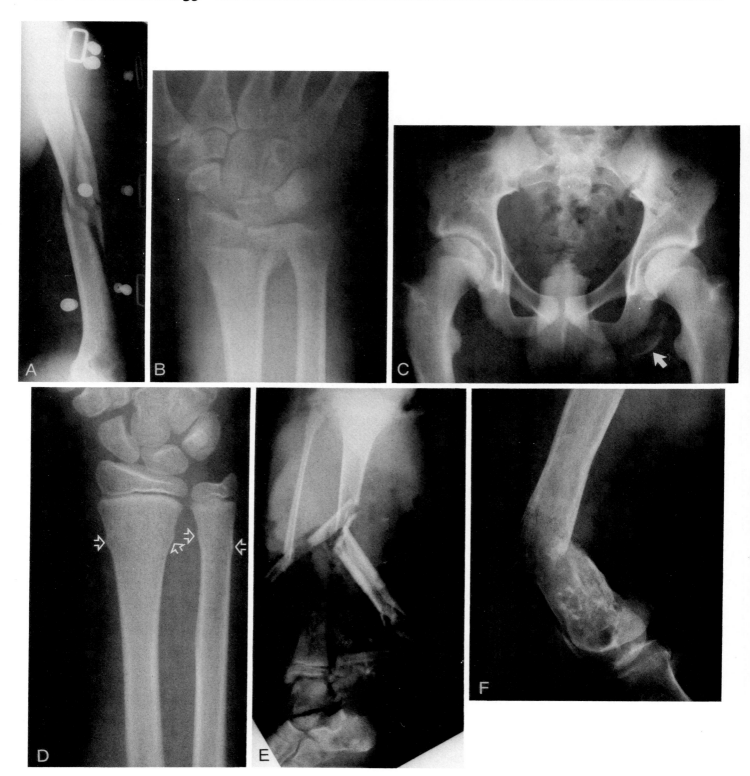

Figure 11.63. Fractures and their descriptive terminology. A, spiral fracture of the midshaft of the humerus. **B,** comminuted compression fracture of the distal radius. There is also a fracture of the ulnar styloid. **C,** avulsion fracture (*arrow*) of the ischial apophysis. **D,** green-stick (torus) fractures of the distal radius and ulna (*arrows*). The torus fracture presents as a bulge along the surface of the otherwise smooth bone. **E,** comminuted open fractures of the distal tibia and fibula. **F,** pathologic fracture of the distal femur in a patient with a malignant bone tumor. Note the bone destruction around the fracture.

11.63 shows several common types of fractures and their descriptive terminology. For a further discussion of terminology, refer to *The Language of Fractures* by Schultz.

Fractures in children occur in two distinct patterns depending on whether the injury is near the growth plate or the shaft. Injuries about the growth plate are classified according to the *Salter-Harris-Ogden* classification, which is based on the degree of involvement of the epiphysis, growth plate, or metaphysis. The type I injury is a pure epiphysiolysis. Type II involves the epiphysis and a small metaphyseal fragment. It is the most common type. The type III injury is a vertical fracture of the epiphysis with epiphysiolysis of the fracture fragment. Type IV is a vertical epiphyseal fracture with metaphyseal involvement. Type V, the rarest, is uniform compression of the epiphyseal plate. Type VI is a compression of part of the epiphyseal plate with lysis of the other. Type VII is an osteochondral fracture of the epiphysis. Figure 11.64 illustrates the Salter-Harris-Odgen classification. Types I and II are said to produce little or no growth disturbance; types III through VI have a higher potential for growth disturbance, and type VII has no potential for disturbance.

Fracture of the shaft of bones may be either complete or of the green-stick variety. Three types of green-stick fractures are recognized: classic green-stick (fracture on one side of the bone, bent on the other), "torus," resembling the base of a Greek column (buckling of cortex on both sides of the bone), and "lead pipe" (one side buckled, one side cracked). Of these, the torus variety (Fig. 11.63**D**) is the most common.

Although an in-depth description of fractures is beyond the scope of this book, you should follow some of the principles listed here when evaluating patients with skeletal trauma. (*a*) Assume a fracture is present if there is pain, swelling, and discoloration over a bony surface in a child. It is best to treat patients for fracture and bring them back in 7 to 10 days for follow-up radiographs rather than to let them depart from your emergency

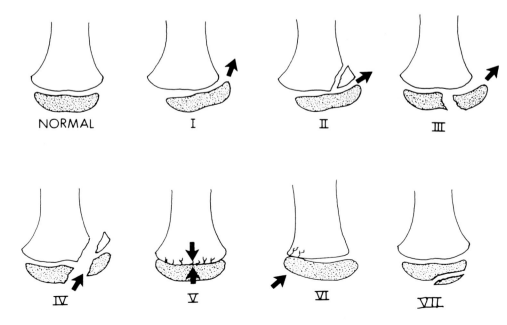

Figure 11.64. Salter-Harris-Ogden classification of growth plate injuries.

NORMAL   I   II   III

IV   V   VI   VII

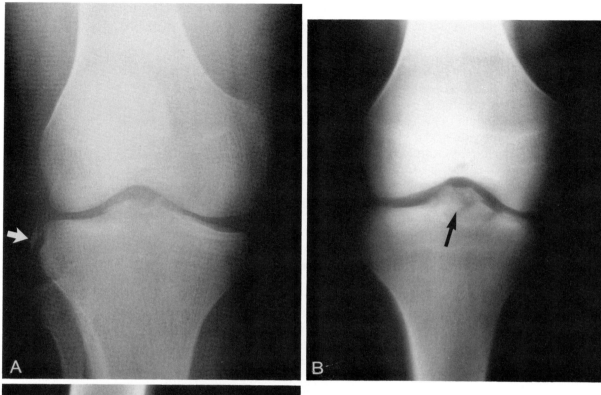

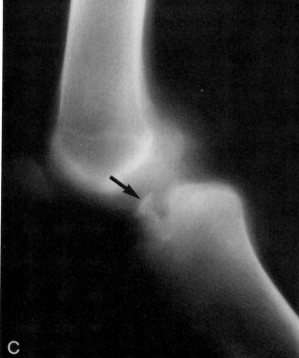

Figure 11.65. Use of tomography in a patient with a Segond fracture complex. A, frontal radiograph shows an avulsion of the lateral aspect of the proximal tibia (*arrow*). Cast material obscures further detail. **B,** frontal tomogram shows avulsion fracture of the intercondylar spines (*arrow*). **C,** lateral tomogram shows avulsed fragments (*arrows*). Comment: The Segond fracture is significant in that there is always damage to the anterior cruciate ligament complex.

department with an untreated fracture. (*b*) Comparison views should be made whenever you are uncertain about the presence or absence of a fracture (particularly in small children whose epiphyseal lines could be confused for a fracture). (*c*) Tomography is often useful in determining whether or not a fracture is present. It also may be used to determine the extent of fracture (Fig. 11.65). (*d*) A CT scan is useful for evaluating fractures of certain joints such as the shoulder and ankle (Fig. 11.66). It is also the best method of assessing pelvic fractures (Fig. 11.67) and in establishing the extent of vertebral fractures. (*e*) Magnetic resonance is useful in assessing the extent of spinal cord compression in vertebral fractures (Fig. 11.68). It is not helpful in routine fracture diagnosis.

Postoperative Changes

A large number of prostheses and appliances are used in orthopaedics today. You should familiarize yourself with the more common of these and their appearance in bone (Fig. 11.69). Furthermore, the sites of previous screw holes, osteotomy, or prostheses may present a variety of bony defects that are easily recognizable if you are familiar with the types of procedures used in orthopaedic surgery (Fig. 11.70).

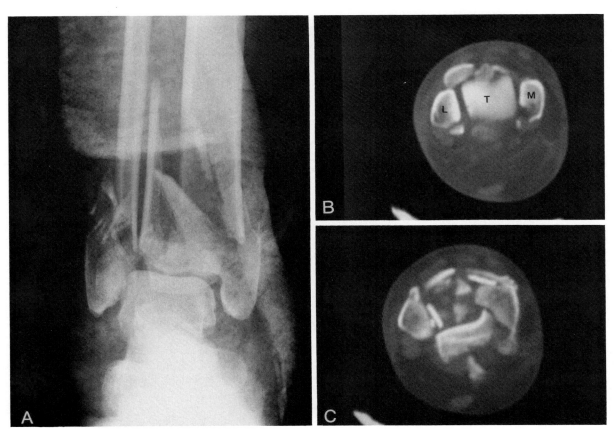

Figure 11.66. Pylon fracture of the ankle. A, frontal radiograph shows a severely comminuted fracture of the distal tibia and fibula. **B,** CT scan at the level of the talus shows the medial (*M*) and lateral (*L*) malleoli to maintain their normal relationship to the talus (*T*). **C,** slightly higher, the severely comminuted nature of the fracture can be appreciated.

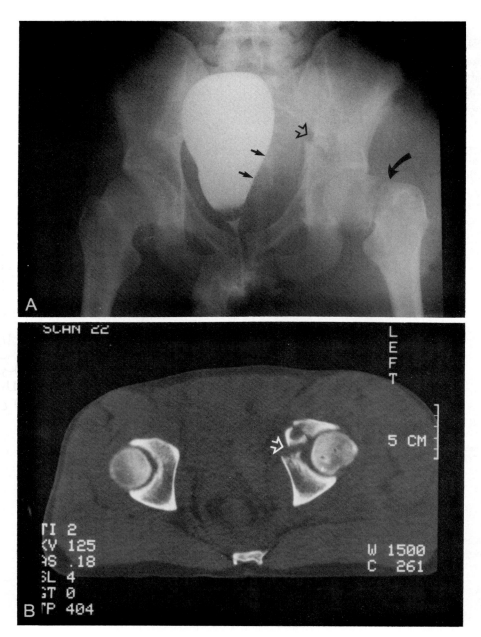

Figure 11.67. Pelvic fracture. A, frontal radiograph shows fractures involving the left acetabulum (*open arrow*) and left femoral neck (*curved arrow*). A large pelvic hematoma compresses and displaces the contrast-filled bladder to the right (*small arrows*). **B,** CT scan through the hips shows the severely comminuted acetabular fracture on the left (*arrow*).

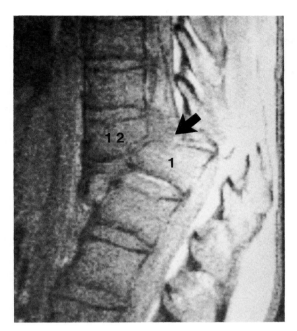

Figure 11.68. Fracture dislocation of T-12 on L-1. An MRI scan shows the dislocation. Note the cord transection (*arrow*).

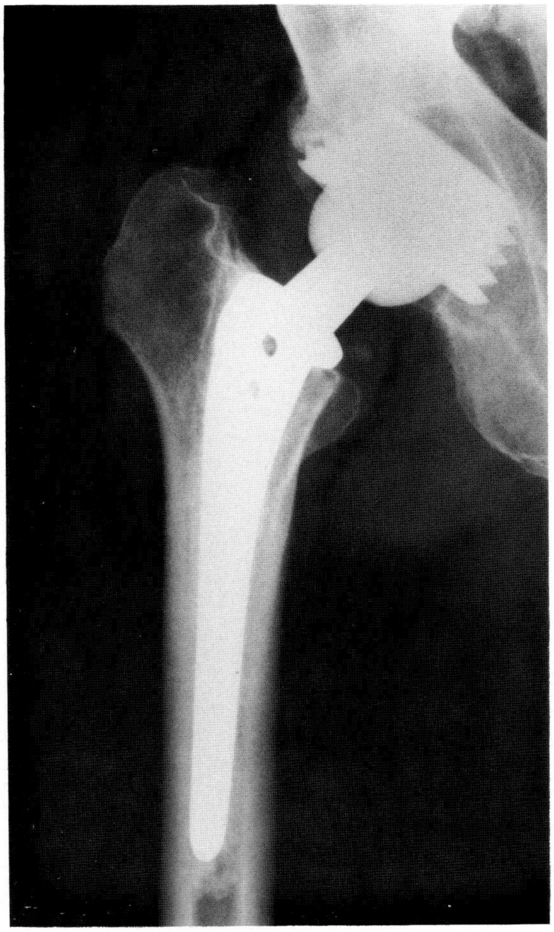

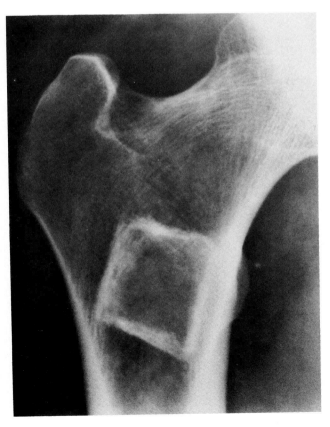

Figure 11.69. Normal posteroperative appearance of a total hip prosthesis. There are a large variety of these devices.

Figure 11.70. Residuum of an excisional bone biopsy. The square margins of this sclerotic lesion are the clue to the iatrogenic nature of the lesion.

Summary

Most bone lesions fall into one of six basic pathologic categories: congenital, inflammatory, metabolic, neoplastic, traumatic, and vascular. By recognizing patterns of destruction and the use of a series of predictor variables, it is possible to reduce the complexities of skeletal radiology to a workable format. The application of the mnemonic *ABCS* was introduced to stress the analysis of bony *A*natomy and alignment, *B*ony mineralization, *C*artilage (joint-space) changes, and *S*oft tissue changes. The principles of fracture diagnosis have been discussed.

Suggested Additional Reading

Bloem JL, Sartoris DJ. MRI and CT of the musculoskeletal system: a text-atlas. Baltimore: Williams & Wilkins, 1991.

Edeiken J, Dalinka MK, Karasick D. Edeiken's roentgen diagnosis of diseases of bone. 4th ed. Baltimore: Williams & Wilkins, 1989.

Greenfield GB. Radiology of bone diseases. 4th ed. Philadelphia: JB Lippincott, 1990.

Kleinman PK. Diagnostic imaging of child abuse. Baltimore: Williams & Wilkins, 1987.

Manaster BJ. Skeletal radiology. St. Louis: Mosby Year Book, 1989.

McCort JJ, ed. Trauma radiology. New York: Churchill Livingstone, 1990.

Resnick D, Niwayama G. Diagnosis of bone and joint disorders. 2nd ed. Philadelphia: WB Saunders, 1988.

Schultz RJ. The language of fractures. 2nd ed. Baltimore: Williams & Wilkins, 1990.

Chapter 12

Cranial Imaging

Neuroradiology is the subspecialty area concerned with radiologic investigation of the brain and spinal cord. It is this area that has been most dramatically changed by the technical developments of the past two decades. Computerized tomography (CT), magnetic resonance (MR) imaging, and digital subtraction angiography have been major breakthroughs in the imaging of the brain and spinal cord. Although abnormalities in other areas of the body may be grossly evident, the changes present on studies of the central nervous system are often subtle. The student or house officer who is confronted with a neuroradiologic study is often frustrated and feels insecure. Remember, however, that neuroradiology is founded on the same principles of anatomy, physiology, and pathology as any other diagnostic area. This chapter will deal with cranial imaging; the following chapter with spinal imaging. Because of the complexity of neuroradiologic examination, detailed description of the various entities is beyond the scope of this book. However, the pertinent aspects of each type of study, their indications, and a basic discussion of the main pathologic entities will be included to provide you with a proper foundation to allow you to select the appropriate study for your patients.

TECHNICAL CONSIDERATIONS

The cranial contents are now imaged primarily by CT, MR, and angiography. In the past, the evaluation of these structures was performed in a manner to display the effects of certain intracranial abnormalities on structures that could be opacified. Hence, skull films were performed primarily to detect shifts in the calcified pineal. Pneumoencephalography was performed to outline not only the cerebral ventricular system, but also to show the effects of neoplasms and other lesions on those structures. Cerebral angiography was a primary tool to detect not only neovascularity (tumor and new vessels), but also to show displacement and encasement of vessels by intracranial mass lesions. Although angiography is still used in busy neuroradiologic practices, the actual number of studies has been diminished dramatically by the use of CT and MR.

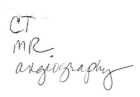

Skull radiography is still a highly overused examination. The yield of positive findings is extremely low compared to the number of examinations made. Skull radiography, as a rule, is generally *not* indicated for head trauma. Any patient who has sustained a significant cranial injury should be evaluated by CT. This tenet makes sense when you realize that a fracture is *a soft tissue injury in which a bone is broken.* The validity of this statement can be seen in the results of a study that we recently performed. At Allegheny General Hospital, two clinical groups deal with trauma patients. The emergency department physicians evaluate patients involved in minor trauma. All major trauma, including patients in whom there is loss of consciousness, are referred to the trauma service. One hundred patients prospectively treated by each group were evaluated. Of the 100 patients seen by the emergency department, all had plain skull radiographs performed. Six of these patients had skull fractures demonstrated by skull radiographs. All six of these underwent subsequent cranial CT evaluation, which showed no intracranial pathology. The skull fractures were demonstrated in all six cases by CT. The 100 patients evaluated by the trauma service were evaluated by CT examination only. Of this group, 32 had skull fractures demonstrated by CT and all had intracranial abnormalities present. An additional 22 patients had intracranial abnormalities *without* evidence of skull fracture. In no instance did the CT examination fail to demonstrate a fracture that was present. More significantly, however, was the fact that the six patients with skull fractures seen by the emergency department had no intracranial abnormalities and, in all likelihood, would have fared just as well with observation only had they not received skull radiographs. The study by Masters et al. supports our observation.

However, there are some indications for radiography of the skull. It should be used for bone diseases or bone abnormalities—penetrating injury, a destructive lesion, metabolic disease, or anomalies of the skull. In addition, the skull may be evaluated for postoperative changes.

A CT examination of the brain and surrounding tissue is usually performed as a first study for evaluation of patients with suspected intracranial abnormalities. This study is generally performed first without and then with intravenous contrast enhancement to demonstrate vascular structures or abnormalities.

Cranial MR imaging has been one of the greatest technological improvements in the evaluation of suspected intracranial lesions. It is rapidly becoming the primary investigative tool for suspected intracranial abnormalities because of its ability to display the brain in exquisite detail. Cranial MR is performed utilizing T1- and T2-weighted spin-echo sequences as well as a variety of gradient echo images. The scanning parameters of these studies may be adjusted to optimize the characteristics of certain intracranial lesions. One of the greatest advances in MR imaging has been the ability to detect the abnormalities produced by multiple sclerosis. Previously, this disease defied early detection by imaging methods.

Cerebral angiography is used to evaluate vascular lesions such as arteriosclerotic occlusive disease, aneurysms, and vascular malformations. It is also used to supplement CT and MR imaging in patients with tumors to aid the surgeon in their removal. The development of digital subtraction angiography allows the neuroradiologist to perform the study using minimal amounts of contrast media.

ANATOMIC CONSIDERATIONS

Skull films will be encountered whenever there is a history of penetrating trauma, facial fracture, sinus disease, destructive lesion, or metabolic problem. You will most often encounter skull films as part of a metastatic or metabolic bone survey. Their analysis should be conducted in a logical, orderly fashion using the *ABCS* method described in the last chapter with the exception of "C," which now stands for calcifications. The order of examination, therefore, should be: bony vault, sella turcica, facial bones, basal foramina, sinuses, calcifications, and soft tissues.

The standard views of the skull are the posterior-anterior (PA), lateral, anterior-posterior (AP), half-axial (Towne), and base. Each view is designed to demonstrate particular areas of the skull. The PA view is designed to demonstrate the frontal bones, frontal and ethmoid sinuses, nasal cavity, superior orbital rims, and mandible (Fig. 12.1). The lateral view demonstrates the frontal, parietal, temporal, and occipital bones, the mastoid region, the sella turcica, the roofs of the orbits, and the lateral aspects of the facial bones (Fig. 12.2). The modified half-axial projection (Towne, occipi-

[handwritten margin notes:]
bony vault
sella turcica
facial bones
basal foramina
sinuses
calcifications
soft tissues

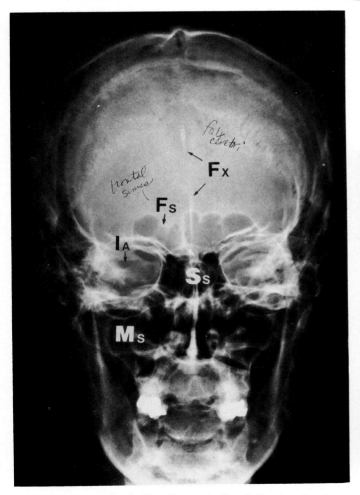

Figure 12.1. A PA skull radiograph. The following structures are visible: *Fx,* falx cerebri; *Fs,* frontal sinus; *Ia,* internal auditory canal; *Ss,* sphenoid sinus; *Ms,* maxillary sinus.

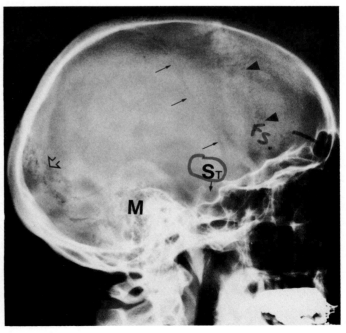

Figure 12.2. Lateral radiograph of the skull. The following structures are visible: coronal suture (*arrowheads*), occipital suture (*open arrow*), middle meningeal vascular grooves (*straight arrows*), sella turcica (*St*), and mastoid air cells (*M*).

tal view) (Fig. 12.3) demonstrates the occipital bone, the mastoid and middle ear regions, the foramen magnum, and the zygomatic arches. The base view (Fig. 12.4) shows the basal structures of the skull, including major foramina. The occipitomental (Waters) projection (Fig. 12.5) is used primarily to study the facial bones and sinuses. Other plain film studies of the skull include internal auditory canal views, views for the optic struts, mastoid series, and studies of the temporomandibular (TM) joint. These areas are best studied by CT and, in the case of the TM joint, MR imaging. Dentists and oral surgeons also use a panoramic type of tomogram to study the mandible and facial bones (Fig. 12.6).

There are a large variety of normal structures and conditions that may cause you diagnostic concern. These include prominent vascular grooves (Fig. 12.7), hyperostosis frontalis interna (Fig. 12.8), calcified falx cerebri (Fig. 12.9), and persistent anomalous sutures (Fig. 12.10). Whenever in doubt, review the films with a radiologist.

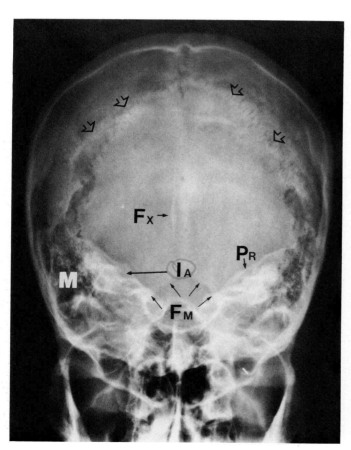

Figure 12.3.   Modified half-axial projection (Towne). The following structures are visible: occipital sutures (*open arrows*), mastoid air cells (*M*), falx cerebri (*Fx*), internal auditory canal (*Ia*), petrous ridge (*Pr*), and foramen magnum (*Fm*).

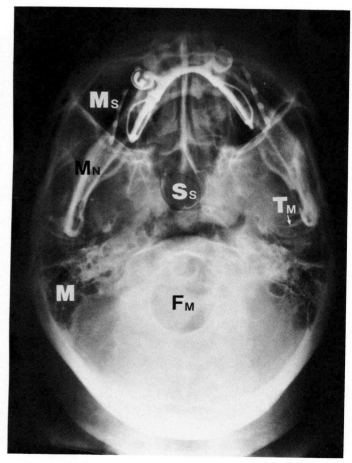

Figure 12.4.   Base view. The following structures are visible: *Ss*, sphenoid sinus; *Fm*, foramen magnum; *Tm*, temporomandibular joint; *M*, mastoid air cells; *Mn*, mandible; *Ms*, maxillary sinus.

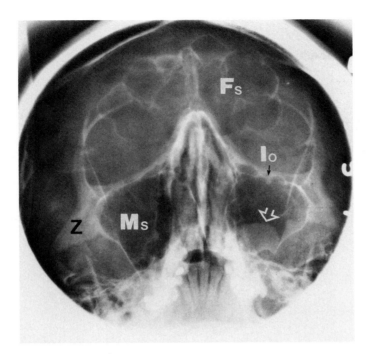

Figure 12.5.   Occipitomental (Waters) projection. The following structures are visible: *Z*, zygomatic arch; *Ms*, maxillary sinus; *Fs*, frontal sinus; *Io*, inferior orbital rim (*small arrow*). There is a mucous retention cyst (*open arrow*) in the left maxillary sinus.

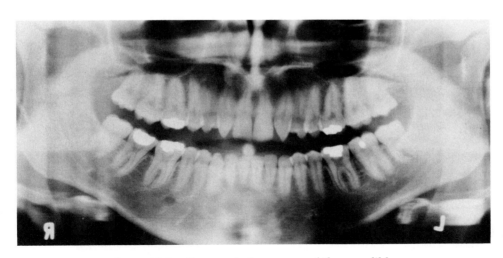

Figure 12.6.   Panoramic tomogram of the mandible.

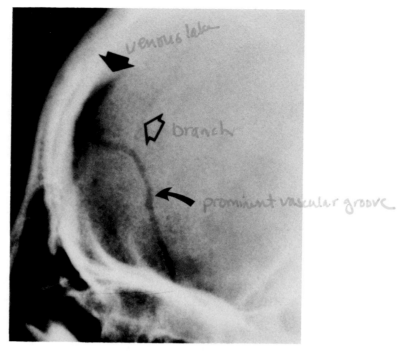

Figure 12.7. **Prominent vascular groove.** The prominent vascular groove (*curved arrow*) ends in a venous lake (*large black arrow*). Note the branch (*open arrow*).

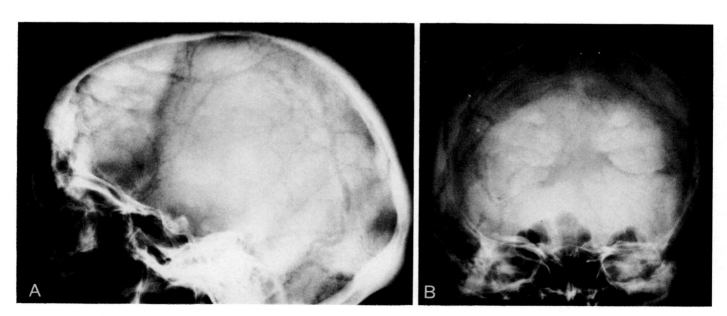

Figure 12.8. **Hyperostosis frontalis interna.** Lateral (**A**) and frontal (**B**) radiographs show the thickened internal table of the skull. This is a normal variant.

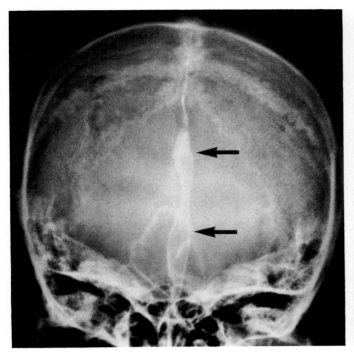

Figure 12.9.   Calcified falx cerebri (*arrows*).

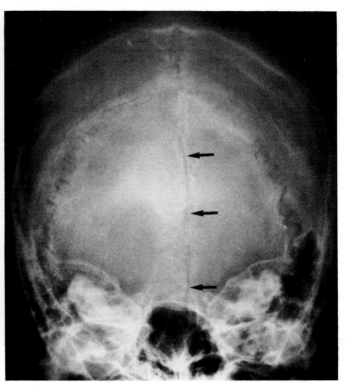

Figure 12.10.   Persistent metopic suture (*arrows*).

Evaluation of the brain with CT and MR produces transverse images that are remarkable in their similarity. Magnetic resonance has the advantage of producing images that clearly distinguish gray from white matter. Enhancement of vascular structures may be accomplished by using intravenous gadolinium- DTPA. Magnetic resonance has the additional advantage of being able to portray the brain in sagittal and coronal planes.

Figures 12.11 through 12.14 show representative CT images and their MR counterparts of the various normal intracranial structures.

When CT is performed for the evaluation of facial structures, particularly trauma, it is performed in transverse plane as well as in direct coronal plane where possible (Fig. 12.15 **A** and **B**). Coronal reconstructions may also be performed. Referring oral and maxillofacial as well as plastic surgeons have found three-dimensional reconstruction of facial images to be extremely useful (Fig. 12.15 **C** and **D**).

PATHOLOGIC CONSIDERATIONS

The four most common pathologic states you will encounter in the nervous system radiologically are trauma, neoplasm, vascular disease, and multiple sclerosis.

Advantages of MR

MR - distinguish gray from white
- Able to portray the brain in sagittal + coronal planes.

CT - facial
transverse + direct coronal planes.

oral maxillofacial
3D reconstruct CT

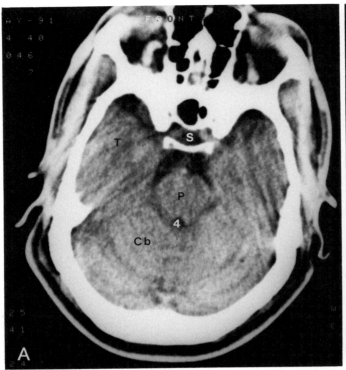

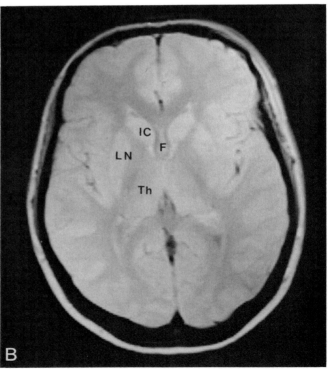

Figure 12.11. Comparable CT and MR images of the brain near the skull base. Note the greater detail on the MR image. **A,** CT. **B,** MR image. The following landmarks are visible: *Cb,* cerebellum; *P,* pons; *T,* temporal lobe; *S,* sella turcica; *4,* fourth ventricle; *ICA,* internal carotid arteries; *I,* infundibulum of the pituitary; *O,* optic nerve; *M,* occular muscles.

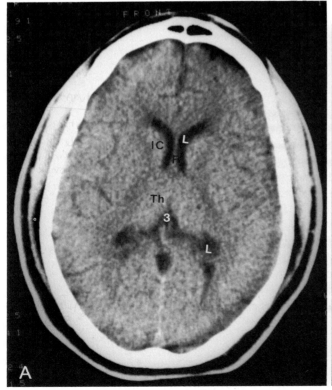

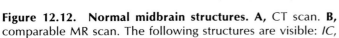

Figure 12.12. Normal midbrain structures. A, CT scan. **B,** comparable MR scan. The following structures are visible: *IC,* internal capsule; *L,* lateral ventricle; *F,* fornix; *LN,* lentiform nucleus; *Th,* thalamus; *3,* third ventricle.

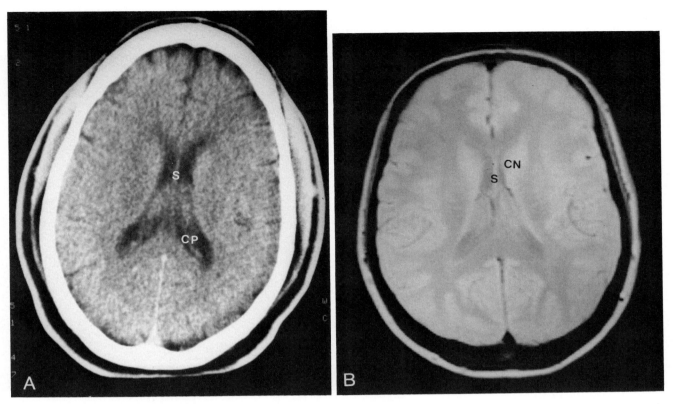

Figure 12.13. Normal cerebral anatomy. These views are slightly higher than those in Figure 12.12. **A,** CT scan. **B,** comparable MR image. The following structures are visible: *S,* interventricular septum; *CP,* choroid plexus; *CN,* caudate nucleus.

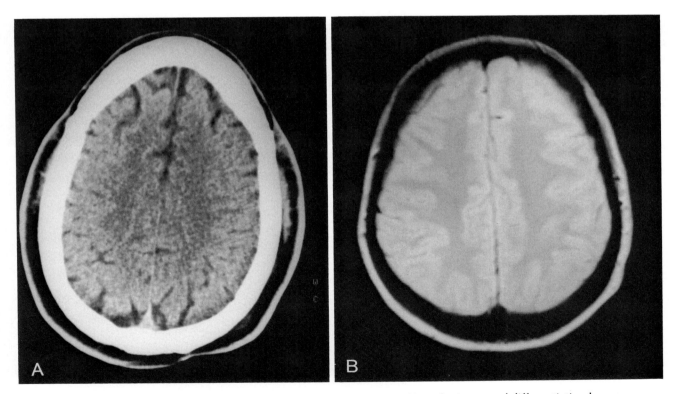

Figure 12.14. High cerebral cortex. A, CT scan. **B,** MR image. Note the improved differentiation between gray matter and white matter by MR.

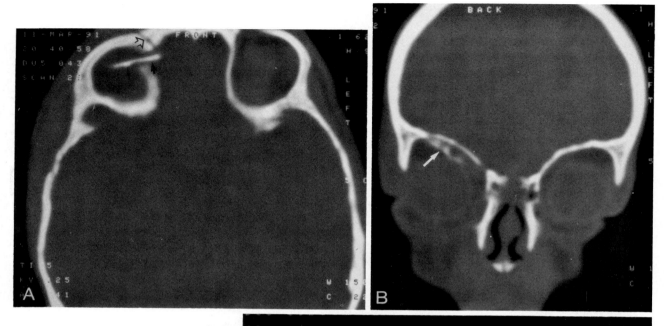

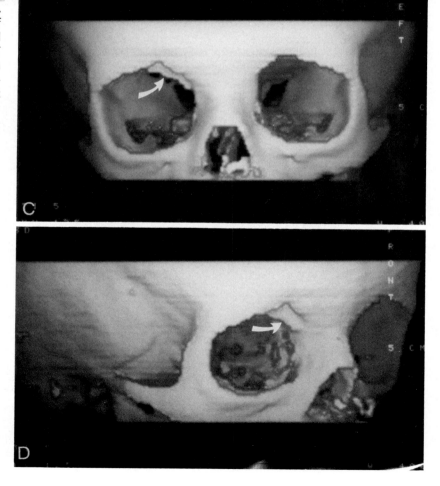

Figure 12.15. Value of three-dimensional CT in a patient with a right orbital roof fracture. **A,** axial CT section shows a fracture of the roof of the right orbit (*open arrow*). Note the intraorbital shard of bone (*solid arrows*). **B,** direct coronal CT shows the shard of bone (*arrow*) impinging upon the globe. **C,** frontal three-dimensional reconstruction shows the displaced bone fragment (*arrow*). **D,** oblique three-dimensional reconstruction shows the deformity of the orbital contour as well as the displaced fragment (*arrow*).

Trauma

As previously mentioned, fractures of the skull and their sequelae are the best example of the statement, "A fracture is a soft tissue injury in which a bone is broken." Indications for CT examination following trauma include signs and symptoms of neurologic abnormality: loss of consciousness and abnormal neurologic findings on examination. Since the treatment of skull fractures, with two notable exceptions, is directed toward treating the neurologic abnormality, the presence or absence of a fracture itself makes little difference in the management of the patient. You will encounter many patients in whom a skull fracture is present without neurologic findings or sequelae, as well as cases of head injury without fracture where significant neurologic damage has occurred.

Two situations in which the skull fracture itself is significant are the depressed fracture and the fracture associated with penetration of a bullet or other foreign object. However, in both these instances there are usually associated neurologic abnormalities that will dictate CT examination prior to corrective therapy. Figures 12.16 to 12.18 illustrate skull fractures and their associated findings.

Facial fractures occur in a variety of recognizable patterns. For example, a blow to the malar region (from a fist) is most likely to produce the so-called "tripod fracture" of the zygoma, wherein the zygoma fractures at the arch, at the frontozygomatic suture, and through the inferior orbital rim. There is also an accompanying fracture of the maxilla. For this reason we call this injury a zygomaticomaxillary complex (ZMC) fracture. Other more severe forms of facial trauma include various degrees of maxillofacial separation (the Le Fort-type fractures). A CT scan is required for complete evaluation of these patients (Fig. 12.19).

An associated abnormality that often occurs in patients with skull or facial trauma is cervical vertebral trauma. A direct blow to the skull or face is usually of sufficient force to produce enough stress on the cervical verte-

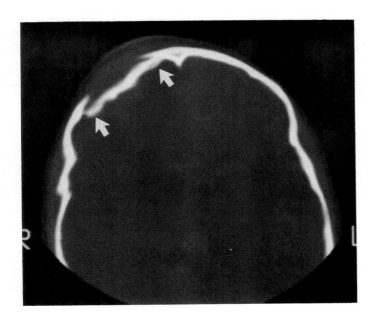

Figure 12.16. Depressed skull fracture. Cranial CT at bone window shows the depressed fragment in the right frontal region (*arrows*).

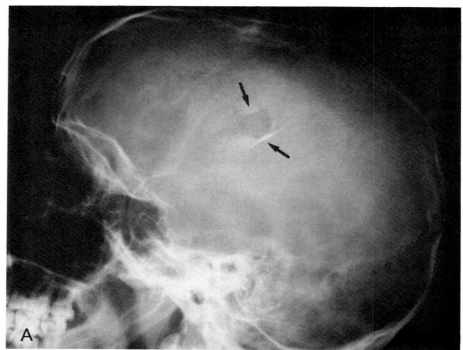

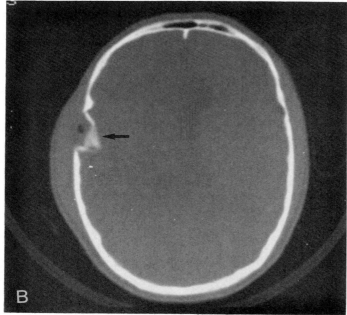

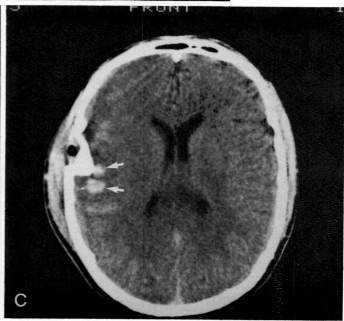

Figure 12.17. Depressed skull fracture with intracerebral hemorrhage. A, lateral radiograph shows a comminuted depressed fracture in the parietal region (*arrows*). **B,** CT image at bone window shows the depressed fragment (*arrow*). **C,** same image using brain windows shows multiple areas of intracranial hemorrhage (*arrows*) adjacent to the fracture.

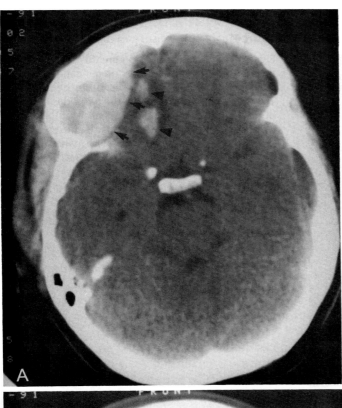

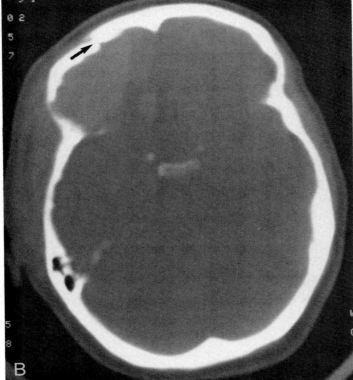

Figure 12.18. Skull fracture in the right frontal region with epidural hematoma. A, CT scan at brain windows shows the lentiform epidural hematoma (*arrows*) as well as intracerebral hemorrhage (*arrowheads*). **B,** same section at bone windows shows the fracture (*arrow*).

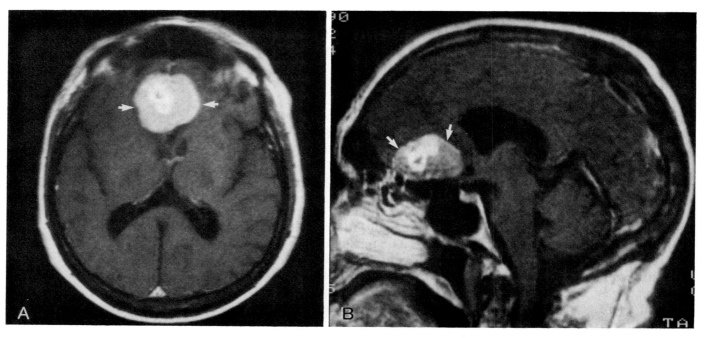

Figure 12.21. **Frontal meningioma.** (This is the same patient as in Fig. 12.20). **A,** axial MR image shows the mass to better advantage (*arrows*). Note the extremely high signal in the center of the mass. **B,** direct sagittal MR image shows similar findings (*arrows*).

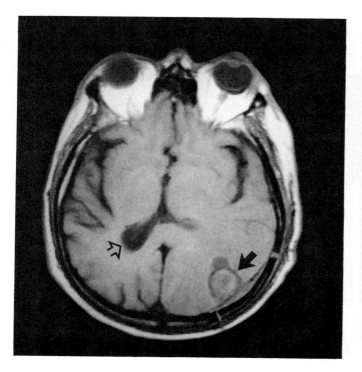

Figure 12.22. **Metastatic lesion showing ventricular compression.** Magnetic resonance shows that the metastatic lesion (*solid arrow*) in the left occipital lobe has compressed the posterior horn of the left lateral ventricle. Compare with the normal right ventricle (*open arrow*).

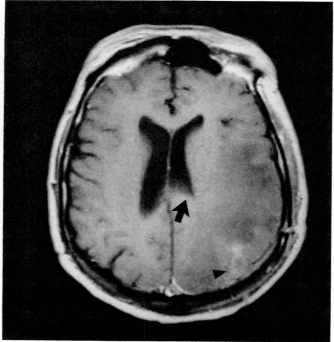

Figure 12.23. **Metastatic lesion showing edema.** This is the same patient as in Figures 12.22 and 12.25. An MR image shows the edema as an area of lower signal than normal brain. Note the loss of convolutional markings on the left, ventricular compression (*arrow*), and the tumor itself (*arrowhead*).

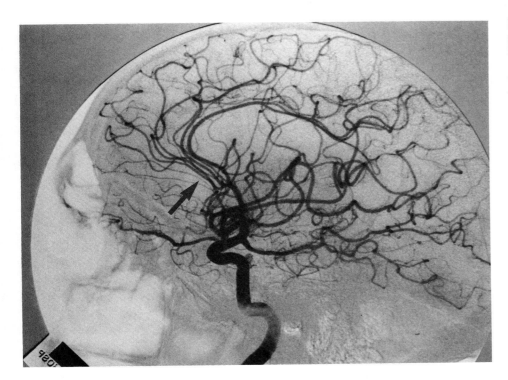

Figure 12.24. Cerebral arteriogram in a patient with frontal meningioma. (The same patient as in Figs. 12.20 and 12.21.) Note the elevation of both anterior cerebral arteries (*arrow*) by the tumor.

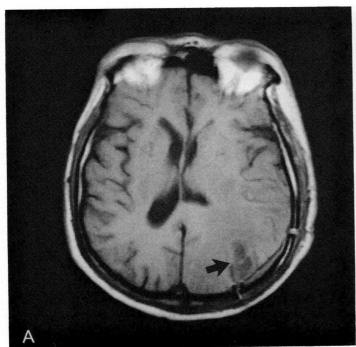
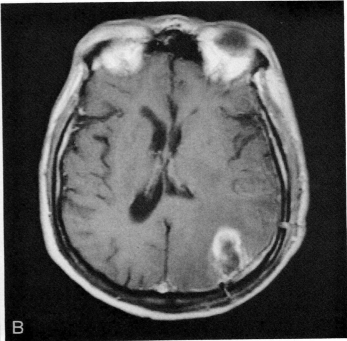

Figure 12.25. Metastatic brain tumor showing contrast enhancement. (The same patient as in Figs. 12.22 and 12.23.) **A,** without contrast, the tumor is seen as a multilobular area of low signal (*arrow*). **B,** following gadolinium contrast enhancement. Note how much more prominent the tumor is following contrast enhancement. The unenhanced portion of the tumor represents necrosis.

Vascular Disease

Vascular lesions probably constitute the most common intrinsic abnormality of the brain and surrounding meninges. These include infarction secondary to atherosclerotic or embolic occlusions (Fig. 12.26), intracerebral hemorrhage (Fig. 12.27), arteriovenous malformations, and extracerebral hematomas (Fig. 12.28). All these are readily diagnosable by CT and MR examinations. Furthermore, examination of the carotid arteries in the neck by Doppler ultrasound is now a method used to evaluate patients with suspected ischemic cerebral problems. Positive studies are followed up with arteriography if carotid angioplasty is contemplated.

Multiple Sclerosis

The development of MR imaging has provided a new method of evaluating patients with suspected multiple sclerosis. This insidious and severely debilitating disease that affects primarily young adults previously defied all imaging methods to establish a correct diagnosis. Magnetic resonance imaging now can demonstrate the plaques that form within the white matter of the brain (Fig. 12.29). Although the disease remains incurable, an earlier accurate diagnosis is essential to first, rule out other significant diseases, and secondly to begin therapy.

Brain Abscess

Abscesses of the brain often present as mass lesions. The clinical history is not always one of acute onset of neurologic symptoms. Nearly all patients have an established focus of infection elsewhere in the body. The findings on CT and MR are those of a mass, usually with an enhancing rim representing the capsule around the mass (Fig. 12.30). They may be difficult to differentiate from a necrotic neoplasm.

Figure 12.26.   Bilateral brain infarct. An MR image shows areas of high signal (*arrows*) on this T2-weighted image. Note the ventricular dilatation in this elderly patient.

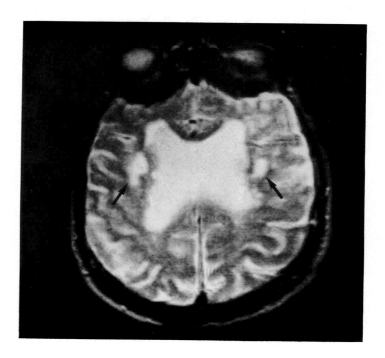

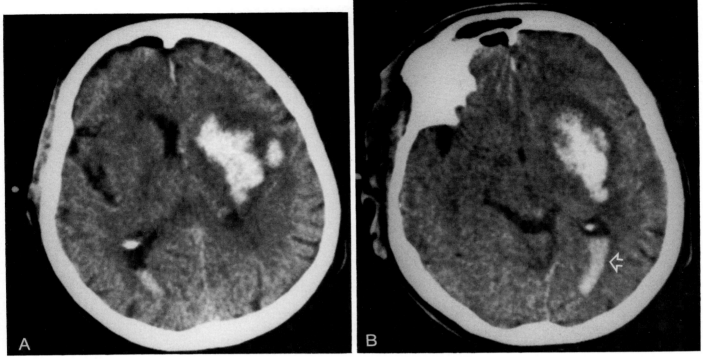

Figure 12.27.   Spontaneous intracerebral hemorrhage in a patient shown to have an aneurysm. A, CT scan shows increased density of the hemorrhage in the left periventricular region. **B,** at a slightly lower level, blood layers out in the posterior horn of the lateral ventricle (*arrow*).

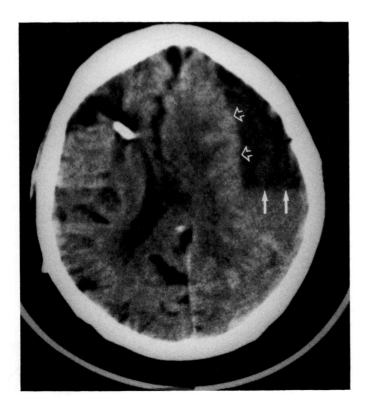

Figure 12.28. Subdural hematoma. A CT scan shows compression of the left side of the brain by a large extracerebral hematoma (*open arrows*). The blood products have separated and a fluid level is visible (*solid arrows*).

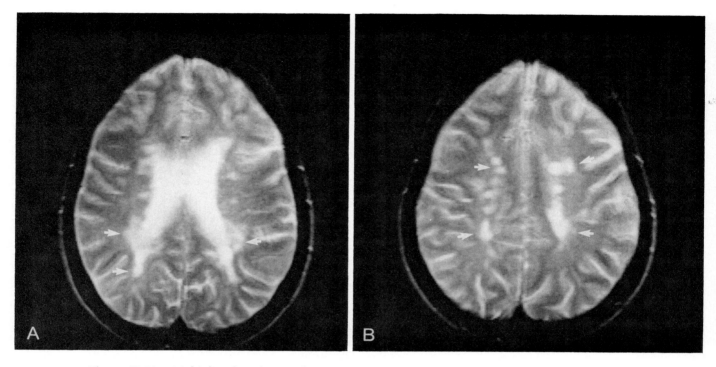

Figure 12.29. Multiple sclerosis. A and **B,** contiguous T2-weighted MR images, show areas of ventricular plaques of high signal (*arrows*).

Figure 12.30. Left frontal brain abscess. This contrast-enhanced CT scan shows the rim of the abscess to enhance (*arrowheads*). Note the surrounding edema (*open arrows*).

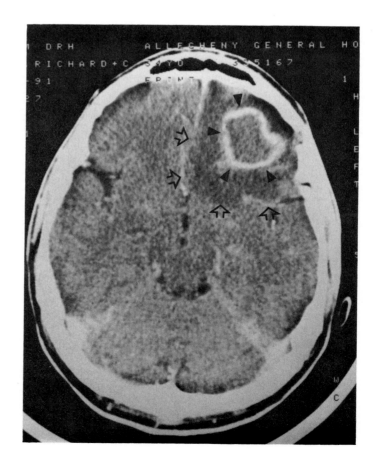

Summary

The pertinent anatomy of the normal skull radiograph has been reviewed. Emphasis was placed on the impact that cranial CT and MR scanning has had on neuroradiology. Four pathologic entities—trauma, tumor, vascular disease, and multiple sclerosis—have been discussed briefly.

Suggested Additional Reading

Grossman CB. Magnetic resonance imaging and computed tomography of the head and spine. Baltimore: Williams & Wilkins, 1991.

Latschaw RE, ed. MR and CT imaging of the head, neck, and spine. 2nd ed. St. Louis: Mosby Year Book, 1991.

Masters SJ, McClean PM, Arcarese JS, et al. Skull x-ray examination after head trauma: recommendations by a multidisciplinary panel and validation study. N Engl J Med 1987;316:84–91.

Osborne AG. Handbook of neuroradiology. St. Louis: Mosby Year Book, 1991.

Schnitzlein HN, Murtagh FR, eds. Imaging anatomy of the head and spine. 2nd ed. Baltimore: Williams & Wilkins, 1990.

Som PM, Bergeron T, eds. Head and neck imaging. 2nd ed. St. Louis: Mosby Year Book, 1991.

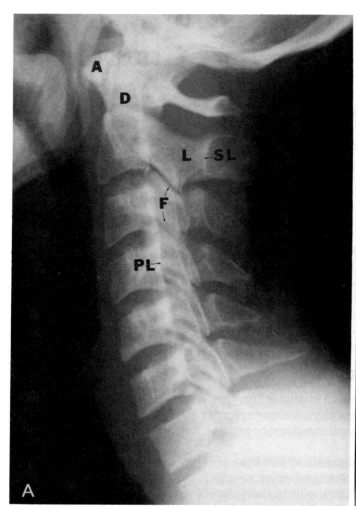

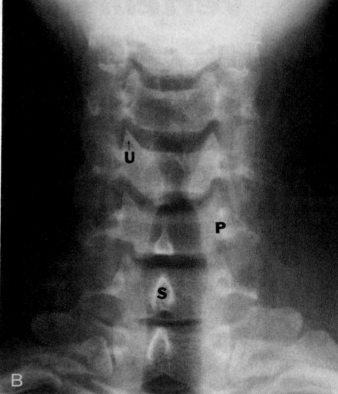

Figure 13.1. Normal cervical spine. A, lateral view. Note the normal alignment of the anterior and posterior portions of the vertebral bodies. The posterior vertebral body line (*PL*) is solid. The spinolaminar line (*SL*) is also aligned. The facet joints (*F*) are uniform and symmetric. The spaces between the laminae (*L*) are fairly uniform with the exception of C2-3, a normal variant. Note the position of the dens (*D*) and its relation to the anterior arch of the atlas (*A*). The width of the body of C-2 does not exceed that of C-3. Note the ring-like structure immediately below the dens. This structure is actually a composite of normal images. Disruption of this "ring" is an important finding in trauma. **B,** frontal view. Note the alignment of the spinous processes (*S*), the pedicles (*P*), and the uncinate processes (*U*).

ally a conglomeration of radiographic shadows from the superior articular facet of C-2 superiorly, the posterior vertebral body line posteriorly, foramen transversarium inferiorly, and the anterior vertebral body anteriorly. This ring is often disrupted in fractures through the body of C-2.

The frontal view shows normal alignment of the lateral margins of the vertebrae. The pedicles are normally aligned, and the distance between them does not vary more than 2 mm from level to level. The interspinous spaces are uniform. The uncinate processes are small, pointed projections along the posterolateral margins of the vertebrae.

Computerized tomography is one of the most frequently used examinations for evaluation of the vertebral column and its contents. It provides transverse images of the vertebrae and shows the surrounding soft tissues. A CT scan provides a further dimension to evaluation of vertebral diseases and injuries (Fig. 13.2). Coronal and sagittal reconstructions may be obtained (Fig. 13.3) as well as three-dimensional reconstructions. A CT scan is also a prime study for evaluation of herniated intervertebral discs (Fig. 13.4). In this regard, it may be combined with myelography to enhance a diagnosis. Computerized tomography is also employed in a variety of infectious and neoplastic disorders to show the extent of destruction of not only the vertebra, but the spread of the lesion into the soft tissues (Fig. 13.5).

Polydirectional tomography is used almost exclusively for the evaluation of suspected vertebral injuries. It is particularly effective in evaluating

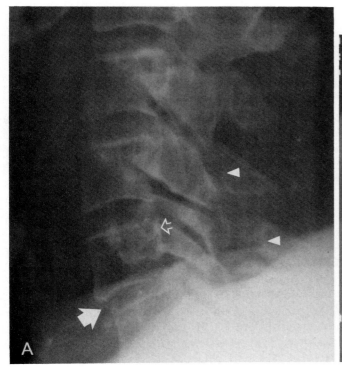 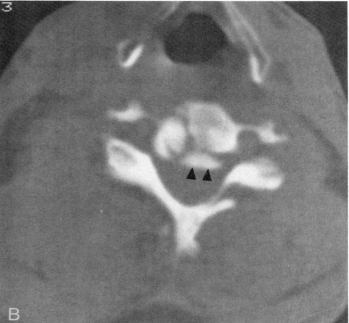

Figure 13.2.   C-5 burst fracture. A, lateral radiograph shows anterolisthesis of C-5 on C-6 (*large arrow*). There is bowing of the posterior vertebral body line (*open arrow*). Note the disruption of the spinolaminar line (*arrowheads*). The fact that the spinolaminar line of C-5 is not forward indicates that there is a bilaminar fracture at that level. **B,** CT scan shows fracture of the body of C-5 with retropulsion of the bone fragment into the vertebral canal (*arrowheads*).

Figure 13.3. Burst fracture of C-4. A CT scan with sagittal reconstruction shows anteriolisthesis of C-4 and C-5 with bone fragments in the vertebral canal (*arrow*). (This is the same patient as in Fig. 13.2.)

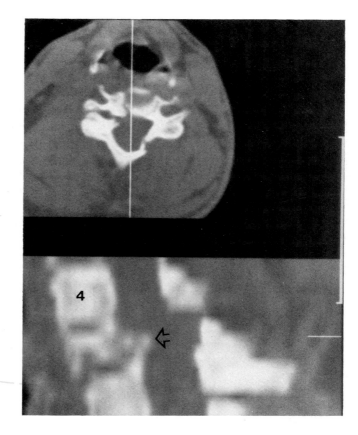

areas that do not lend themselves to either plain film, CT, or MR examinations (Fig. 13.6).

Magnetic resonance imaging is used for vertebral abnormalities almost as much as it is used for cranial abnormalities. The advantage of MR over CT and plain radiography is its ability to actually demonstrate the spinal cord. Thus, it is useful for demonstrating herniated intervertebral discs (Fig. 13.7), infections (Fig. 13.8), and tumors (Fig. 13.9), as well as trauma (Fig. 13.10).

Myelography was used more extensively before the development of MR for the evaluation of compressive lesions involving the spinal cord. Myelography is performed by the introduction of water-soluble, low osmotic contrast media into the subarachnoid space. Conventional films are then made after the patient is placed in the appropriate position to allow the contrast to fill the area of interest. It is used most often to evaluate herniated nucleus pulposus (Fig. 13.4**B**). In this regard, it is most often combined with CT examination (Figs. 13.4**C** and 13.11). Myelography is also useful in patients following trauma to evaluate those with suspected nerve root avulsions (Fig. 13.12).

Diagnostic ultrasound is used only intraoperatively to evaluate spinal cord lesions. This new technique allows a special ultrasound transducer to be placed directly on the dura to determine the exact location of a spinal cord tumor.

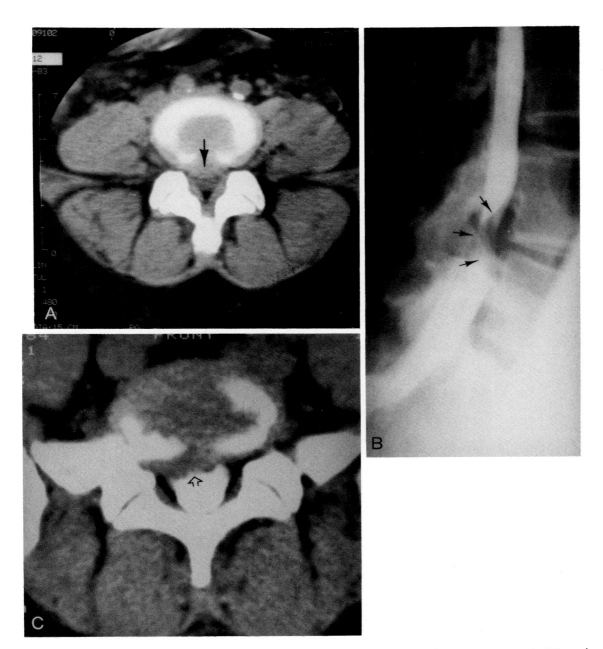

Figure 13.4.   Herniated nucleus pulposus. A, CT scan shows a soft tissue density (*arrow*) encroaching the thecal sac. **B,** myelogram shows extradural compression of the contrast-filled thecal sac (*arrows*) in the same patient. **C,** CT myelogram in a different patient shows herniated disc material compressing the contrast-filled thecal sac (*arrow*).

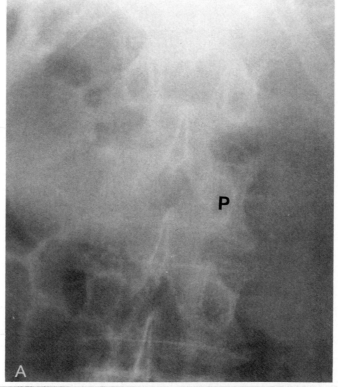

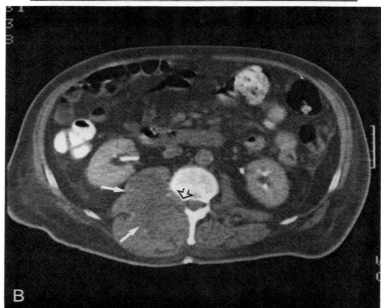

Figure 13.5.   Metastatic carcinoma with cord compression. A, frontal radiograph shows destruction of the pedicle and body of L-2 on the right. The normal pedicle (*P*) is seen on the left. **B,** CT scan through the same area shows a large paraspinal mass (*solid arrows*). Note the destroyed pedicle on the right (*open arrow*).

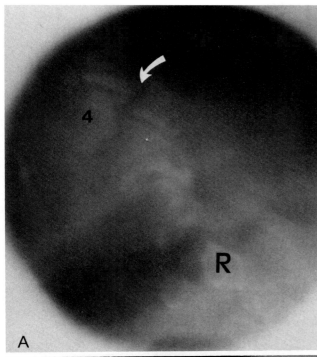

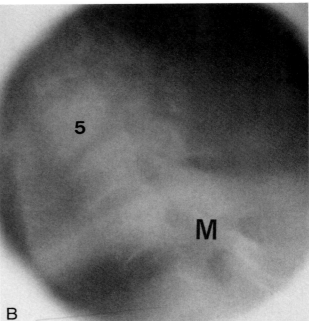

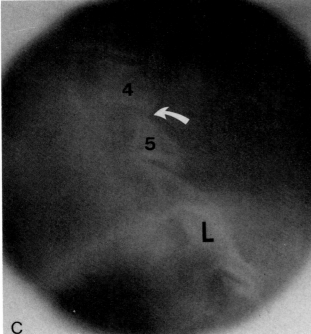

Figure 13.6. Tomograms showing facet locking. (This is the same patient as in Fig. 13.2.) **A,** on the right side there is a fracture through the articular pillar of C-4. The pillar of C-3 locks on this C-4 fractured pillar (*arrow*). **B,** midline (*M*) section shows slight anterolisthesis of C-5 (*5*) on C-6. **C,** a section through the left-sided pillars (*L*) show anterolisthesis of the pillar of C-4 (*4*) on C-5 (*5*) (*arrow*).

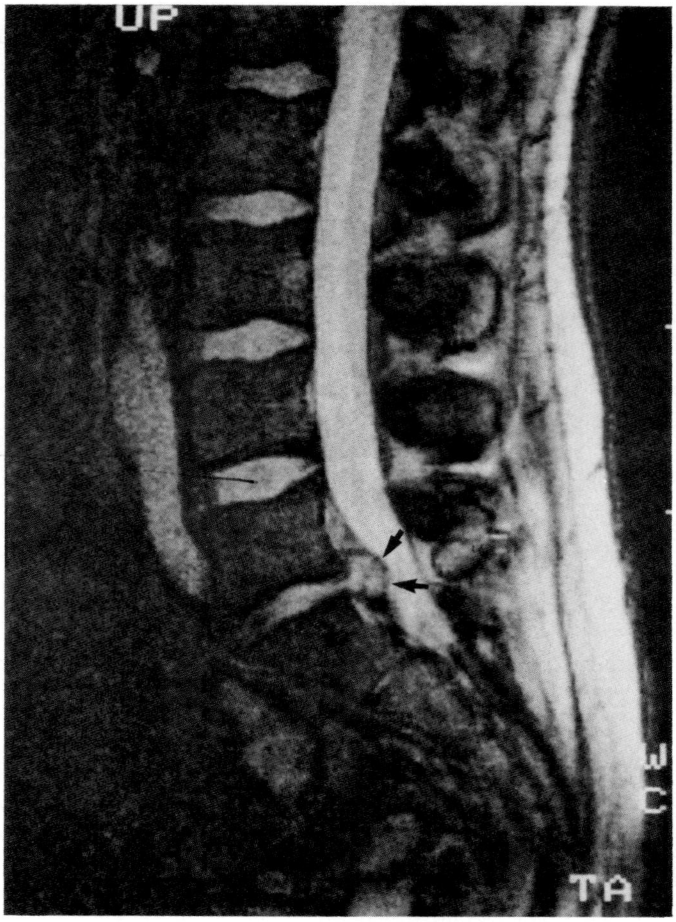

Figure 13.7. **Herniated nucleus pulposus.** Sagittal gradient echo MR image shows the herniated nuclear material (*arrows*) impinging the thecal sac.

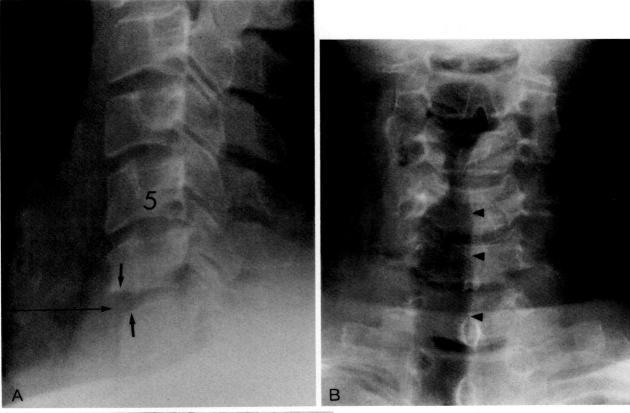

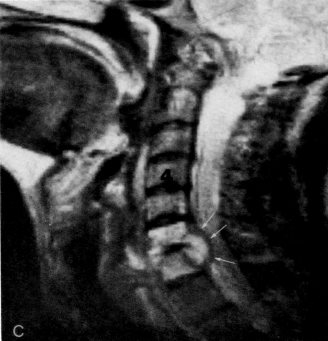

Figure 13.8. Disc space infection. A, lateral radiograph shows erosions along the C-6 disc space (*single arrows*). Note the increased width of the paravertebral soft tissues (*double-ended arrow*). **B,** frontal radiograph shows displacement of the trachea (*arrowheads*) to the right of the large prevertebral soft tissue mass. **C,** MRI shows an epidural abscess (*arrows*) compressing the thecal sac at C-6 and C-7.

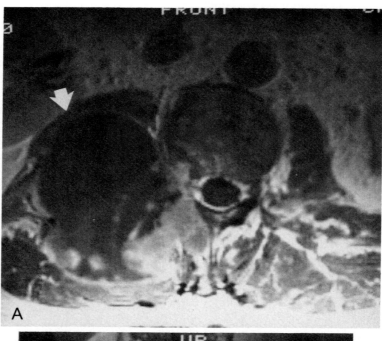

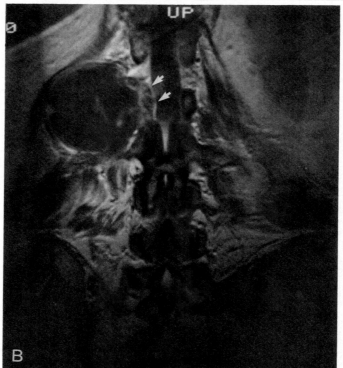

Figure 13.9. **Metastatic tumor invading vertebral canal.** (This is the same patient as in Fig. 13.5.) **A,** axial MR image shows a large paraspinal mass (*arrow*). **B,** direct coronal image shows compression of the epidural space (*arrows*) by the large mass. Magnetic resonance has the ability to image in direct sagittal and coronal planes.

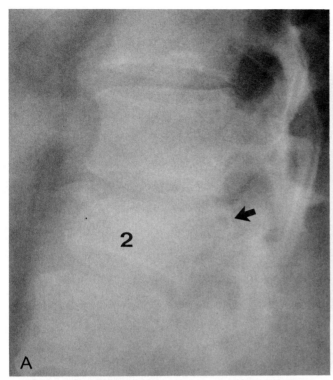

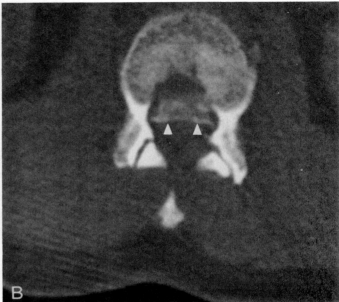

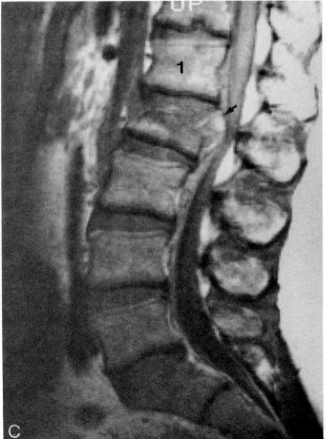

Figure 13.10. Burst fracture of L-2. A, lateral radiograph shows compression of the body of L-2 (*2*). There is posterior displacement of a large fragment (*arrow*) into the vertebral canal. **B,** CT scan shows the large fragment in the vertebral canal narrowing that structure (*arrowheads*). **C,** MR image shows the fragment (*arrow*) compressing the thecal sac.

Figure 13.11.   Herniated Intervertebral Disc. A CT myelogram showing herniated disc compressing the contrast-filled thecal sac (*arrow*).

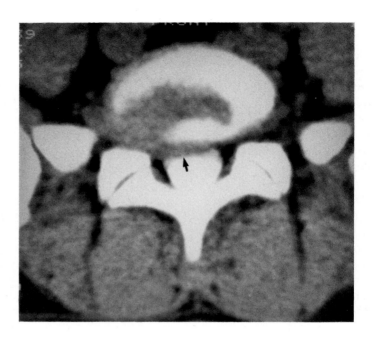

Figure 13.12.   Nerve root avulsion following trauma. This myelogram shows extravasation of contrast along the root sheath (*arrows*).

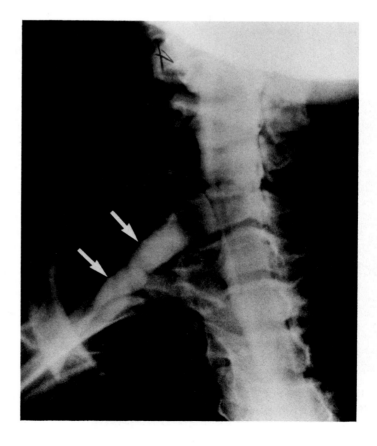

ANATOMIC CONSIDERATIONS

The vertebral column is a collection of 33 irregular bones extending from the base of the skull through the entire length of the neck and trunk. Because of the attached muscles, ligaments, and intervertebral discs, the vertebral column is a strong flexible support for the body that also protects the spinal cord. The upper 24 presacral vertebrae remain separate throughout life. The remaining five sacral and four coccygeal segments are called the fixed vertebrae, because they are fused.

There are certain common characteristics of all the moveable presacral vertebrae. With the exception of the atlas (C-1) and the axis (C-2), all these "typical" vertebrae include a body, located anteriorly that serves a weight-bearing function, and a vertebral arch located posterior to the body that acts as a protective shell for the spinal cord, meninges, peripheral nerves, and blood vessels (Fig. 13.13). The vertebral arch comprises two pedicles and two laminae. The pedicles join the arch to the vertebral body; the laminae join the pedicles to form the posterior wall of the vertebral foramen, which encloses the spinal cord. Seven projections or processes are attached to the vertebral arch: two transverse processes, one spinous process, and four articular processes. The transverse processes and spinous process serve as the attachment points for muscles. The articular processes determine the direction and degree of motion allowed by the particular segment of the vertebral column.

There are differences in the structure of the vertebrae at each level. All cervical vertebrae have, as distinguishing features, transverse foramina in each transverse process. The atlas, C-1, has no body. The axis, on

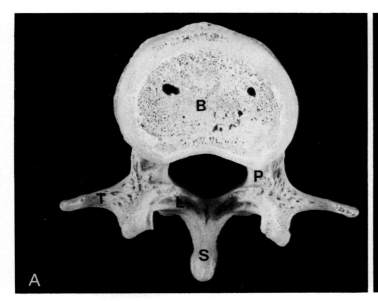 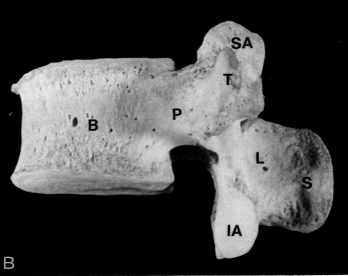

Figure 13.13. "Typical" vertebra (L-2). **A,** top view. **B,** side view. The following structures are visible: *B,* vertebral body; *P,* pedicle; *L,* lamina; *T,* transverse process; *S,* spinous process; *SA,* superior articular facet; *IA,* inferior articular facet. All vertebrae, with the exception of C-1, have these structures.

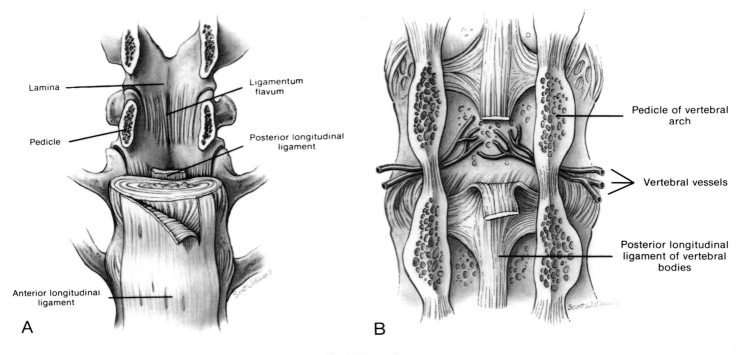

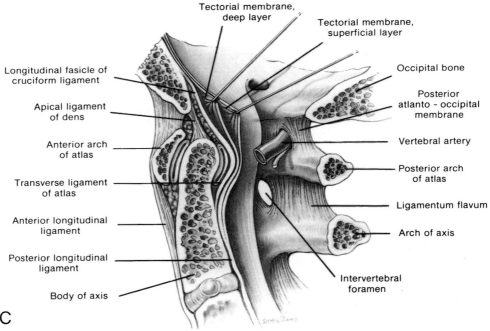

Figure 13.14. Normal vertebral ligaments. A, typical arrangement as viewed from the front. **B,** as viewed from behind. **C,** sagittal view of the craniovertebral junction. Reproduced with permission from Daffner RH. Imaging of vertebral trauma. Rockville, MD: Aspen Publishers, 1988.

the other hand, has a tooth-like protuberance from the upper portion of its body, the dens or odontoid process. The C3-7 also have uncinate processes along the posterolateral margin of the upper surface of the vertebral body that develop during adolescence and provide additional stabilization. Degenerative changes along the articulations that these uncinate processes make with the vertebrae above are a common cause of neck pain in older individuals.

The thoracic vertebrae all have one or more paired facets to accept the ribs. The upper thoracic vertebrae more closely resemble cervical vertebrae and the lower thoracic vertebrae more closely resemble lumbar vertebrae. The spinous processes of the thoracic vertebrae point downward.

Lumbar vertebrae lack both the transverse foramina and costal facets. Their spinous processes are large and rectangular. Their main function is support.

The vertebrae are separated and articulated by a series of joints and supporting ligaments. There are basically two types of joints: slightly moveable, symphyseal joints (the intervertebral discs), and freely moveable synovial (apophyseal or facet) joints. Motion in these joints is of a gliding nature. The intervertebral disc comprises a laminated outer portion, the anulus fibrosis, and an inner portion, the nucleus pulposus. The nucleus pulposus is eccentrically located with the shorter distance toward the vertebral canal. This accounts for the more common herniation of this material into this canal than anteriorly. The supporting ligaments (Fig. 13.14) serve to stabilize the vertebral column and restrict motion.

Motion permitted in the cervical region is flexion, extension, and rotation. Most rotation occurs with lateral flexion. The thoracic region is relatively restricted by the attached ribs. A minimal amount of flexion occurs in the upper thoracic vertebrae. However, at the thoracolumbar junction (T11-L2), a greater degree of flexion and minimal extension is allowed. In the lumbar region, flexion and extension, to a lesser degree than that in the cervical region, is also allowed. There is also a minor degree of rotation permitted predominantly at the thoracolumbar junction. The fact that motion is allowed in the cervical region as well as the thoracolumbar junction accounts for the high incidence of injuries to these levels.

PATHOLOGIC CONSIDERATIONS

There are five categories of abnormalities involving the vertebral column that you will encounter in your practice: (1) developmental, (2) degenerative, (3) traumatic, (4) neoplastic, and (5) postoperative.

Developmental Abnormalities

Developmental abnormalities occur commonly within the vertebral column. It is estimated that 1 in every 1,000 live births results in a significant developmental abnormality of the vertebral column. These may range from nothing more serious than an unfused spinous process (spina bifida occulta) (Fig. 13.15) to a severe form of spinal dysraphism, usually with multiple associated abnormalities (Fig. 13.16). Very often, these anomalies produce scoliosis. Other anomalies include hemivertebra, congenital fu-

Figure 13.15. Spina bifida occulta. There is failure of fusion of the laminae of L-5, producing a cleft (*arrow*). This is a normal variant with no associated neurologic or clinical findings.

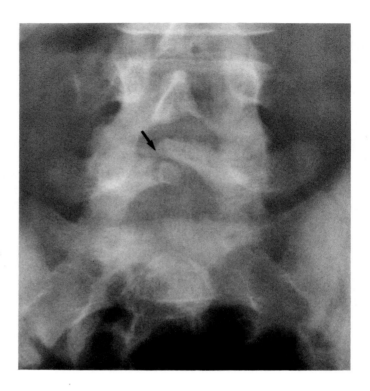

Figure 13.16. Lumbosacral spinal dysraphism (severe spina bifida). There is wide dysraphism with congenital absence of the laminae of L-3, L-4, and L-5 (*double-ended arrows*). This anomaly is usually associated with a myriad of neurologic abnormalities including hydrocephalus. Note the ventriculoperitoneal shunt catheter (*small arrows*).

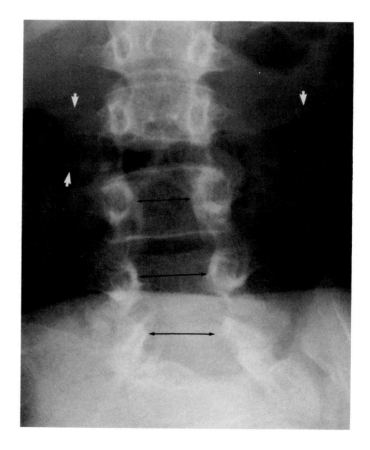

sions, and cervical ribs. Advancements in medical and surgical therapy for patients with severe spinal abnormalities have now made it possible for these unfortunate individuals to survive into adulthood.

Degenerative Abnormalities

Degenerative disease (spondylosis) of the vertebral column is one of the most common entities that you will encounter. The extent of degenerative disease may range from mild disc space narrowing and spur formation (Fig. 13.17) to severe spondylosis deformans, in which there is disc space narrowing, facet joint narrowing, and spur formation (Fig. 13.18). These spurs may encroach on either the intervertebral foramina or the vertebral canal to produce stenosis of those structures. Impingement on the spinal cord or peripheral nerves is best evaluated by CT, MR, or myelography (Fig. 13.19). Degeneration of the intervertebral disc frequently results in herniation of the semisolid nucleus pulposus into the vertebral canal.

Spondylosis, considered a normal complication of aging, is extremely common. Herniated intervertebral discs in the lumbar region are found very commonly as incidental findings in asymptomatic patients. However, once a patient becomes symptomatic, evaluation with CT, MR, and/or

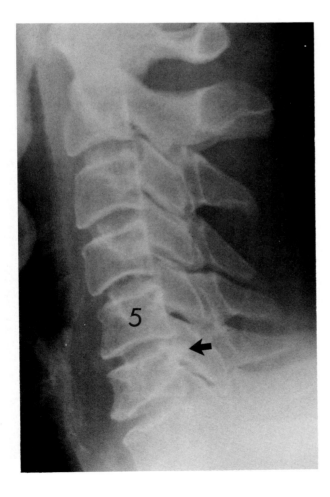

Figure 13.17. Mild cervical spondylosis. Lateral view shows a narrowing of the C-5 (*5*) disc space. Posterior spurs (*arrow*) intrude on the vertebral canal.

Figure 13.18. Severe spondylosis. A, lateral view shows narrowing of all the disc spaces below C-4 (*4*). Spurs encroach the vertebral canal at the disc level. Note the sclerosis of the facet joints. **B,** oblique view shows spurs encroaching the intervertebral foramina at multiple levels (*arrows*).

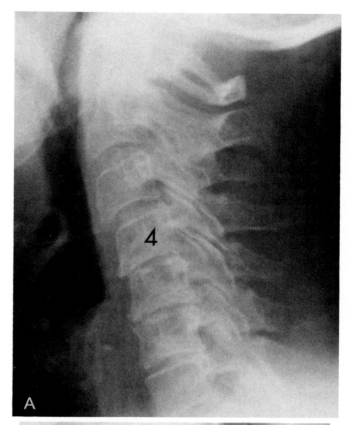

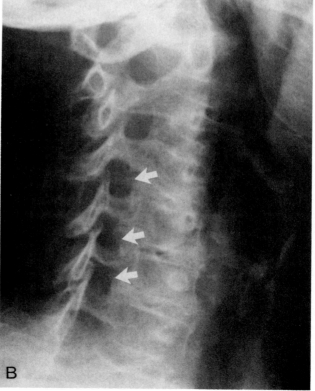

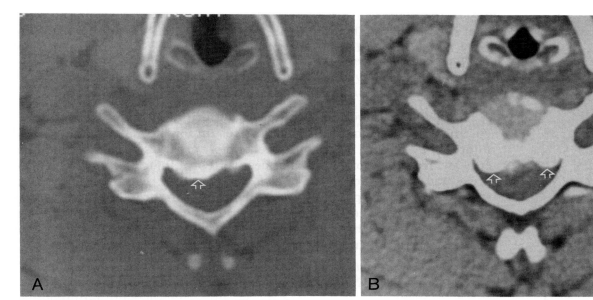

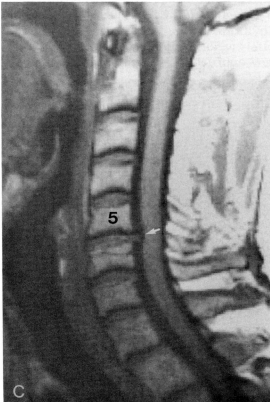

Figure 13.19. Cervical spondylosis. (This is the same patient as in Fig. 13.17.) **A,** CT scan at bone window shows large osteophyte narrowing of the vertebral canal (*arrow*). **B,** CT scan at soft tissue windows shows bilateral narrowing at a level slightly lower than **A** (*arrows*). **C,** sagittal MR image shows encroachment of the vertebral canal by herniated disc and spurs at C-5 (*5*) (*arrow*). The cord is not compressed in this view.

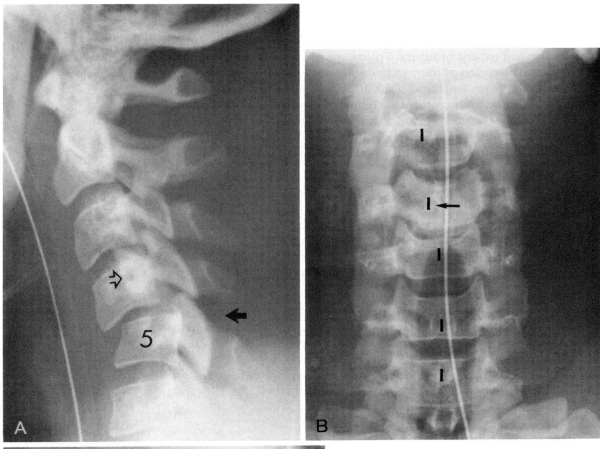

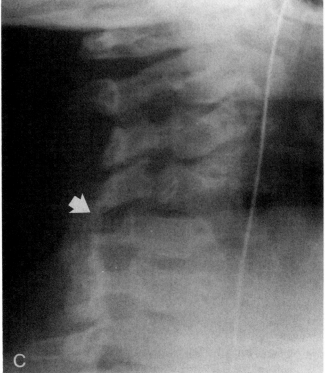

Figure 13.22. Unilateral facet lock. A, lateral radiograph shows anterolisthesis of C-4 on C-5 (*5*). Note the widening of one facet joint (*solid arrow*). The rotated pillar of C-4 (*open arrow*) may be seen through the body of C-4. **B,** frontal radiograph shows malalignment of the spinous processes (*solid vertical lines*). The spinous processes of C-3 and C-4 are displaced to the right (*arrow*), indicating that it is the right facet that is locked. **C,** trauma oblique view shows the locked facet (*arrow*).

mm is the normal upper limits of difference for the following measurements: interspinous or interlaminar space, interpediculate distance (transverse or vertical), unilateral or bilateral atlantoaxial offset, anterolisthesis or retrolisthesis with flexion or extension, facet joint width, and the difference in the height of the anterior and posterior thoracic and lumbar vertebral bodies. This important "rule of 2s" will hold you in good stead in most instances.

Abnormalities of bony integrity include any obvious fracture, disruption of the "ring" of C-2 (Fig. 13.23), widening of C-2—the so-called "fat" C-2 sign—widening of the interpediculate distance, and disruption of the posterior vertebral body line.

Cartilage or joint space abnormalities include widening of the predental space, abnormally wide intervertebral disc space (Fig. 13.24), widening of the facet joints (Fig. 13.25), or "naked" facets, and widening of the interspinous or interlaminar distance.

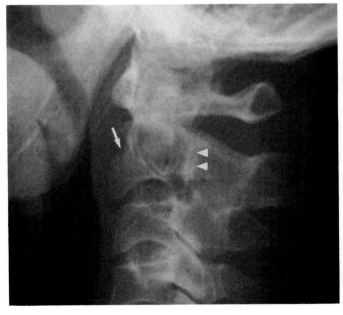

Figure 13.23. C-2 fracture. There is apparent widening of the body of C-2 in relation to C-3. Note the fracture along the anterior margin (*arrow*). The posterior vertebral body line is displaced posteriorly (*arrowheads*). Note the disruption of the spinolaminar line.

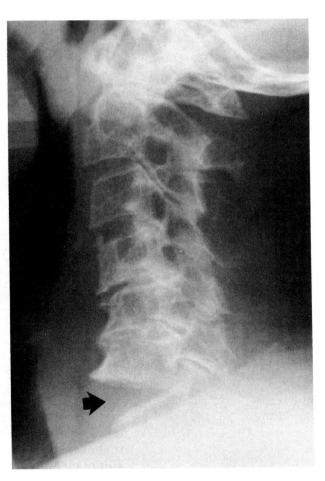

Figure 13.24. Wide disc space (*arrow*) in a patient with an extension injury.

Figure 13.28. Metastases invading the vertebral canal. Sagittal T1-weighted MR image (*T1*) shows destructive process involving C-3. There is extradural compression of the spinal cord (*arrows*). Additional metastatic lesions are present at C-6 and C-7 as evidenced by the low signal (darkness) in those vertebrae.

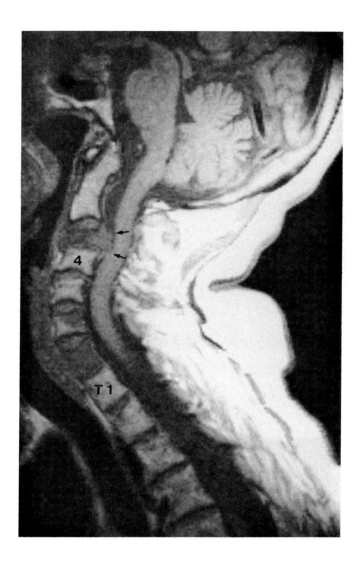

Plain films are not as sensitive as MR or radionuclide bone scanning. It has been estimated that up to 50% of cancellous bone must be destroyed before the lesion is visible on plain films. In this regard, CT has some advantages.

Infections

Infection often affects the vertebral column either as a direct consequence of surgery or from hematogenous seeding. The region adjacent to the intervertebral discs is most commonly involved. For most infections, plain films will reveal bony destruction along both sides of bony margins of disc space. A CT scan will show the lytic areas to better advantage and may delineate an associated soft tissue mass. An MR image shows the inflammatory mass as well as any involvement of the vertebral canal with epidural abscess. Figure 13.29 shows a typical disc space infection.

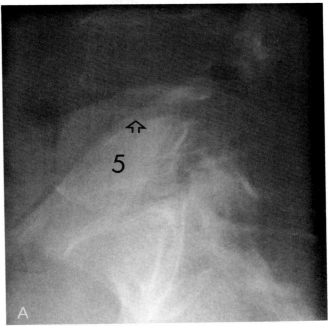

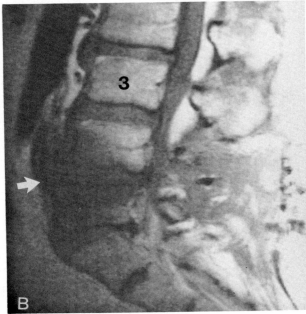

Figure 13.29.   Disc space infection. A, lateral radiograph shows loss of the superior disk margin of L-5 (*5*) (*arrow*). **B,** sagittal T1-weighted image shows areas of low signal involving L-4 and L-5. The disc margin of L-5 is indistinct; it is still preserved in L-4. Note the anterior paraspinal mass (*arrow*).

Mirvis SE, Young JWR. Imaging in trauma and critical care. Baltimore: Williams & Wilkins, 1991.

Postoperative Changes

Index

Page numbers followed by t and f indicate tables and figures, respectively.